ESSENTIALS OF FOOD SCIENCE

SECOND EDITION

VICKIE A. VACLAVIK, PH.D., R.D.
The University of Texas Southwestern Medical Center, Dallas, TX

ELIZABETH W. CHRISTIAN, PH.D.
Texas Woman's University, Denton, TX

Kluwer Academic/Plenum Publishers
New York, Boston, Dordrecht, London, Moscow

Library of Congress Cataloging-in-Publication Data

Vaclavik, Vickie.
  Essentials of food science/Vickie A. Vaclavik and Elizabeth W. Christian–2nd ed.
    p. cm.
  Includes bibliographical references and index.
  ISBN 0-306-47363-1
  1. Food–Analysis. 2. Food-Composition. 3. Nutrition. I. Christian, Elizabeth W. II.
  Title.

  TX531 .V33 2003
  664–de21   2002028280

ISBN: 0-306-47363-1

©2003 Kluwer Academic/Plenum Publishers, New York
233 Spring Street, New York, N.Y. 10013

10 9 8 7 6 5 4 3 2 1

A C.I.P. record for this book is available from the Library of Congress.

Printed in the United States of America

bn.

ESSENTIALS
OF FOOD
SCIENCE

D

FOOD SCIENCE TEXT SERIES

The Food Science Text Series provides faculty with the leading teaching tools. The Editorial Board has outlined the most appropriate and complete content for each food science course in a typical food science program, and has identified textbooks of the highest quality, written by leading food science educators.

Editorial Board

Food Science Text Series

Principles of Food Chemistry, Third Edition (1999), John M. deMan
Principles of Food Processing (1997), Dennis R. Heldman and Richard W. Hartel
Modern Food Microbiology, Sixth Edition (2000), James M. Jay
Sensory Evaluation of Food: Principles and Practices (1998), Harry T. Lawless and Hildegarde Heymann
Essentials of Food Sanitation (1997), Norman G. Marriott
Principles of Food Sanitation, Fourth Edition (1999), Norman G. Marriott
Food Analysis, Third Edition (2003), S. Suzanne Nielsen
Food Science, Fifth Edition (1995), Norman N. Potter and Joseph H. Hotchkiss
Fundamentals of Food Process Engineering, Second Edition (1990), Romeo T. Toledo
Essentials of Food Science, Second Edition (2003), Vickie A. Vaclavik and Elizabeth W. Christian
Elementary Food Science, Fourth Edition (1996), Ernest R. Vieira
Food Analysis Laboratory Manual (2003), S. Suzanne Nielsen
Introduction to Food Process Engineering (2003), Peter G. Smith

C O N T E N T S

PREFACE

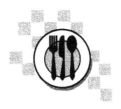

PURPOSES

Essentials of Food Science (now in its second edition) is designed to present principles of food science for the nutrition, dietetics, hospitality, and culinary arts student enrolled in an introductory food science course in their curriculum.

There are many, very good textbooks dedicated to furthering the knowledge of food science. Yet, the approach to writing this text is different. This is not intended to be a textbook for food science majors, who must have a more rigorous, scientific teaching approach to food science concepts. Rather, this book was designed primarily for use by non-majors, who themselves have rigorous coursework outside the field of Food Science, yet who would benefit from a knowledge of the science of foods.

As educators, we thoroughly enjoy the subject matter and our intent continues to be to present concepts in a ready-friendly manner. As in the first edition, the chapters in this text follow the order of the USDA Food Guide Pyramid—which is familiar and useful to practitioners in food-related professions.

The presentation of food science principles begins with an introduction to food components—evaluation of quality factors in food and water. It continues with a study of carbohydrates, including starches, pectins, gums, and foods at the base of the Food Guide Pyramid—bread, cereal, rice, and pasta foods, as well as vegetables and fruits.

Discussion progresses to chapters on proteins—meat, poultry, fish, dry beans, eggs, and milk. These are followed by chapters covering emulsions and foams, fats and oils, and lastly, sugars and sweeteners that appear at the top of the Food Guide Pyramid.

After discussing the various food ingredients, a chapter on baked products covers batters and doughs. It builds upon information in earlier chapters regarding carbohydrates, proteins, fats, oils, and sweeteners.

Chapters on aspects of food production—safety, processing, preservation, packaging, and use of additives in food—include application to retail and commercial manufacturing operations. The discussion of food science in this text is completed with a view of government regulation of the food supply and labeling.

What is new: In part due to advances in the field of new technology, and for student clarification, this edition includes an expansion of concepts relating to material in all chapters, including quality, pectins and gums, organic food, irradiation, biotechnology, sugar substitutes, fat replacers, packaging, health claims, food security, USDA dietary guidelines and more. There is also a new chapter dedicated to a discussion of emulsification and foams. An improvement may be noted in a new index that allows the reader to more quickly find his/her topics of interest!

Nutrition and food safety continue to be important issues for consumers, therefore, as applicable, individual chapters contain sections on nutritive value and safety concerns regarding the foods discussed. Additionally, each chapter contains a glossary and helpful references useful for further study.

THANKS

We would both like to thank the Lord for providing wisdom for each challenge along the path of publication and great joy in the process!

We would like to thank the faculty, staff, students, and friends at our respective Universities for their input and encouragement.

We are appreciative to numerous sources, credited in each chapter, whose provision of materials in the text assist in offering better explanations.

Thanks to the Vaclavik family: to my husband, Frank, and to our three school-age sons who gave up their "turns" on the computer, and could not imagine that I was working on a new edition already!

Thanks also to the Christian family: to my husband, Joe, for his constant love, support and understanding, and daughters Rebecca and Laura for their patience when Mom was working on the computer again!

FOR MORE INFORMATION

More information is available in texts relating to such topics as food chemistry, food engineering, food packaging, food preparation, food safety, food technology, nutrition and quantity foods, product evaluation, and in references cited at the end of each chapter. **Bold, *italicized*** words appearing in the text of each chapter are defined in a glossary at the completion of each chapter.

V. A. Vaclavik (vä-klä′-vik)
E. W. Christian

Food Guide Pyramid
A Guide to Daily Food Choices

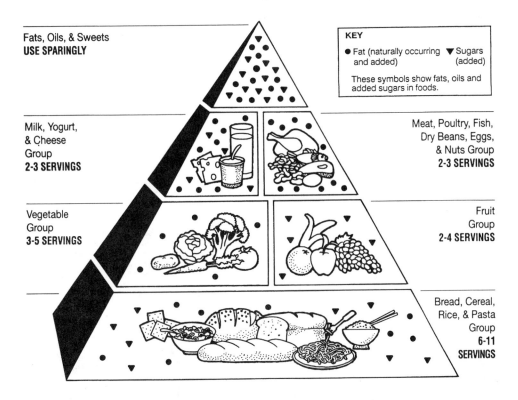

Fats, Oils, & Sweets
USE SPARINGLY

KEY
● Fat (naturally occurring ▼ Sugars
 and added) (added)

These symbols show fats, oils and
added sugars in foods.

Milk, Yogurt,
& Cheese
Group
2-3 SERVINGS

Meat, Poultry, Fish,
Dry Beans, Eggs,
& Nuts Group
2-3 SERVINGS

Vegetable
Group
3-5 SERVINGS

Fruit
Group
2-4 SERVINGS

Bread, Cereal,
Rice, & Pasta
Group
**6-11
SERVINGS**

Use the Food Guide Pyramid to help you eat better every day...the Dietary Guidelines way. Start with plenty of Breads, Cereals, Rice, and Pasta; Vegetables; and Fruits. Add two to three servings from the Milk group and two to three servings from the Meat group.

Each of these food groups provides some, but not all, of the nutrients you need. No one food group is more important than another – for good health you need them all. Go easy on fats, oils, and sweets, the foods in the small tip of the Pyramid.

To order a copy of "The Food Guide Pyramid" booklet, send a $1.00 check or money order made out to the Superintendent of Documents to: Consumer Information Center, Department 159-Y, Pueblo, Colorado 81009.

U.S. Department of Agriculture, Human Nutrition Information Service, August 1992, Leaflet No. 572

Additional multicultural Food Guide Pyramids for African-American, Chinese, Indian, Jewish, Mexican, Navajo, Puerto Rican and Vietnamese cultures are available from: Penn State Nutrition Center, University Park, PA.

How to Use The Daily Food Guide

What counts as one serving?

Breads, Cereals, Rice and Pasta
1 slice of bread
1/2 cup of cooked rice or pasta
1/2 cup of cooked cereal
1 ounce of ready-to-eat cereal

Vegetables
1/2 cup of chopped raw
    or cooked vegetables
1 cup of leafy raw vegetables

Fruits
1 piece of fruit or melon wedge
3/4 cup of juice
1/2 cup of canned fruit
1/4 cup of dried fruit

Milk, Yogurt and Cheese
1 cup of milk or yogurt
1 1/2 to 2 ounces of cheese

Meat, Poultry, Fish, Dry Beans, Eggs and Nuts
2 1/2 to 3 ounces of cooked lean
    meat, poultry, or fish
Count 1/2 cup of cooked beans,
    or 1 egg, or 2 tablespoons of
    peanut butter as 1 ounce of
    lean meat (about 1/3 serving)

Fats, Oils and Sweets
LIMIT CALORIES FROM THESE
especially if you need to lose weight

> The amount you eat may be more than one serving. For example, a dinner portion of spaghetti would count as two or three servings of pasta.

How many servings do you need each day?

	Women & some older adults	Children, teen girls, active women, most men	Teen boys & active men
Calorie level*	about 1,600	about 2,200	about 2,800
Bread group	6	9	11
Vegetable group	3	4	5
Fruit group	2	3	4
Milk group	2–3**	2–3**	2–3**
Meat group	2 for a total of 5 ounces	2 for a total of 6 ounces	3 for a total of 7 ounces

* These are the calorie levels if you choose lowfat, lean foods from the 5 major food groups and use foods from the fats, oils and sweets group sparingly.

** Women who are pregnant or breastfeeding, teen-agers and young adults to age 24 need 3 servings.

A Closer Look at Fat and Added Sugars

The small tip of the Pyramid shows fats, oils and sweets. These are foods such as salad dressings, cream, butter, margarine, sugars, soft drinks, candies and sweet desserts. Alcoholic beverages are also part of this group. These foods provide calories but few vitamins and minerals. Most people should go easy on foods from this group.

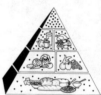

Some fat or sugar symbols are shown in the other food groups. That's to remind you that some foods in these groups can also be high in fat and added sugars, such as cheese or ice cream from the milk group, or french fries from the vegetable group. When choosing foods for a healthful diet, consider the fat and added sugars in your choices from all the food groups, not just fats, oils and sweets from the Pyramid tip.

A number of countries have developed/revised their own Food Guide illustrations. They "have different food availabilities, food preferences, dietary patterns, and cultural definitions of foods". Universal dietary recommendations do not exist.

EXAMPLE

Australia, Canada, China, Germany, Great Britain, Korea, Mexico, Philippines, Portugal, Puerto Rico, Sweden, US[1].

---

[1] Painter J, Rah J, Lee Y. Comparison of international food guide pictorial representations. *J. Am. Diet Assoc.* 2002; 102: 483–489.

WORLD WIDE WEB (WWW) SITES

FDA—http://www.fda.gov

FDA Code of Federal Regulations—http://www.access.gpo.gov/nara/cfr

USDA—http://www.usda.gov

USDA database—http://www.nal.usda.gov.fnic/foodcomp

The American Dietetic Association—http://www.eatright.org

The Institute of Food Technologists—http://www.ift.org

The National Restaurant Association—http://www.restaurant.org

PART 1

Introduction to Food Components

CHAPTER 1

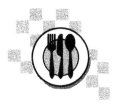

Evaluation of Food Quality

INTRODUCTION

Food quality is an important concept, because the food people choose depends largely on quality. Consumer preference is important to the food manufacturer, who wants to gain as wide a share of the market for the product as possible. Quality is difficult to define precisely, but it refers to the degree of excellence of a food and includes all the characteristics of a food that are significant and that make the food acceptable.

Whereas some attributes of a food, such as nutritional quality, can be measured by chemical analysis, food acceptability is not easy to measure as it is very subjective. In fact, consumers make subjective judgments using one or more of the five senses every time they select or eat any food. For example, potato chips, celery, and some cereals have a crunchy sound when they are eaten; the taste and smell of foods can be highly appealing or unacceptable; and the appearance and feel of a food are also important in determining its acceptability.

Food quality must be monitored on a regular day-to-day basis to ensure that a uniform product is produced and that it meets the required quality control standards. Companies must also monitor the quality of their products during storage while changing ingredients and developing new lines. Objective tests using laboratory equipment are useful for routine quality control, but they cannot measure consumer preference. The only sure way to determine what a population thinks about any food is to ask them! This is done using sensory testing and asking panelists to taste a food and give their opinion on it. Both sensory and objective tests are important in evaluating food quality, and ideally, they should correlate with or complement each other.

ASPECTS OF FOOD QUALITY

Food quality has both subjective and nonsubjective aspects. Appearance, texture, and flavor are largely subjective attributes, whereas nutritional and bacterial quality

3

are not. The last two qualities can be measured objectively, either by chemical analysis, by measuring bacterial counts, or using other specific tests (1,2). They will only be mentioned briefly in this chapter, and the subjective qualities will be discussed in detail.

Appearance

The appearance of a food includes its size, shape, color, structure, transparency or turbidity, dullness or gloss, and degree of wholeness or damage. While selecting a food and judging its quality, a consumer takes these factors into account, as they are indeed an index of quality. For example, the *color* of a fruit indicates how ripe it is, and color is also an indication of strength (as in tea or coffee), degree of cooking, freshness, or spoilage (3,4). Consumers expect foods to be of a certain color, and if they are not, it is judged to be a quality defect. The same is true for *size,* and one may choose large eggs over small ones, or large peaches over small ones, for example.

Structure is important in baked goods. For example, bread should have many small holes uniformly spread throughout, and not one large hole close to the top. *Turbidity* is important in beverages; for example, orange juice is supposed to be cloudy because it contains pulp, but white grape juice should be clear and without any sediment, which would indicate a quality defect.

Texture

Texture refers to those qualities of a food that can be felt with the fingers, tongue, palate, or teeth. Foods have different textures, such as crisp crackers or potato chips, crunchy celery, hard candy, tender steaks, chewy chocolate chip cookies, and creamy ice cream, to name but a few.

Texture is also an index of quality. The texture of a food can change as it is stored, for various reasons. If fruits or vegetables lose water during storage, they wilt or lose their turgor pressure, and a crisp apple becomes unacceptable and leathery on the outside. Bread can become hard and stale on storage. Products like ice cream can become gritty due to precipitation of lactose and growth of ice crystals if the freezer temperature is allowed to fluctuate, allowing thawing and refreezing.

Evaluation of texture involves measuring the response of a food when it is subjected to forces such as cutting, shearing, chewing, compressing, or stretching. Food texture depends on the rheological properties of the food (5). **Rheology** is defined as the science of deformation and flow of matter or, in other words, reaction of a food when a force is applied to it. Does it flow, bend, stretch, or break? From a sensory perspective, the texture of a food is evaluated when it is chewed. The teeth, tongue and jaw exert a force on the food, and how easily it breaks or flows in the mouth determines whether it is perceived as hard, brittle, thick, runny, and so on. The term **mouthfeel** is a general term used to describe the textural properties of a food as perceived in the mouth.

Subjective measurement of texture gives an indirect evaluation of the *rheological* properties of a food. For example, a sensory panel might evaluate *viscosity* as the consistency or mouthfeel of a food. However, viscosity can be measured directly using a viscometer. Rheological properties are therefore discussed in more detail in section "Objective Evaluation" of this chapter.

Flavor

Flavor is a combination of taste and smell and is largely subjective. If a person has a cold, food usually seems to be tasteless. However, it is not the taste buds that are affected but the sense of smell. Taste is detected by the taste buds at the tip, sides, and back of the tongue, whereas aromas are detected by the olfactory epithelium in the upper part of the nasal cavity. For any food to have an aroma, it must be volatile, but volatile substances can be detected in very small amounts (vanillin can be detected at a concentration of 2×10^{-10} mg/liter of air). Aroma is a valuable index of quality. A food will often smell bad before it looks bad, and old meat can be easily detected by its smell. (However, foods that are contaminated with pathogens may have no off-odor, so the absence of bad smell is not a guarantee that the food, such as meat, is safe to eat.)

The taste of a food is a combination of five major tastes—salt, sweet, sour, bitter, and **umami**. It is complex and hard to describe completely. *Sweet* and *salt* tastes are detected primarily on the tip of the tongue, and so they are detected quickly, whereas *bitter* tastes are detected mainly by taste buds at the back of the tongue. It takes longer to perceive a bitter taste, and it lingers in the mouth; thus bitter foods are often described as having an aftertaste. *Sour* tastes are mainly detected by the taste buds along the side of the tongue.

Sugars, alcohols, aldehydes, and certain amino acids taste sweet to varying degrees. Acids (such as vinegar, lemon juice, and the many organic acids present in fruits) contribute the sour taste, saltiness is due to salts, including sodium chloride, and bitter tastes are due to alkaloids such as caffeine, theobromine, quinine, and other bitter compounds.

Umami is a taste that has recently been added to the other four. It is a savory taste given by ingredients such as monosodium glutamate (MSG) and other flavor enhancers. The umami taste is significant in Japanese foods and in snack foods such as taco-flavored chips.

TASTE SENSITIVITY

People vary in their sensitivity to different tastes. Sensitivity depends on the length of time allowed to taste a substance. Sweet and salt tastes are detected quickly (in less than a second), because they are detected by taste buds on the tip of the tongue; in addition, they are usually very soluble compounds. Bitter compounds, on the other hand, may take a full second to be detected because they are detected at the back of the tongue. The taste may linger, producing a bitter aftertaste.

Sensitivity to a particular taste also depends on the concentration of the substance responsible for the taste. The **threshold** concentration is defined as the concentration required for identification of a particular substance. The threshold concentration may vary from person to person; some people are more sensitive to a particular taste than others and are, therefore, able to detect it at a lower concentration. Below the threshold concentration, a substance would not be identified but may affect the perception of another taste. For example, *subthreshold* salt levels *increase* perceived sweetness and *decrease* perceived acidity, whereas subthreshold sugar concentrations make a food taste *less* salty than it actually is. Although it is not clear why, flavor enhancers such as MSG also affect taste sensitivity by intensifying a particular taste in a food.

Temperature of a food also affects its flavor. Warm foods generally taste stronger and sweeter than cold foods. For example, melted ice cream tastes much sweeter than frozen ice cream. There are two reasons for the effects of temperature on flavor. The volatility of substances is increased at higher temperatures, and so they smell stronger. Taste bud receptivity is also an important factor. Taste buds are most receptive in the region between 68 and 86°F (20 and 30°C), and so tastes will be more intense in this temperature range.

Psychological factors also affect taste sensitivity and perception. Judgments about flavor are often influenced by preconceived ideas based on the appearance of the food or on previous experience with a similar food. For example, strawberry-flavored foods would be expected to be red. However, if colored green, because of the association of green foods with flavors such as lime, it would be difficult to identify the flavor as strawberry unless it was very strong. Color intensity also affects flavor perception. A stronger color may cause perception of a stronger flavor in a product, even if the stronger color is simply due to the addition of more food coloring! Texture can also be misleading. A thicker product may be perceived as tasting richer or stronger simply because it is thicker, and not because the thickening agent affects the flavor of the food. Other psychological factors that may come into play when making judgments about the flavor of foods include time of day (for example, certain tastes are preferred at breakfast time), general sense of well-being, health, and previous reactions to a particular food or taste.

SENSORY EVALUATION

Sensory evaluation has been defined as a scientific method used to evoke, measure, analyze, and interpret those responses to products as perceived through the senses of sight, smell, touch, taste, and hearing (7). This definition has been accepted and endorsed by sensory evaluation committees within both the Institute of Food Technologists and the American Society for Testing and Materials. For more detailed information on sensory evaluation, the reader is referred to the books by Lawless and Heymann (8), and by Stone and Sidel (7).

Sensory testing utilizes one or more of the five senses to evaluate foods. *Taste panels*, comprising groups of people, taste specific food samples under controlled conditions and evaluate them in different ways depending on the particular sensory test being conducted. This is the *only* type of testing that can measure consumer preference and acceptability. When it comes to public opinion of a product, there is no substitute for tasting by individual consumers.

In addition to a taste-panel evaluation, objective tests can be established that correlate with sensory testing, which give an indication of consumer acceptability, but this may not always be sufficient. In the development of *new* foods or when changing an *existing* product, it is necessary to determine consumer acceptance directly, and objective testing is not sufficient, even though it may be a reliable, objective indication of food quality.

Sensory methods may be used to determine:

1) whether foods differ in taste, odor, juiciness, tenderness, texture, and so on

2) to what extent foods differ

3) to ascertain consumer preferences and to determine whether a certain food is acceptable to a specific consumer group.

Three types of sensory testing are commonly used, each with a different goal. ***Discrimination or difference tests*** are designed to determine whether there is a difference between products; ***descriptive tests*** determine the extent of difference in specific sensory characteristics; and ***affective or acceptance/preference tests*** determine how well the products are liked, or which products are preferred. There are important differences between these three types of tests. It is important to select the appropriate type of test so that the results obtained are able to answer the questions being asked about the products, and are useful to the manufacturer or product developer.

The appropriate tests must be used under suitable conditions, in order for results to be interpreted correctly. All testing must be carried out under controlled conditions, with controlled lighting, sound (no noise), and temperature to minimize distractions and other adverse psychological factors.

Sensory Testing Procedure

Sensory testing is carried out by members of a taste panel, preferably in individual testing booths under controlled conditions. All distractions, bias, and adverse psychological factors must be minimized so that the evaluation is truly an evaluation of the sample being tested, and not a reaction to adverse circumstances, cultural prejudice, or the opinions of other testers. The noise level must be controlled to avoid distractions, temperature and humidity should be within an acceptable range, and lighting within the booth must also be monitored. In addition, there should be no extraneous smells, which may distract people from making judgments about the product under test.

Because color has a significant effect on subjective evaluation of a product, color differences may need to be masked. This is achieved by using red lights in the booths when necessary. It is important that people rate samples that may have different color intensities on *flavor* and not simply on the fact that they *look* different. For example, two brands of cheese puffs may look different because one is a deeper shade of orange than the other, and so one could tell the difference between them simply because of their color. However, there may not be a difference in the taste. If the color difference is masked by conducting the tests under red light, any differences detected could then be attributed to flavor differences, and not to color differences.

The samples are usually placed on a tray, and passed to each panelist through a hatch in front of the testing booth. The tray should contain a **ballot** that gives specific instructions on how to evaluate the samples and a place for the panelist's response. A cracker and water are provided, in order to cleanse the palate before tasting the samples. It is important that tasters have not eaten spicy or highly flavored food before tasting food samples, or their judgment may be impaired. Preferably, panelists should not have eaten anything immediately prior to carrying out a taste test.

Additionally, it is important that panelists cannot identify the products they are tasting and that they do not know which sample is the same as their neighbor's sample, so that there is no room for bias in the results. This is accomplished by assigning 3-digit random numbers to each product. For example, if two products are being tested (denoted product 1 and 2), each product is given at least two different random numbers. Panelists sitting next to each other will not be given samples with the same number, so that they cannot compare notes and agree with each other and introduce bias into the results that way.

If two products are being tested, 50% of the panelists must test product 1 first, and the rest must test product 2 first, but the order of testing must be randomized. This eliminates bias due to sample order, and also due to any changes in experimental conditions that may occur from the beginning to the end of the test. The specific product order and random numbers seen by each panelist are detailed on a **master sheet** to ensure that the test design is carried out correctly.

Sensory Tests

Discrimination or difference tests are used to determine if there is a perceivable difference between products. Such tests would be used if a company was changing the source of one of its ingredients or substituting one ingredient for another. Difference tests can also be used to see if the quality of a product changes over time or to compare the shelf life of a particular product packaged in different packaging materials. For example, a difference test could be used to determine if juices keep their flavor better when stored in glass bottles rather than in plastic ones.

A *small* group of panelists may be used to conduct such tests and they may be trained to recognize and describe the differences likely to occur in the products being tested. For example, if trained panelists are testing different tea blends or flavor bases, they have more experience than an average consumer in recognizing particular flavors associated with such products, and they are more sensitive to differences, and are able to describe them better. This is partly because they have been trained to identify such flavors. However, they are likely to be experienced tea drinkers (or tea connoisseurs) with a liking for different teas before they are trained for taste-panel work. Such people may be employees of the company doing the testing or members of a university research group. They would be expected to detect small differences in the product flavor that

```
TEST # _____                          Panelist # _____

                   TRIANGLE DIFFERENCE TEST

PRODUCT _____

INSTRUCTIONS: Proceed when you are ready. (Quietly so as not to distract others.)
FOR EACH SAMPLE:
1)  Take a bite of the cracker and a sip of water to rinse your mouth.
2)  Two of the samples are the same and one is different. CIRCLE the ODD sample. If
    you can not tell, guess.


    _____        _____            _____
3)  Describe the reason why the ODD sample is DIFFERENT. (Please be specific.)
```

FIGURE 1.1.   Ballot for triangle sensory test (obtained from Dr. Clay King at the
Sensory Testing Laboratory at Texas Woman's University, Denton, Texas).

would go unnoticed by most of the general population. Thus, their evaluation would be important in trying to keep a tea blend constant or in determining if there is a significant flavor difference when the source of an ingredient is changed.

It may also be important to know if small differences in a product can be detected by untrained consumers, who simply like the product and buy it on a regular basis. For this reason, difference tests are often conducted using larger panels of untrained panelists.

Two of the most frequently used difference tests are the triangle test and the duo–trio test. Typical ballots for these tests are given in Figures 1.1 and 1.2. These ballots and the one shown in Figure 1.3 were developed at the sensory evaluation laboratory at Texas Woman's University, Denton, Texas by Dr. Clay King, in

```
TEST # _____                          Panelist # _____

                   DUO-TRIO DIFFERENCE TEST

PRODUCT _____

INSTRUCTIONS: Proceed when you are ready. (Quietly so as not to distract others.)
FOR EACH SAMPLE:
1)  Take a bite of the cracker and a sip of water to rinse your mouth.
2)  CIRCLE the number of the sample which is THE SAME as the reference R. If you
    can not tell, guess.

    R            _____           _____
3)  Why are R and the sample you chose the same?
```

FIGURE 1.2.   Ballot for duo–trio sensory test (obtained from Dr. Clay King at the
Sensory Testing Laboratory at Texas Woman's University, Denton, Texas).

TEST # _____   **Panelist #** _____

LIKEABILITY RATING AND PAIRED PREFERENCE TEST

PRODUCT _____

INSTRUCTIONS: Proceed when you are ready. (Quietly so as not to distract others.)
Evaluate one sample at a time, working from top to bottom.

FOR EACH SAMPLE:

1) Take a bite of the cracker and a sip of water to rinse your mouth.

2) Taste the sample then **CIRCLE** the number which best expresses your opinion of
   the sample.

SAMPLE CODE: _____

Likeability   1   2   3   4   5   6   7   8   9
Scale   Dislike   Like
             Extremely   Extremely

SAMPLE CODE: _____

Likeability   1   2   3   4   5   6   7   8   9
Scale   Dislike   Like
             Extremely   Extremely

Describe the DIFFERENCES between the two samples. (Please be specific.)

Taste the samples again, then circle the one you prefer.

_____   _____

Describe the reasons why you prefer the one you chose.

FIGURE 1.3. Ballot for likeability and paired preference sensory tests (obtained from Dr. Clay King at the Sensory Testing Laboratory at Texas Woman's University, Denton, Texas).

conjunction with Coca-Cola Foods. The ballots have been used for consumer testing of beverages and other foods at the university sensory facility.

In the ***triangle test***, each panelist is given three samples, two of which are alike, and is asked to indicate the *odd* sample. The panelists are asked to taste the samples from left to right, cleansing their palate before each sample by taking a bite of cracker and a sip of water. Then they circle the number on the ballot sheet that corresponds to the sample they believe to be different. If they cannot tell, they must guess. Statistics are applied to the results to see if there is a significant difference among the products being tested. Because the panelists have to guess which is the odd one if they cannot detect a difference, one-third of them would pick the correct sample as being odd just by guessing. Therefore, more than one-third of the panelists must choose the correct answer for there to be a significant difference among the products. For example, if there are 60 members on a taste panel, 27 would need to choose the correct answer for the results to be significant at a probability level of 0.05, and 30 correct answers would be needed for significance at a probability level of 0.01. A probability level (or **p value**) of 0.05 means that out of 100 trials, the same result would be obtained 95 times, indicating 95% confidence that the result is valid. A probability of 0.01 is equivalent to 99% confidence in the significance of the results, because the same result would be expected in 99 out of 100 trials. Statistical tables are available to determine the number of correct answers required for significance at different probability levels (9).

In the **duo–trio test**, each panelist is given a reference and two samples. He or she is asked to taste the reference first, and then each sample, working from left to right, and circle on the ballot the sample that is the same as the reference. Again, if a panelist cannot tell which sample is the same as the reference, he or she must guess, and statistics must be applied to the results to determine whether there is a significant difference among the products. If everyone guessed, 50% of the panelists would get the correct answer, and so for the results to be significant, more than 50% must choose the correct answer. For a panel of 60 people, 40 must give the correct answer for the results to be significant at the 0.01 probability level. Again, tables are available to determine if results are statistically significant (9).

Affective, acceptance, or **preference** tests are used to determine whether a specific consumer group likes or prefers a particular product. This is necessary for the development and marketing of new products, as no laboratory test can tell whether the public will accept a new product or not. A *large* number of panelists, representing the general public must be used; thus, consumer testing is expensive and time-consuming. A relevant segment of the population needs to test the product. For example, if it is being aimed at over-50s, senior citizens must make up the taste panel, and not mothers with young children. The opposite would apply if the product was aimed at young children. (Products aimed at children would have to be acceptable to mothers as well, because they would be the ones to buy it.) Ethnic products must be tested either by the group for which they are aimed, or by a wide cross section of the public if the aim is to introduce the products to a broader market than is currently interested.

Panelists are not trained for this type of sensory testing. All that is required from them is that they give their opinion of the sample(s). However, they are normally screened to make sure that they are users or potential users of the product to be tested. Typically, they are asked to fill out a *screening sheet*, and answer questions about how much they like the product (or similar products), and how often they consume it. Anyone who does not like the product is asked not to take the test. The screening sheet may also ask for demographic information, such as gender and age range of the panelists. The specific questions for each screening sheet are determined by whoever sets up the test, based on the consumer group they aim to target with their product.

The simplest preference tests are **ranking tests**, where panelists are given two or more samples and asked to rank them in order of preference. In the *paired preference* test, panelists are given two samples and asked to circle the one they prefer. Often, the panelists are asked to taste a sample and score it on a nine-point hedonic scale from "dislike extremely" to "like extremely". This type of test is called a **likeability test**.

Sometimes panelists are asked to test more than one sample, to score each on the nine-point likeability scale, and then to describe the differences between the samples. This would not be a difference test, as differences in this case are usually obvious, and the point of the test is to see which product is preferred. In fact, the differences may be considerable. An example might be comparison of a chewy brand of chocolate chip cookies with a crunchy variety. The difference is obvious, but consumer preference is not obvious and would not be known without carrying out preference tests on the two products. A paired preference or ranking test may be included on a same ballot, and carried out along with a likeability test. An example of a typical ballot is given in Figure 1.3.

Descriptive tests are usually carried out by a small group of highly trained panelists. They are specialized difference tests, where the panelists are not simply asked whether they can determine differences between the two products, but are asked to *rate* particular aspects of the flavor of a particular product on a scale. Flavor aspects vary depending on the type of product being studied. For example, flavor notes in tea may be bitter, smoky, and tangy, whereas flavor notes in yogurt may be acid, chalky, smooth, and sweet. A descriptive "flavor map" or profile of a product is thus developed. Any detectable changes in the product would result in changes in the flavor map. The training required to be able to detect, describe, and quantify subtle changes in specific flavor notes is extensive. Therefore, establishment of such panels is costly. When trained, the panelists function as analytical instruments, and their evaluation of a product is not related to their like or dislike of it. The descriptive taste panel work is useful to research and development scientists, because it gives detailed information on the types of flavor differences between products.

OBJECTIVE EVALUATION

Objective evaluation of foods involves *instrumentation*, and use of physical and chemical techniques to evaluate food quality. *Objective testing* uses equipment to evaluate food products instead of variable human sensory organs. Such tests of food quality are essential in the food industry, especially for routine quality control of food products.

An objective test measures one particular attribute of a food rather than the overall quality of the product. Therefore, it is important to choose an objective test for food quality that measures a key attribute of the product being tested. For example, orange juice is both acidic and sweet; thus, suitable objective tests for this product would be measurement of pH and measurement of sugar content. These tests would be of no value in determining the quality of a chocolate chip cookie. A suitable test for cookie quality might include moisture content or the force required to break the cookie.

There are various objective tests available for monitoring food quality. Fruits and vegetables may be graded for size by passing them through apertures of a specific size. Eggs are also graded in this manner, and consumers may choose among six sizes, including small, large, or jumbo-sized eggs. Flour is graded according to particle size, which is required to pass through sieves of specific mesh size.

Color may be measured objectively by several methods, ranging from simply matching the product to colored tiles to using the **Hunterlab color and color difference meter**. The color meter measures the intensity, chroma, and hue of the sample and generates three numbers for the sample under test. Thus, small changes in color can be detected. This method of color analysis is appropriate for all foods. For liquid products, such as apple juice, a **spectrophotometer** can be used to measure color. A sample is placed in the machine and a reading is obtained, which is proportional to the color and/or the clarity of the juice.

Food Rheology

Many objective methods for measurement of food quality involve measurement of some aspect of texture, such as hardness, crispness, or consistency. As mentioned already, texture is related to the rheological properties of food, which determine how it responds when subjected to forces such as cutting, shearing, or pulling.

Rheological properties can be divided into three main categories. A food may exhibit *elastic* properties, *viscous* properties, or *plastic* properties, or a combination. In reality, rheological properties of most foods are extremely complex and they do not fit easily into one category.

Elasticity is a property of a solid and is illustrated by a rubber band or a coiled spring:

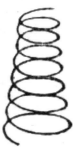

If a force or *stress* is applied, the material will deform (stretch or be compressed) in proportion to the amount of force applied, and when the force is removed, it will immediately return to its original position. If sufficient force is applied to a solid, it will eventually break. The force required to break the material is known as the *fracture stress*.

Some solids are more elastic than others; examples of very elastic solids are springs and rubber bands. Bread dough also has elastic properties, although its rheology is complex, and includes viscous and plastic components as well. All solid foods exhibit elastic properties to some degree.

Viscosity is a property of a liquid and is illustrated by a piston and cylinder (or a dashpot), or by a syringe:

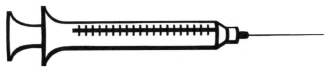

Viscosity is a measure of the resistance to flow of a liquid when subjected to a shearing force. The thicker the liquid, the greater is its viscosity or resistance to flow. For example, water has a low viscosity and flows readily, whereas catsup is considered "thick," has a higher viscosity, and flows relatively slowly.

Liquids can be separated into **Newtonian** and **non-Newtonian** fluids. In the case of a Newtonian liquid, the shear stress applied to the fluid is proportional to the shear rate or shear velocity of the flowing liquid. This means that the viscosity is independent of the shear rate. Therefore, viscosity will be the same, even if the viscometer used to measure it is operated at different speeds. A graph of shear stress against shear rate would give a straight line, and the viscosity could be calculated from the gradient of the line (see Figure 1.4). The steeper the line, the greater the resistance to flow, and the greater the viscosity of the liquid.

Examples of Newtonian liquids include water, sugar syrups, and wine. However, most liquid foods are non-Newtonian, in which case the consistency or apparent viscosity depends on the amount of shear stress applied. This can be seen with catsup, which appears fairly solid, and is hard to get out of the bottle if it has been standing for a while. However, after shaking (applying a shear stress), the catsup becomes almost runny, and will flow out of the bottle much more easily. If the bottle is again left to stand, the consistency of the undisturbed catsup will be regained after a short period of time. Shaking the bottle causes the molecules to align so that they flow over each other more easily, and the apparent viscosity decreases. A graph of shear stress against shear rate would not give a straight line for catsup, since the apparent viscosity is not constant. (Strictly speaking, the term "apparent viscosity" should be used for non-Newtonian liquids, whereas the term "viscosity" should be reserved for Newtonian liquids.)

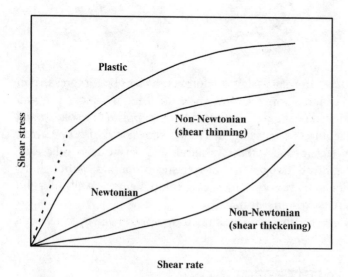

FIGURE 1.4. Schematic representation of flow behavior of Newtonian and non-Newtonian liquids [Modified from Bowers, 1992 (6)].

Some non-Newtonian liquids appear to get thicker when a shear stress is applied. In this case, the particles in the liquid tend to aggregate and trap pockets of liquid, thus making it harder for the molecules to flow over each other. Examples of such liquids include starch slurries and dilute solutions of some gums, such as alginates, carboxymethylcellulose, and guar gum.

The viscosity of both Newtonian and non-Newtonian liquids is affected by temperature. Higher temperatures cause liquids to flow more readily, thus decreasing viscosity, whereas lower temperatures cause an increase in viscosity. For this reason, it is important to make measurements of viscosity at a constant temperature and to specify that temperature.

A *plastic* substance can be molded, because it contains a liquid, but only after a certain minimum force (the *yield stress*) is applied. At forces below the yield stress, it behaves as an elastic solid, but above the yield stress, it behaves as a liquid. Examples of plastic substances include modeling clay, and foods such as warm chocolate, and hydrogenated vegetable shortenings that can be creamed easily.

Some foods exhibit both elastic and viscous properties at the same time. They are termed *viscoelastic*. Bread dough is a good example of a viscoelastic material. When a force is applied, the material first deforms like an elastic solid, but then starts to flow. When the force is removed, it only partly regains its original shape.

The rheological properties of a food affect its texture and sensory properties. For example, brittleness, shortness, and hardness are related to the fracture stress of a solid food, whereas thickness and creaminess are related to the consistency or apparent viscosity of a liquid food. The rheological properties of many foods can be modified by adding stabilizers such as gums. These are added to increase viscosity, which in turn restricts movement of everything in the system, and may delay undesirable changes, such as precipitation of solids or separation of emulsions.

Objective Measurement of Texture

Many objective methods for measurement of food quality involve measurement of some aspect of texture. For example, viscometers are used to measure viscosity or consistency of foods ranging from thin liquids such as oil to thick sauces such as catsup. The sophistication of these instruments also varies widely. The **Bostwick consistometer** is a simple device that involves filling a reservoir with the sample to be tested. A stopwatch is started, the gate holding the product in the reservoir is lifted, and the product is timed to flow a certain distance along the consistometer trough. At the other end of the scale, **Brookfield viscometers** are sophisticated instruments that may be used to measure viscosity under controlled temperature and when the sample is subjected to shearing forces of different magnitudes.

The **Instron Universal Testing Machine** has various attachments that allow it to measure different aspects of texture, including compressibility of bread and the force required to break a cookie or to shear a piece of meat.

The **Brabender amylograph** (Chapter 4) is an instrument that was developed to measure the viscosity of starch mixtures as they are heated in water. Another instrument with a very specific use is the mixograph, which is used to measure the ease of mixing of bread doughs.

Sophisticated equipment, such as the **mass spectrophotometer**, **gas chroma-tography**, and **high-performance liquid chromatography** equipment are available in research and analytical laboratories for analysis of specific products or components.

The list of equipment used in the food industry for evaluating food quality would fill a complete textbook! Certain principles must be emphasized when considering objective tests to evaluate the quality of a food product:

- The objective test must be appropriate for the food product being tested. In other words, it must measure an attribute of the food that has a major effect on quality.

- Ideally, the objective test results should correlate with sensory testing of similar food products to make sure that the test is a reliable index of quality of the food.

- Most objective tests used to assess food quality are empirical; that is, they do not measure an absolute property of the food. However, the results are still meaningful, as long as instruments are calibrated with materials that have similar properties to the foods under test.

- Objective tests include all types of instrumental analysis, including laboratory tests to determine chemical composition, nutrient composition, and bacterial composition.

- Objective tests are repeatable and are not subject to human variation. If the equipment is properly maintained and is used correctly, it should give reliable results from day to day.

Objective tests are necessary to identify contaminants in foods and to reveal faulty processing methods as well as testing for deterioration such as rancidity in fats and oils. Objective tests are essential for routine quality control of foods and food products. However, they must correlate with sensory testing, because no single objective test can measure the overall acceptability of a specific food or food product.

An in-depth study of analysis of foods by objective methods is beyond the scope of this book. For more information, the reader is referred to Food Analysis by S. Suzanne Nielsen (10), and to the many other textbooks available on the subject.

COMPARISON OF SUBJECTIVE AND OBJECTIVE EVALUATION

Both *sensory evaluation* and *objective evaluation* of food quality are essential in the food industry in order to routinely monitor food quality and to ensure that the foods being produced are acceptable to consumers. The two methods of evaluation complement each other.

Sensory testing is expensive and time-consuming, because many panelists are required to test a single product in order for the results to be meaningful. On the other hand, objective testing is efficient and, after the initial purchase of the necessary equipment, relatively inexpensive. One person can usually perform an objective test on many samples in a day, whereas it may take a day to perform a complete sensory test on one or two samples. Objective tests give repeatable results, whereas sensory tests may give variable results due to variation of human responses and opinions.

While sensory evaluation gives a judgment of the overall acceptability of a product, an objective method of evaluation is only able to measure one aspect of the food, and this may not always be sufficient to determine whether the quality of the product is acceptable. The only true judge of acceptability of a food product is a consumer! Therefore, objective tests must correlate with sensory tests to give a reliable index of food quality.

Objective tests are essential for routine quality control of food products. However, sensory evaluation is essential for product research and development. Only consumers can tell whether there is a perceivable difference in a product when the formulation or packaging is changed, and only consumers can determine whether a new product is acceptable or preferred over another brand.

SUBJECTIVE VS. OBJECTIVE ANALYSIS—OVERVIEW

Subjective/Sensory Analysis	*Objective Analysis*
Uses individuals	Uses equipment
Involves human sensory organs	Uses physical and chemical techniques
Results may vary	Results are repeatable
Determines human sensitivity to changes in ingredients, processing, or packaging	Need to find a technique appropriate for the food being tested
Determines consumer acceptance	Cannot determine consumer acceptance unless correlated with sensory testing
Time-consuming and expensive	Generally faster, cheaper, and more efficient than sensory testing
Essential for product development and for marketing of new products	Essential for routine quality control

---

CONCLUSION

Food quality can be defined as the degree of excellence of a food and includes factors such as taste, appearance, and nutritional quality, as well as its bacteriological or keeping quality. Food quality goes hand in hand with food acceptability, and it is important that quality is monitored, both from a food safety standpoint and to ensure that the public likes a particular product and will continue to select it. Both sensory and objective methods are important in evaluation of food quality and the two methods complement one another. Sensory analysis is essential for development of new products, because only consumers can tell whether they like a product or not.

However, objective testing is also important, especially for routine quality control of food products.

GLOSSARY

Affective or acceptance/preference tests: Used to determine whether a specific consumer group likes or prefers a particular product.

Ballot: Sheet of paper on which the panelist receives pertinent sample information and instructions, and on which observations are recorded during a sensory test.

Descriptive tests: Specialized difference tests used to describe specific flavor attributes of a product, or to describe degree of difference between products.

Discrimination or difference tests: Used to determine if there is a perceivable difference between samples.

Duo–trio test: Samples include a reference food and two samples, one of which is the same as the reference.

Elasticity: Ability of a material to stretch when a force is applied and to return to its original position when the force is removed.

Likeability test: Panelists rate a sample on a hedonic scale from "dislike extremely" to "like extremely."

Master sheet: Details the specific three-digit product numbers and positions for every panelist in a sensory test. Used to ensure that each product is seen an equal number of times in each position, so that bias is avoided.

Mouthfeel: Textural qualities of a food as perceived in the mouth.

Newtonian liquid: The viscosity is independent of the shear rate. Stirring or shaking does not make the liquid runnier or thicker. Examples are water, sugar syrups, and wine.

Non-Newtonian liquid: Apparent viscosity depends on the shear rate. Catsup gets thinner with increasing shear rate, whereas some gums thicken with increasing shear rate.

Objective evaluation: Involves use of physical and chemical techniques to evaluate food quality, instead of variable human sensory organs.

Plasticity: Material flows when subjected to a certain minimum force; material can be molded.

p-Value: Statistical probability that a result is significant. A p value of 0.01 indicates 99% confidence that a result is significant. In other words, out of 100 trials, the same result would be expected 99 times. The probability of the opposite result occurring is only 1 in 100 trials.

Ranking test: Panelists rank two or more samples in order of preference or intensity for a particular attribute.

Rheology: Science of the deformation and flow of matter, how a food reacts when force is applied; includes elasticity, viscosity, and plasticity.

Sensory testing: Use of senses to evaluate products; involves consumer opinion.

Threshold: Concentration required for identification of a particular substance.

Triangle test: Three samples, two of which are alike, one is odd.

Umami: Savory taste, given by substances such as monosodium glutamate.

Viscosity: Resistance to flow of a liquid when a shear force is applied. Liquids with a low viscosity flow readily, whereas liquids with a high viscosity flow slowly.

REFERENCES

1. Giese J. Measuring physical properties of foods. *Food Technology*. 1995; 49(2): 54–63.
2. Szczesniak AS. Physical properties of foods: What they are and their relation to other food properties. In: Peleg M, Bagley EB, eds. *Physical Properties of Foods*. Westport, CT: AVI, 1983.
3. Gullet EA. Color and food. In: Hui YH, ed. *Encyclopedia of Food Science and Technology*. New York: John Wiley and Sons, 1992.
4. Mabron TJ. Color measurement of food. *Cereal Foods World*. 1993; 38(1): 21–25.
5. Bourne ML. *Food Texture and Rheology*. New York: Academic Press, 1982.
6. Bowers J. Characteristics of food dispersions. In: Bowers J, ed. *Food Theory and Applications*, 2nd ed. New York: MacMillan, 1992, p 30.
7. Stone H, Sidel JL. *Sensory Evaluation Practices*, 2nd ed. San Diego, CA: Academic Press, 1993.
8. Lawless HT, Heymann H. *Sensory Evaluation of Food. Principles and Practices*. Gaithersburg, MD: Aspen Publishers, 1999.
9. Roessler EB, Pangborn RM, Sidel JL, Stone H. Expanded statistical tabels for estimating significance in paired-preference, paired-difference, duo–trio and triangle tests. *Journal of Food Science*. 1978; 43: 940–942.
10. Neilsen SS. *Food Analysis,* 2nd ed. Gaithersburg, MD: Aspen Publishers, 1998.

CHAPTER 2

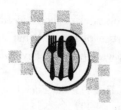

Water

INTRODUCTION

Water is abundant in all living things and, consequently, in almost all foods, unless steps have been taken to remove it. It is essential for life, even though it contributes no calories to the diet. Water also greatly affects the texture of foods, as can be seen when comparing grapes and raisins (dried grapes), or fresh and wilted lettuce. It gives crisp texture or turgor to fruits and vegetables, and it also affects perception of the tenderness of meat. For some food products, such as potato chips, salt, or sugar, lack of water is an important aspect of their quality, and keeping water *out* of such foods is important to maintain quality.

Almost all food processing techniques involve the use of water or modification of water in some form: freezing, drying, emulsification (trapping water in droplets), breadmaking, thickening of starch, and making pectin gels are a few examples. Further, because bacteria cannot grow without water, the water content has a significant effect on maintaining quality of the food. This explains why freezing, dehydration, or concentration of foods increases shelf life and inhibits bacterial growth.

Water is important as a solvent or dispersing medium, dissolving small molecules to form true solutions and dispersing larger molecules to form colloidal solutions. Acids and bases ionize in water; water is also necessary for many enzyme-catalyzed and chemical reactions to occur, including hydrolysis of compounds such as sugars. It is also important as a heating and cooling medium and as a cleansing agent.

Because water has so many functions that are important to a food scientist, it is important to be familiar with some of its unique properties. When modifying the water content of a food, it is necessary to understand these functions in order to predict the changes that are likely to occur during processing of such foods.

Drinking water is available to the consumer in convenient bottled, canned and aseptic containers.

CHEMISTRY OF WATER

The chemical formula for water is H_2O. Water contains strong **covalent bonds** that hold the two hydrogen atoms and one oxygen atom together. The oxygen can be regarded to be at the center of a tetrahedron, with a bond angle of 105° between the two hydrogen atoms in *liquid water* and a larger angle of 109° 6′ between the hydrogens in *ice* (Figure 2.1).

The bonds between oxygen and each hydrogen atom are polar bonds, having a 40% partial ionic character. This means that the outer-shell electrons are unequally shared between the oxygen and hydrogen atoms, the oxygen atom attracting them more strongly than each hydrogen atom. As a result, each hydrogen atom is slightly positively charged and each oxygen atom is slightly negatively charged. Therefore they are able to form **hydrogen bonds**.

A hydrogen bond is a *weak* bond between polar compounds where a hydrogen atom of one molecule is attracted to an electronegative atom of another molecule (Figure 2.2). It is a weak bond relative to other types of chemical bonds such as covalent or ionic bonds, but it is very important because it usually occurs in large numbers and, therefore, has a significant cumulative effect on the properties of the substance in which it is found. Water can form up to four hydrogen bonds (oxygen can hydrogen bond with two hydrogen atoms).

Water would be expected to be gas at room temperature if compared with similar compounds in terms of their positions in the periodic table, but because of the many hydrogen bonds it contains, it is liquid. Hydrogen bonds between hydrogen and oxygen are common, not just between water molecules, but between many other types of molecules that are important in foods, such as sugars, starches, pectins, and proteins.

Due to its V-shape, each molecule of water can form up to four hydrogen bonds with its nearest neighbors. Each hydrogen atom can form one hydrogen bond, but the oxygen atom can form two, which results in a three-dimensional lattice in ice. The structure of ice is dynamic, and hydrogen bonds are continually breaking and re-forming between different water molecules. Liquid water also contains hydrogen

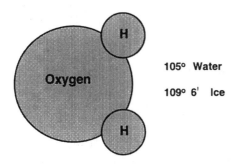

FIGURE 2.1 Bond angle of water and ice.

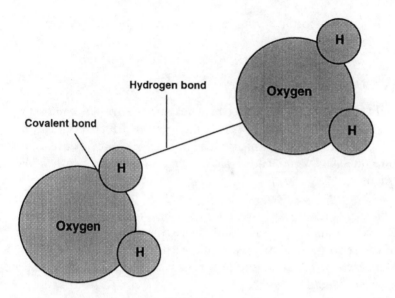

FIGURE 2.2 Hydrogen and covalent bonds in water molecules.

bonds and, therefore, has a variety of ordered structures that are continually changing as hydrogen bonds break and re-form. In liquid water, it is estimated that about 80% of water molecules are involved in hydrogen bonding at any one time at 212°F (100°C), whereas 90% are involved in liquid water at 32°F (0°C).

Because liquid water has a smaller bond angle than ice, the molecules can be packed together more tightly, and so the *coordination number* or, in other words, the average number of nearest neighbors is higher for water than for ice. The average distance between water molecules is also affected by temperature and increases with temperature as the molecules have more kinetic energy and can move around faster and further at higher temperatures. Both of these affect the density of water, but the coordination number has a much more dramatic effect. Ice is less dense than water because the molecules have a smaller coordination number and cannot be packed together as tightly as water. Therefore, ice floats.

As water freezes, its density decreases and its volume increases by about 9%. This is very significant when freezing foods with high water content. Containers and equipment must be designed to accommodate the volume increase when the product freezes, for example, molds for popsicles must allow room for expansion. This volume increase also contributes to the damage to the structure of soft fruits on freezing. This is discussed in Chapter 7. As water is heated above 39°F (4°C), the increase in the average distance between molecules causes a slight decrease in density.

SPECIFIC HEAT AND LATENT HEAT OF WATER

When ice is heated, the temperature increases in proportion to the amount of heat applied. The **specific heat** of water is the energy (in calories or in joules) required to raise the temperature of 1 g of water by 1°C, and is the same whether heating water or ice. It is relatively high compared to other substances due to the hydrogen bonds. The specific heat of water is 1 cal/g/°C. This means that it takes 100 cal to raise the temperature of 1 g of water from 0 to 100°C.

Once ice has reached 0°C, energy needs to be put in to break the hydrogen bonds and enable ice to change to the liquid form. Until the ice has been converted to liquid, there is no further change in temperature. The **latent heat of fusion** is the energy required to convert 1 g of ice is to water at 0°C and is 80 cal; that is, 1 g of ice at the freezing point absorbs approximately 80 cal as it changes to the liquid state.

The **latent heat of vaporization** is the energy required to convert 1 g of water into vapor at 100°C and is 540 cal; that is, 1 g of water at the boiling point absorbs approximately 540 cal as it becomes steam.

The specific heat and latent heat for water are all fairly high compared with most substances, and this is an important consideration when water is used as a medium of heat transfer. It takes considerable energy to heat water, and that energy is then available to be transferred to the food. Foods *heated* in water are slow to heat. Water also must take up considerable heat to evaporate. It takes heat from its surroundings, thus, it is a good *cooling* agent.

When ice is subjected to vacuum and then heated, it is converted into vapor without going through the liquid phase. This phenomenon is known as **sublimation**, and is the basis for the food processing method known as **freeze drying**. Coffee is an example of a food product that is freeze-dried. The process is expensive and is only used for foods that can be sold at a high price, such as coffee. The coffee beans are frozen and then subjected to a high vacuum, after which radiant heat is applied until almost all of water is removed by sublimation. Freezer burn is also the result of sublimation.

VAPOR PRESSURE AND BOILING POINT

Vapor Pressure

If a puddle of water is left on the ground for a day or two, it will dry up because the liquid evaporates. The water does not boil, but individual water molecules gain enough energy to escape from the liquid as vapor. Over a period, an *open*, small pool of water will dry up in this way. If the liquid is in a *closed* container, at equilibrium, some molecules are always evaporating and vapor molecules are condensing, so there is no overall change in the system. The *vapor* (gaseous) molecules that have escaped from the *liquid* state exert a pressure on the surface of the liquid known as the **vapor pressure**.

When the vapor pressure is *high*, the liquid evaporates (is vaporized) easily and *many* molecules exist in the vapor state; the boiling point is low. Conversely, a *low* vapor pressure indicates that the liquid does not vaporize easily and that there are few molecules existing in the vapor state. The boiling point for these liquids is higher. The liquid boils when the vapor pressure reaches the external pressure.

The vapor pressure increases with increasing temperature. At higher temperatures, the molecules have more energy and it is easier for them to overcome the forces holding them within the liquid and to vaporize, and so there are more molecules in the vapor state.

The vapor pressure decreases with addition of solutes, such as salt or sugars. In effect, the solutes dilute the water; therefore, there are less water molecules (in the same volume) available for vaporization and, thus, there will be fewer molecules in the vapor state, and the vapor pressure will be lower. Attraction to the solute also limits evaporation.

Boiling Point

Anything that lowers the vapor pressure (pressure by gas above the liquid) increases the boiling point. This is due to the fact that as the vapor pressure is lowered at a particular temperature, more energy must be put in; in other words, the temperature must be raised to increase the vapor pressure again. The external pressure does not change if salts or sugars are added, but it is harder for the molecules to vaporize and so the temperature at which the vapor pressure is the same as the external pressure (boiling point) will be higher. One mole of sucrose elevates the boiling point by 0.52°C, and one mole of salt elevates the boiling point by 1.04°C. Salt has double the effect of sucrose because it is ionized, and for every mole of salt, there is 1 mol of sodium ions and 1 mol of chloride ions. Salts and sugars depress the freezing point of water in a similar fashion.

If the external pressure is increased by heating in a pressure cooker or retort (commercial pressure cooker), the boiling point increases and a shorter time than normal is required to cook a particular food (the basis of preserving foods by canning). For example, food may be heated in cans in retorts, and the steam pressure is increased to give a boiling point in the range 239–250°F (115–121°C). Conversely, if the external pressure is decreased, for example, at high altitude, water boils at a lower temperature and so food may require a longer time to cook.

WATER AS A DISPERSING MEDIUM

Substances are dissolved, dispersed, or suspended in water depending on their particle size and solubility. Water is the usual dispersion medium.

Water *dissolves* small molecules such as salts, sugars, or water-soluble vitamins to form a true **solution**, which may be either **ionic** or **molecular** (A discussion of unsaturated, saturated, and supersaturated solutions appears in Chapter 14.).

Solution

An ionic solution is formed by dissolving substances that ionize in water, such as salts, acids, or bases. Taking sodium chloride as an example, the solid contains sodium (Na^+) and chloride (Cl^-) ions held together by ionic bonds. When placed in water, the water molecules reduce the attractive forces between the oppositely charged ions, the ionic bonds are broken, and the individual ions become surrounded by water molecules, or **hydrated**. Each ion is usually surrounded by six water molecules; the ions move independently of each other.

Polar molecules, such as sugars, which are associated by hydrogen bonding, dissolve to form **molecular solutions**. When a sugar crystal is dissolved, hydrogen-bond interchange takes place and the hydrogen bonds between the polar hydroxyl groups on the sugar molecules are broken and replaced by hydrogen bonds between water and the sugar molecules. Thus, the sugar crystal is gradually hydrated; each sugar molecule being surrounded by water molecules.

Water molecules bind to polar groups on the sugar molecules by hydrogen bonds. The sugar molecules are removed from the sugar crystal and hydrated as water molecules surround them and bind to them by hydrogen bonds.

When a hydrogen-bond interchange is involved, solubility increases with increasing temperature. Heating disrupts hydrogen bonds and reduces water–water and sucrose–sucrose attraction, thus facilitating formation of hydrogen bonds between water and sucrose, and hydration of sucrose molecules. Therefore, sucrose is much more soluble in hot water than in cold water. Solutes increase the boiling point of water, and the dramatic increase in sucrose solubility with temperature, particularly at temperatures above 100°C (the boiling point of pure water), makes it possible to determine the sucrose concentration by measuring the boiling point of sucrose solution (Chapter 13). This is important when making candies or pectin jellies.

Colloidal Dispersion

Molecules that are too big to form true solutions can be dispersed in water, depending on their size. Those with a particle size range 1–100 nm are dispersed to form a ***colloidal dispersion*** or ***sol***. Examples of such molecules include cellulose, *cooked* starch, pectic substances, gums, and some food proteins. Colloidal dispersions are often unstable; thus, food scientists must take care to stabilize them where necessary if they occur in food products. They are particularly unstable to factors such as heating, freezing, or pH change. Changing the conditions in a stable dispersion can cause precipitation or gelation; this is desirable in some cases, for example, when making pectin jellies.

(The reader is referred to Chapter 4 for a discussion of sols and gels, but *sol* is a colloid that pours—a two-phase system with a solid dispersed phase in a liquid continuous phase, for example a hot sauce. A ***gel*** is also a two-phase system, containing an elastic solid with a liquid dispersed phase in a solid continuous phase.)

Colloid science is important to food scientists as many convenient or packaged foods have colloidal dimensions, and their stability and sensitivity to certain types of reactions can only be understood with knowledge of colloid science.

Suspension

Particles that are larger than 100 nm are too large to form a colloidal dispersion. These form ***suspension*** when mixed with water. The particles in a suspension separate out over a period, whereas no such separation is observed with colloidal dispersions. An example of a suspension would be *uncooked* starch grains in water. They can be suspended throughout the liquid by stirring, but if left undisturbed, they settle down, and a sediment is observed at the bottom of the container.

FREE, BOUND, AND ENTRAPPED WATER

Water is abundant in all living things and, consequently, in almost all foods, unless steps have been taken to remove it. Most natural foods contain water up to 70% of their weight or greater unless they are dehydrated, and fruits and vegetables contain water up to 95% or greater. Water that can be extracted easily from foods by squeezing or cutting or pressing is known as *free water*, whereas water that cannot be extracted easily is termed as **bound water**.

Bound water is usually defined in terms of the ways it is measured; different methods of measurement give different values for bound water in a particular food. Many food constituents can bind or hold onto water molecules, such that they cannot be easily removed and they do not behave like liquid water. Some characteristics of bound water include:

- It is not free to act as a solvent for salts and sugars.
- It can be frozen only at very low temperatures (below the freezing point of water).
- It exhibits essentially no vapor pressure.
- Its density is greater than that of free water.

Bound water has more structural bonding than liquid or free water, thus it is unable to act as a solvent. As the vapor pressure is negligible the molecules cannot escape as vapor; and the molecules in bound water are more closely packed than in the liquid state, so the density is greater. An example of bound water is the water present in cacti or pine tree needles—the water cannot be squeezed or pressed out; extreme desert heat or a winter freeze does not negatively affect bound water and the vegetation remains alive. Even upon dehydration, food contains bound water.

Water molecules bind to polar groups or ionic sites on molecules such as starches, pectins, and proteins. Water closest to these molecules is held most firmly, and the subsequent water layers are held less firmly and are less ordered, until finally the structure of free water prevails. A more detailed discussion of bound water is given in Food Chemistry books, for example, Fennema (1).

Water may also be **entrapped** in foods such as pectin gels, fruits, vegetables, and so on. Entrapped water is immobilized in capillaries or cells, but if released during cutting or damage, it flows freely. Entrapped water has properties of free water and no properties of bound water.

Freshness of any produce is evaluated in part by the presence of water. Food items appear more wilted when free water is increasingly lost through dehydration (Chapter 7).

WATER ACTIVITY (A_W)

Water activity, or A_w, is a ratio of the vapor pressure of water in a solution (P_s) to the vapor pressure of pure water (P_w):

$$A_w = P_s/P_w$$

A_w must be high as living tissues require sufficient level of water to maintain turgor. However, microorganisms such as bacteria, mold, and yeast multiply at a high A_w. Because their growth must be controlled, preservation techniques against spoilage due to these microorganisms take into account the water activity of the food. Less bacterial growth occurs if the water level is lowered to less than 0.85 (FDA Model Food Code). Of course, there are other factors in addition to the water that must be present for bacterial growth to occur (food, optimum pH, etc.).

Jams, jellies, and preserves are prepared using high concentrations of sugar and brines, which contain high concentrations of salt that are used to preserve hams. Sugar and salt are both effective preservatives as they lower down A_w. Salt lowers down A_w even more effectively than sugar due to its chemical structure that ionizes and attracts water.

Foods are also dehydrated or frozen to reduce the available water. Drying or freezing are common food preservation techniques.

ROLE OF WATER IN FOOD PRESERVATION AND SHELF LIFE OF FOOD

The control of water level in foods is an important aspect of food quality as water content affects the shelf life of food. For example, foods may be more desirable either crispy or dry. Freezing and drying are common food preservation processes that are used to extend the shelf life of foods because they render water unavailable for pathogenic or spoilage bacteria. If the water in foods is frozen quickly, there is less damage to the food at the cellular level. Preservatives (Chapter 16) may be added to a formulation to prevent mold or yeast growth. Humectants, which have an affinity for water, are added to retain moisture in foods.

WATER HARDNESS AND TREATMENTS

The hardness of water is measured in parts per million or in "grains," with one grain equivalent to 0.064 g of calcium carbonate. *Soft water* contains 1–4 grains per gallon some organic matter, and has no mineral salts. *Hard water* contains 11–20 grains per gallon. Water may exhibit *temporary* hardness due to iron or calcium and magnesium bicarbonate ions [$Ca(HCO_3)_2$ and $Mg(HCO_3)_2$]. The water may be softened by boiling (soluble bicarbonates precipitate when boiled and leave deposits or scales) and insoluble carbonates may be removed from the water.

Permanently hard water *cannot* be softened by boiling as it contains either calcium or magnesium sulfates ($CaSO_4$ or $MgSO_4$) as well as other salts that are not precipitated by boiling. Permanent hard water may only be softened by the use of chemical softeners. Hard water exhibits less cleaning effectiveness than soft water due to the formation of insoluble calcium and magnesium salts with soap, which could be prevented by the use of detergents.

Water has a pH of 7 or neutral; tap water displays a variance on either side of neutral. It may be slightly alkaline or slightly acidic depending on the source and so forth. Hard water has a pH of up to 8.5. Chlorinated water is that which has had chlorine added to kill or inhibit the growth of microorganisms. Manufacturing or processing plants may require chemically pure water to prevent turbidity, off-color, and off-flavor. Tap water may not be sufficiently pure for use in food products.

CONCLUSION

Water is essential for life and makes up the major part of living tissue. The nature of hydrogen bonds allows water to bond with other water molecules as well as with sugar, starches, pectins, and proteins. Water absorbs energy as it changes from frozen to liquid to vapor state, and is an effective cooling medium. If water is easily extracted from foods by squeezing, or pressing, it is known as free water. Inversely, water that is not easily removed from foods and that is not free to act as a solvent is known as bound water; water in foods imparts freshness. A measure of water activity is the ratio of the vapor pressure of water in a solution to the vapor pressure of pure water. If water is unavailable for pathogenic or spoilage-causing bacteria to multiply, food is better preserved and has a longer shelf life.

GLOSSARY

Bound water: Water that cannot be extracted easily; it is bound to polar and ionic groups in the food.

Colloidal dispersion: Molecules, larger than those in solution, dispersed in the surrounding medium.

Covalent bonds: Strong bonds that hold the two hydrogen atoms and one oxygen atom together in a water molecule.

Free water: Water that can be extracted easily from foods by squeezing, cutting, or pressing.

Freeze drying: A food processing method that converts ice to vapor without going through the liquid phase (sublimation).

Gel: Elastic solid; a two-phase system that contains a solid continuous phase and a liquid dispersed phase.

Hard water: Contains 11–20 grains per gallon. Hardness is due to calcium and magnesium bicarbonates or sulfates, which results in less effective cleaning.

Hydrogen bonds: Weak bonds between polar compounds where a hydrogen atom of one molecule is attracted to an electronegative atom of another molecule.

Latent heat of fusion: The energy required to convert 1 g of ice to water at 0°C—requires 80 cal.

Latent heat of vaporization: The energy required to convert 1 g of water to vapor at 100°C—requires 540 cal.

Sol: A two-phase system with a solid dispersed in a liquid continuous phase; pourable.

Soft water: Contains one to four grains per gallon, no mineral salts, some organic matter.

Solution: (ionic or molecular) small molecules dissolved in water.

Sublimation: When ice is subjected to vacuum and then heated, it gets converted to vapor without going through the liquid phase; basis for freeze drying; occurs in freezer burn.

Specific heat: The energy required to raise the temperature of 1 g of water by 1°C whether heating water or ice; requires 1 cal/g/°C.

Suspension: Molecules larger than those in a solution or dispersion that are mixed with the surrounding medium. A *temporary* suspension settles upon standing.

Vapor pressure: The pressure vapor molecules exert on the liquid.

Water activity (A$_w$): The ratio of the vapor pressure of water in a solution to the vapor pressure of pure water.

REFERENCES

1. Fennema O. Water and Ice. In: Fennema O, ed. *Food Chemistry*, 3rd ed. New York: Marcel Dekker, 1996.

BIBLIOGRAPHY

Simatros D, Karel M. Characterization of the condition of water in foods: Physiochemical aspects. In: Seow CC, ed. *Food Preservation by Moisture Control*. London: Elsevier Applied Science Publishers, 1988.

Rockland LB, Stewart GF. *Water Activity: Influences on Food Quality*. New York: Academic Press, 1981.

PART II

Carbohydrates in the Food Guide Pyramid

CHAPTER 3

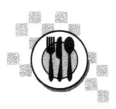

Carbohydrates in Food—An Introduction

INTRODUCTION

Carbohydrates are organic compounds containing carbon, hydrogen, and oxygen, and they may be simple or complex molecules. Historically, the term "carbohydrate" has been used to classify all compounds with the general formula $C_n(H_2O)_n$ as the hydrates of carbon. Important food carbohydrates include simple sugars, dextrins, starches, celluloses, hemicelluloses, pectins, and gums. They are an important source of energy or fiber in the diet, and they are also important constituents of foods because of their functional properties. Carbohydrates may be used as sweeteners, thickeners, stabilizers, gelling agents, and fat replacers. The simplest carbohydrates are known as monosaccharides or sugars, and they have the general formula $C_nH_{2n}O_n$. The most common ones contain six carbon atoms. Disaccharides contain two sugar units, trisaccharides contain three, oligosaccharides contain several units, and polysaccharides are complex polymers containing as many as several thousand units linked together to form a molecule.

MONOSACCHARIDES

Monosaccharides are simple carbohydrates containing between three and eight carbon atoms, but only those with five or six carbon atoms are common. Two of the most important ones in foods are the six-carbon sugars glucose and fructose. These have the general formula $C_6H_{12}O_6$.

Examples of Monosaccharides

Glucose.   Glucose is known as an ***aldose sugar*** because it contains an aldehyde group (CHO) located on the first carbon atom of the chain:

Glucose and an aldehyde group:

$$
\begin{array}{c}
_1CHO \\
| \\
H-_2C-OH \\
| \\
HO-_3C-H \\
| \\
H-_4C-OH \\
| \\
H-_5C-OH \\
| \\
_6CH_2OH
\end{array}
\qquad \text{glucose}
\qquad
\begin{array}{c}
H \\
| \\
-C=O
\end{array}
\qquad \text{aldehyde group}
$$

It is conventional to number the carbon atoms along the chain so that the carbon atom with the highest number is farthest away from the aldehyde (or functional) group. The aldehyde group is therefore located on carbon one in glucose (and in all other aldose sugars). The numbering of the carbon atoms in glucose is shown above.

Two isomers of glucose exist, which are mirror images of each other, D-glucose and L-glucose. D-glucose is the isomer that occurs naturally.

In fact, there are two series of aldose sugars, known as the D-series and the L-series, each formed by adding CHOH groups to build the carbon chain, starting from the smallest aldose sugar, which is D- or L-glyceraldehyde:

$$
\begin{array}{c}
H \quad O \\
\backslash \quad // \\
C \\
| \\
H-C-\boxed{OH} \\
| \\
CH_2OH
\end{array}
\qquad
\begin{array}{c}
H \quad O \\
\backslash \quad // \\
C \\
| \\
\boxed{OH}-C-H \\
| \\
CH_2OH
\end{array}
$$

D-glyceraldehyde   L-glyceraldehyde

Each H–C–OH group within the chain is asymmetrical (since the H and OH groups are different). The highest-numbered asymmetric carbon atom of each D-series sugar has the same configuration as D-glyceraldehyde, rather than its L-isomer. In glucose, the highest-numbered asymmetric carbon atom is carbon-5. This is termed the **reference carbon atom**, because its configuration determines whether the sugar belongs to the D series or to the L series. The hydroxyl group attached to it is called the **reference hydroxyl group**. This group is always on the right side in a D-series sugar.

The straight-chain configuration of glucose (and of other monosaccharides) does not account for all the properties of the molecule. In reality, the straight-chain form exists in equilibrium with several possible ring configurations. In other words, the different configurations exist together in solution in a delicate balance. Glucose can exist in four ring structures: two pyranose or six-membered ring forms, and two furanose or five-membered ring forms. These exist along with the straight-chain form, as shown in Figure 3.1.

The most common configurations for glucose are the **pyranose** structures, drawn according to the Haworth convention in Figure 3.2. These are **anomers**,

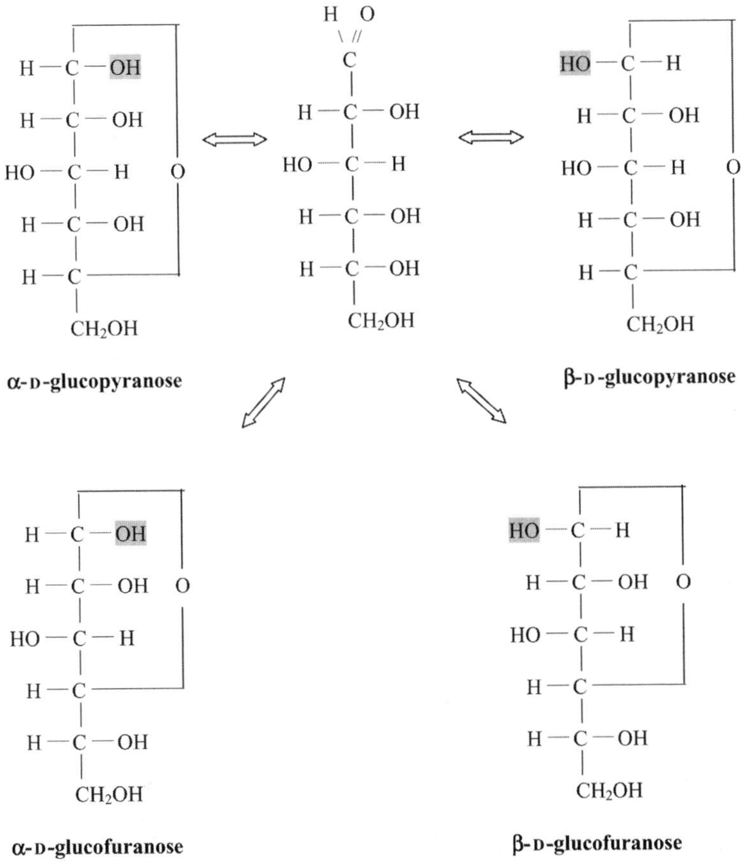

α-D-glucopyranose

β-D-glucopyranose

α-D-glucofuranose

β-D-glucofuranose

FIGURE 3.1   The main isomers of D-glucose (Fischer projections).

and are designated **alpha** (α) and **beta** (β). They are formed when the hydroxyl group on the fifth carbon reacts with the carbonyl group (located on C1). As the ring closes, a new hydroxyl group is formed on C1. This is termed the **anomeric hydroxyl group,** and the carbon atom to which it is attached is termed the **anomeric carbon atom.** For glucose and the other aldoses, the anomeric carbon atom is always the first carbon atom of the chain.

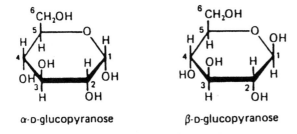

α-D-glucopyranose   β-D-glucopyranose

FIGURE 3.2   The D-glucopyranose anomers, drawn according to the Haworth convention.

The anomeric hydroxyl group can project towards either side of the ring, as shown in Figure 3.2. Hence, there are two possible pyranose structures.

For glucose and all the hexoses, the α-anomer has the anomeric hydroxyl group on the *opposite* face of the ring to carbon-6 (i.e., pointing in the opposite direction to carbon-6), when drawn according to the Haworth convention, whereas the β-anomer has the anomeric hydroxyl group on the *same* face of the ring as carbon-6 (i.e., pointing in the same direction as carbon-6). For the D-series sugars, when the ring closes, carbon-6 is always located above the plane of the ring. Therefore, in the case of the α-anomer, the anomeric hydroxyl group points *down*, or *below* the plane of the ring, whereas in the case of the β-anomer, the anomeric hydroxyl group points *up*, or *above* the plane of the ring.

---

alpha anomer—anomeric hydroxyl group is on the **opposite** face of the ring to carbon-6 D **series sugars**—anomeric hydroxyl group points **down**

beta anomer—anomeric hydroxyl group is on the **same** face of the ring as carbon-6 D **series sugars**—anomeric hydroxyl group points **up**

[For the chemists who prefer to define the alpha- and beta-configurations according to the reference carbon, when the anomeric hydroxyl group is formed on the same side of the ring as the reference hydroxyl group (as seen in the Fischer projection formula), the anomer is denoted alpha, whereas, when it is formed on the opposite side, it is denoted beta.]

In solution, the alpha- and beta-forms are in equilibrium, but the configuration can be fixed if the molecule reacts to form a disaccharide. It is important to know whether the configuration is fixed as the alpha- or beta-configuration, because this affects properties of the molecule, including digestibility. For example, starch contains α-D-glucose molecules, and so can be digested, but cellulose contains β-D-glucose molecules and is indigestible.

Although the ring structures are drawn with flat faces in the Haworth formulae, in reality they are not planar rings, but are bent, and could be visualized more as a boat or a chair configuration.

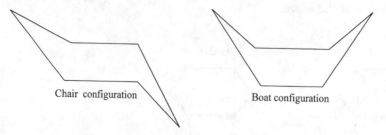

Chair configuration   Boat configuration

The different configurations of glucose and the relationships between them are complex, and are beyond the scope of this book. For a more in-depth treatment, interested readers are referred to books such as Food Chemistry, edited by Owen Fennema, or to basic biochemistry textbooks.

Glucose is the most important aldose sugar. Two other aldose sugars important in foods include galactose and mannose. Galactose is important as a constituent of milk sugar (lactose), and mannose is used to make the sugar alcohol mannitol, which is used as an alternative sweetener in chewing gum and other food products. These are both D-series sugars. In fact, almost all naturally occurring monosaccharides belong to the D-series.

Fructose.   Fructose is a six-carbon sugar, like glucose, but it is a **ketose sugar**, not an aldose, because it contains a ketone group, and not an aldehyde group:

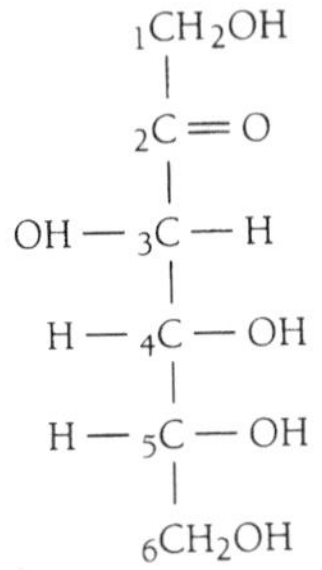

$$
\begin{array}{l}
_1CH_2OH \\
| \\
_2C = O \\
| \\
OH - _3C - H \\
| \\
H - _4C - OH \\
| \\
H - _5C - OH \\
| \\
_6CH_2OH
\end{array}
\qquad \text{fructose}
\qquad\qquad
\begin{array}{l}
| \\
C = O \\
|
\end{array}
\qquad \text{ketone group}
$$

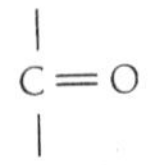

Like the aldose sugars, there is a D-series and an L-series of ketose sugars, but D-fructose is the only ketose of importance in foods. All **ketose sugars** contain a ketone group, not an aldehyde group.

In fructose, the ketone group is located on the second carbon of the chain. The second carbon atom is therefore the anomeric carbon in fructose. Fructose occurs mainly in the α- and β-**furanose**, or five-membered ring configurations, as shown in Figure 3.3.

Both the ketone groups of a ketose sugar and the aldehyde group of an aldose sugar may be called a **carbonyl group**. A carbonyl group contains a carbon atom double-bonded to an oxygen atom, but the other atoms are not specified. Hence, an aldehyde group is a specific type of carbonyl group, with both a hydrogen atom and an oxygen atom attached to the carbon atom. A ketone group is also a carbonyl group, because it contains an oxygen atom double-bonded to a carbon atom located within a hydrocarbon chain.

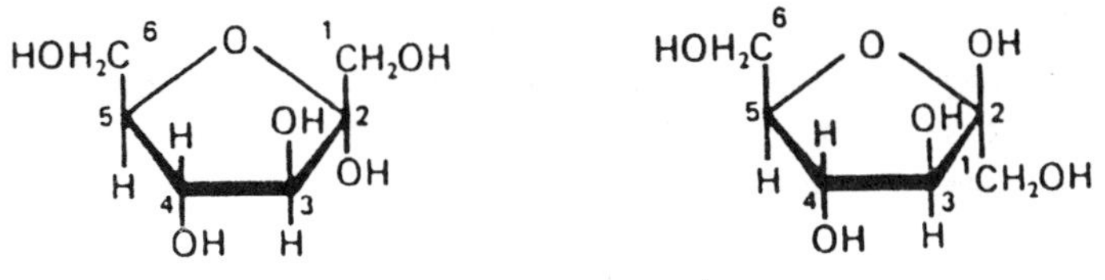

α-D-fructofuranose   β-D-fructofuranose

FIGURE 3.3   The main configurations of D-fructose.

Disaccharides

Disaccharides contain two monosaccharides joined together with a special linkage, called a **glycosidic** bond. Several disaccharides are important in foods—sucrose or table sugar is the most common and contains glucose and fructose. There are other important disaccharides, such as maltose containing two glucose units, and lactose with glucose and galactose. Lactose is also known as milk sugar because it is found in milk. It is the least sweet and least soluble of the sugars.

Glycosidic Bonds

A **glycosidic bond** is formed when the carbonyl group of one monosaccharide reacts with a hydroxyl group of another molecule and water is eliminated (see Figure 3.4).

Formation of a glycosidic link fixes the configuration of the monosaccharide containing the involved carbonyl group in either the α- or β-position. Therefore, it is necessary to specify whether the link is an α- or a β-link. The position of the bond must also be specified. For example, when two glucose molecules are joined to make maltose, the glycosidic link occurs between carbon-1 of the first glucose molecule and carbon-4 of the second, and the configuration of the first glucose molecule is fixed in the α-position. Maltose therefore contains two glucose units linked by an α-1,4-glycosidic bond. The anomeric hydroxyl group that is not involved in the glycosidic bond (i.e., the one on the second glucose molecule) remains free to assume either the α- or β-configuration. Therefore, there are two forms of the disaccharide in equilibrium with each other.

Glycosidic bonds are stable under normal conditions but can be hydrolyzed by acid and heat, or by enzymes such as sucrase, invertase, or amylases.

Glycosidic Bond

- Formed between the free carbonyl group of one monosaccharide and a hydroxyl group of another monosaccharide

- Fixes the configuration of the monosaccharide containing the involved carbonyl group in either the α- or β-position

- It is necessary to specify
  - The **configuration** of the link—whether it is an α-link or a β-link
  - The **position** of the link—it is numbered according to the respective positions of the two carbon atoms it links together. For example, an α-1,4 link glycosidic link would occur between carbon-1 of the first monosaccharide and carbon-4 of the second monosaccharide, as in maltose

- Readily hydrolyzed by
  - Heat and acid
  - Certain enzymes, such as sucrase, invertase, amylases, and so forth

---

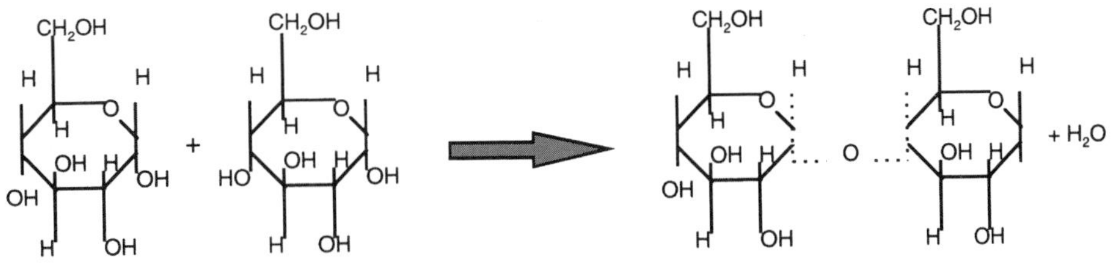

FIGURE 3.4   A glycosidic bond between the carbonyl and hydroxyl groups of monosaccharides.

Examples of Disaccharides

Maltose and Cellobiose.   As has already been mentioned, maltose contains two glucose units linked by an α-1,4-glycosidic bond. When two glucose molecules are joined together and the configuration of the first glucose molecule is fixed in the β-position, cellobiose is formed. Cellobiose contains a β-1,4-glycosidic bond. The chemical formulas for maltose and cellobiose are shown in Figure 3.5.

Maltose is the building block for *starch*, which contains α-1,4-glycosidic bonds. Alpha links can be broken down by the body, so starch is readily digested. Cellobiose is the building block for *cellulose*, which contains β-1,4-glycosidic bonds. Cellulose cannot be digested in the human body because the β-linkages cannot be broken down by the digestive enzymes. Therefore, cellulose is known as dietary fiber. (The glycosidic bonds in cellulose cross the plane of the monosaccharide units they join together, and so they may be termed cross-planar bonds. It is because they are cross-planar that they are not digestible. In reality, because of the orientation of the bonds, the monosaccharide units tend to twist or flip over, as drawn in Figure 3.5, which results in a twisted ribbon effect for the polymer chain.)

Sucrose.   Sucrose is the most common disaccharide, and it contains glucose and fructose joined together by an α-1,2-glycosidic link (see Figure 3.6). The carbonyl groups of both the glucose and the fructose molecule are involved in the glycosidic bond; thus, the configuration of each monosaccharide becomes fixed. Glucose is fixed in the α-configuration, whereas fructose is fixed in the β-configuration. Sucrose can be hydrolyzed to glucose and fructose by heat and acid, or by the enzymes invertase or sucrase. The equimolar mixture of glucose and fructose produced in this way is called ***invert sugar***. Production of invert sugar is important during the formation of candies

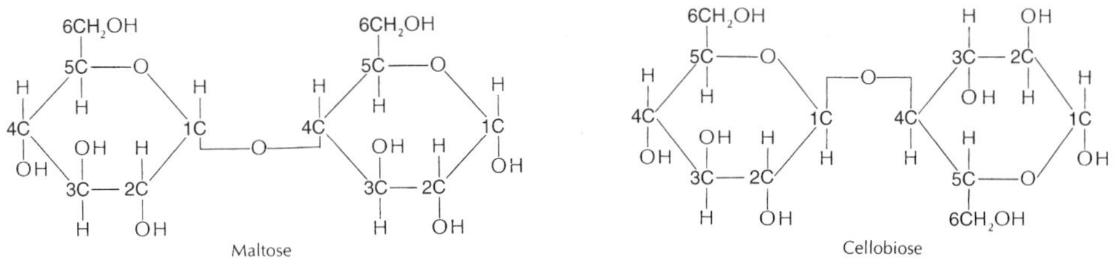

FIGURE 3.5   Maltose and cellobiose.

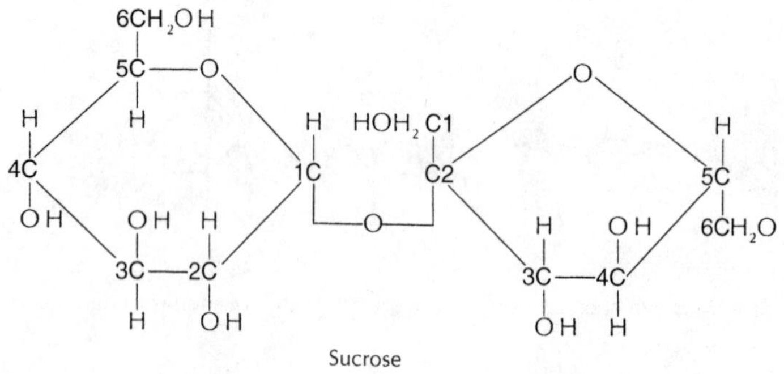

FIGURE 3.6   Sucrose.

and jellies, as invert sugar prevents unwanted or excessive crystallization of sucrose. (For further discussion of crystallization of sucrose, see Chapter 14.)

SOME PROPERTIES OF SUGARS

Sweetness

The most obvious sensory property of sugars such as glucose, fructose, and sucrose is their **sweetness**, which varies depending on the specific sugar. Lactose (milk sugar) is the least sweet, whereas fructose is the sweetest sugar. Sugars are used as sweeteners in candies and many other food products.

Formation of Solutions and Syrups

Sugars are soluble in water and readily form syrups. If water is evaporated, crystals are formed. Sugars form **molecular solutions** due to hydrogen-bond interchange. When sugar is placed in water, the water molecules form hydrogen bonds with the sugar molecules, thus hydrating them and removing them from the sugar crystals. Solubility increases with temperature; thus, a hot sucrose solution may contain more solute than a cold one. (For a discussion of molecular solutions, see Chapter 2.)

If a hot saturated sucrose solution is cooled without disturbance, it will supercool, and a supersaturated solution will be obtained. A *supersaturated solution* contains more solute than could normally be dissolved at that temperature. It is unstable, and if stirred or disturbed, the extra solute will rapidly crystallize out of solution. Supersaturated solutions are necessary in candymaking. For more detail on sugar crystallization and candies, see Chapter 14.

Body and Mouthfeel

Sugars contribute body and "mouthfeel" to foods. In other words, the addition of sugar makes a food more viscous or gives it a less runny consistency. If sugar is replaced by a non-nutritive or high-intensity sweetener such as aspartame or saccharin, the consistency of the food will be watery and thin. To prevent this, another substance has to be added to give the expected body or mouthfeel to the food. Modified starches or gums are usually added to such food products to give the desired consistency without addition of sugar.

Fermentation

Sugars are readily digested and metabolized by the human body and supply energy (4 cal/g). They are also metabolized by microorganisms. This property is important in breadmaking, where sugar is fermented by yeast cells. The yeast feeds on the sugar, producing carbon dioxide, which is the leavening agent and causes bread dough to rise before and during baking.

Preservatives

At high concentrations, sugars prevent growth of microorganisms, because they reduce the water activity of food to a level below which bacterial growth cannot be supported. Sugars can, therefore, be used as preservatives. Examples of foods preserved in this manner include jams and jellies.

Reducing Sugars

Sugars that contain a free carbonyl group are known as *reducing sugars*. All monosaccharides are reducing sugars. Disaccharides are reducing sugars only if they contain a free carbonyl group. Sucrose is not a reducing sugar because it does not contain a free carbonyl group. The carbonyl groups of glucose and fructose are both involved in the glycosidic bond and are, therefore, not free to take part in other reactions. Maltose, on the other hand, has one carbonyl group involved in the glycosidic bond, and the other carbonyl group is free; thus, maltose is a reducing sugar.

Reducing sugars give brown colors to baked goods when they combine with free amino acid groups of proteins in a browning reaction called the *Maillard reaction* (this reaction is discussed further in Chapter 8).

Caramelization

Sugars *caramelize* on heating giving a brown color. Caramelization is caused by the decomposition of the sugars and occurs at extremely high temperatures. A variety of compounds are formed as a result, including organic acids, aldehydes, and ketones. The reaction does not involve proteins and should not be confused with the Maillard browning reaction.

Sugar Alcohols

Reduction of the carbonyl group to a hydroxyl group gives **sugar alcohols** such as xylitol, sorbitol, and mannitol. These compounds are sweet, although not as sweet as sucrose. However, they are not fermented as readily as sugar by microorganisms in the mouth, and so they are noncariogenic. (In other words, they do not cause tooth decay.) Therefore, they are used in chewing gum, breath mints, and other products that may be kept in the mouth for a while. Although products containing sugar alcohols may be labeled as "sugar free," it is important to realize that sugar alcohols are not free of calories. They are not metabolized as efficiently as sugars, and have a lower caloric value (between 1 and 3 kcal/g). Sugar alcohols may be used as a low-energy bulk ingredient (in place of sugar) in many food products. Because sorbitol is mostly transformed to fructose in the body rather than glucose, it is tolerated by diabetics. Hence, it can be used to replace sugar in diabetic foods. The use of sugar alcohols is discussed further in Chapters 14 and 18.

OLIGOSACCHARIDES

Oligosaccharides contain a few (3–10) monosaccharide residues linked together by glycosidic bonds. Common ones include raffinose and stachyose. Raffinose is a **trisaccharide** and contains galactose, glucose, and fructose. Stachyose contains glucose, fructose, and two galactose units. Both occur in legumes such as dry beans and peas. They are not hydrolyzed or digested by the human digestive system, and become food for bacteria in the large intestine. The bacteria metabolize the carbohydrates and produce gas, causing varying degrees of discomfort.

POLYSACCHARIDES

The most important food **polysaccharides** are the starches, pectins, and gums. All are complex carbohydrate polymers with different properties, which depend on the sugar units that make up the molecule, the type of glycosidic linkages, and the degree of branching of the molecules. Starches are discussed in Chapter 4 and pectins and other polysaccharides are covered in Chapter 5.

Dextrins and Dextrans

Dextrins are intermediate-chain length glucose polymers formed when starch is broken down or hydrolyzed. They are larger than oligosaccharides, but considerably shorter than starch molecules. Dextrins contain glucose molecules joined by α-1,4-glycosidic bonds, and they are linear polymers. They are found in corn syrups, produced by hydrolysis of starch.

    Dextrans are also intermediate-chain length glucose polymers, but they contain α-1,6-glycosidic bonds. They are produced by some bacteria and yeasts.

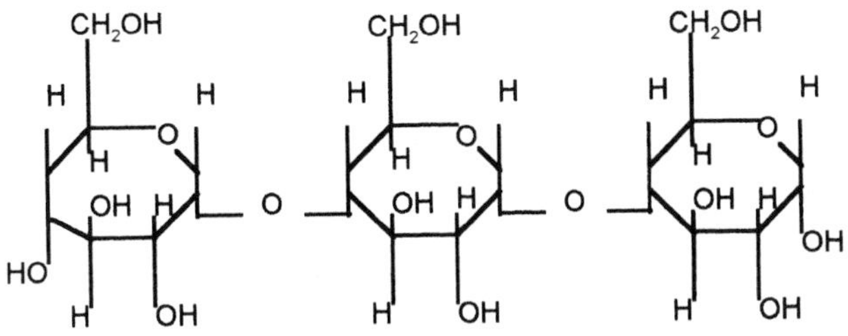

α-1,4-glycosidic linkages of amylose

FIGURE 3.7 Amylose.

Starch

Starch is a glucose polymer that contains two types of molecules, known as amylose and amylopectin. These are shown in Figures 3.7 and 3.8, respectively. Both are long chains of glucose molecules joined by α-1,4-glycosidic bonds; however, amylose is a linear chain, whereas amylopectin contains branches. For every 15–30 glucose residues there is a branch, joined to the main chain by an α-1,6-glycosidic link. The branches make amylopectin less soluble in water than amylose. Usually, the two types of starch occur together, but starches may contain only amylose or only amylopectin. They have different properties, which are discussed in Chapter 4.

Starches can also be modified to give specific functional properties in food products, so knowledge of the properties of different starches is important in the food

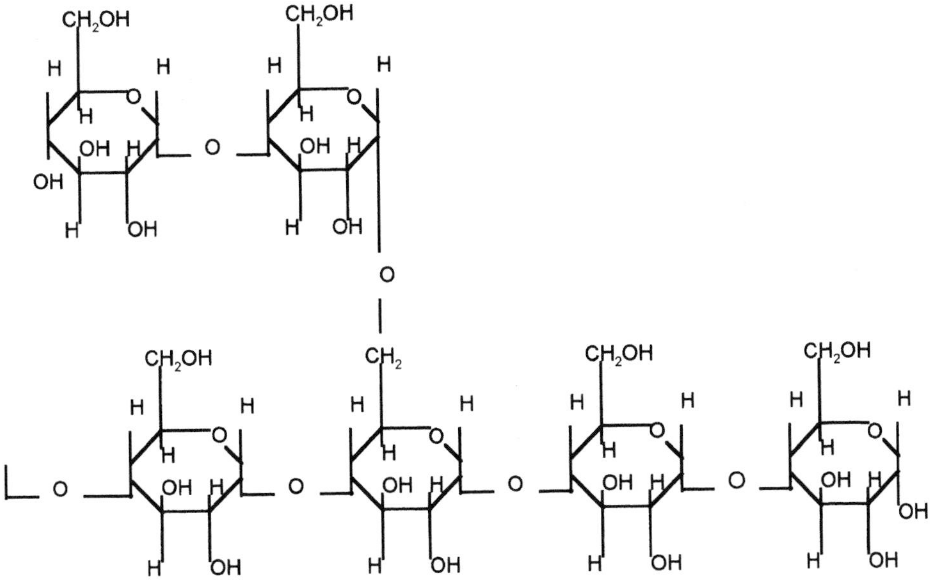

α-1,6-branching of amylopectin

FIGURE 3.8 Amylopectin.

industry. Chapter 4 gives detailed information on characteristics of different starches and their uses in foods.

Pectins and Other Polysaccharides

Pectins, gums, and seaweed polysaccharides are also important carbohydrates used in food products. They are discussed further in Chapter 5. Pectins occur naturally in plant food products, but gums and seaweed polysaccharides do not come from edible plant sources. They are extracted and purified and then added to food products.

Pectins are used mainly as gelling agents in jellies, jams, and other products. They are also used as stabilizers and thickeners. They are found in fruits and vegetables, and they help to hold the plant cells together. Structurally, they are long-chain polymers of α-D-galacturonic acid, which is an acid derived from the simple sugar galactose. They are soluble in water, and under appropriate conditions, they form gels. Their structure and properties are discussed in Chapter 5.

Gums are mainly plant extracts and include gum tragacanth and guar gum. They are highly branched polysaccharides that form very viscous solutions, trapping large amounts of water within their branches. Most do not form gels because of the high level of branching. They are useful as thickeners and stabilizers, particularly in reduced-fat salad dressings and in other convenience foods.

Seaweed polysaccharides include the agars, alginates, and carrageenans. They are classified as gums, although they are able to form gels, unlike most gums. They are useful as gelling agents, thickeners, and stabilizers in foods.

Cellulose and *hemicellulose* are structural polysaccharides that provide support in plant tissues. They are not digested in the body, so they do not supply energy. However, they provide insoluble dietary fiber, which is an important part of a healthy, balanced diet.

CONCLUSION

Carbohydrates come in various shapes and sizes, from small sugar molecules to complex polymers containing thousands of simple sugar units. The digestible carbohydrates provide energy (4 cal/g), whereas the indigestible ones are an important source of dietary fiber. In addition to their nutritional value, carbohydrates are important as thickeners, stabilizers, and gelling agents. They are used in a wide spectrum of convenience foods, and without them, the range of food products relished today would be greatly diminished.

GLOSSARY

Aldose: Sugar containing an aldehyde group monosaccharide—single sugar unit.
Alpha-anomer: The anomeric hydroxyl group is on the opposite face of the ring from carbon-6 (i.e., the two groups point in opposite directions).
Anomeric carbon atom: The carbon atom that is part of the free carbonyl group in the straight-chain form of a sugar.

Anomers: Isomers that differ only in the orientation of the hydroxyl group on the anomeric carbon atom; there are two forms—alpha (α) and beta (β).

Beta-anomer: The anomeric hydroxyl group is on the same face of the ring as carbon-6 (i.e., the two groups point in the same direction).

Carbonyl group: Contains an oxygen atom double-bonded to a carbon atom. The aldehyde group and the ketone group can both be described as a carbonyl group.

Caramelization: Decomposition of sugars at very high temperatures resulting in brown color.

Cross-planar bond: Formed when the hydroxyl groups on the carbon atoms involved in the formation of a glycosidic bond are oriented on opposite faces of the sugar rings. Cross-planar bonds occur in cellobiose and in cellulose. They also occur in pectin. They are not digested in the human digestive system.

Dextrans: Glucose polymers joined by α-1,6-glycosidic bonds. Produced by some bacteria and yeasts.

Dextrins: Glucose polymers joined by α-1,4-glycosidic bonds. Product of starch hydrolysis. Found in corn syrups.

Disaccharide: Two sugar units joined together by a glycosidic bond.

Furanose: Five-membered ring.

Glycosidic bond: Bond that links two sugar units together; it is formed between the free carbonyl group of one sugar and a hydroxyl group of another sugar; the orientation (α or β) and position (e.g., 1,4) of the link must be specified.

Hydroxyl group: The –OH group on the carbon atom.

Invert sugar: An equimolar mixture of glucose and fructose, formed by hydrolysis of sucrose, either by acid and heat, or by enzymes such as invertase or sucrase.

Ketose: Sugar containing a ketone group.

Maillard reaction (Maillard browning reaction): Nonenzymatic browning reaction involving a reducing sugar and a free amino acid group on a protein.

Monosaccharide: Single sugar unit.

Oligosaccharide: Several (3–10) sugar units joined together by a glycosidic bond.

Polysaccharide: Many (hundreds or thousands of) sugar units joined together.

Pyranose: Six-membered ring.

Reducing sugar: Sugar that contains a free carbonyl group.

Reference carbon atom: The highest numbered asymmetric carbon atom; C5 in glucose and fructose.

Reference hydroxyl group: The hydroxyl group attached to the reference carbon atom.

Sugar alcohol: The result of reduction of carbonyl group to a hydroxyl group.

Supersaturated solution: Solution that contains more solute than could normally be dissolved at a particular temperature.

Trisaccharide: Three sugar units joined together by a glycosidic bond.

BIBLIOGRAPHY

BeMiller JN, Whistler RL. Carbohydrates. In: Fennema O, ed. *Food Chemistry,* 3rd ed. New York: Marcel Dekker, 1996.

Charley H, Weaver C. *Foods. A Scientific Approach*, 3rd ed. New York: Merrill/Prentice-Hall, 1998.

Garrett RH, Grisham CM. *Biochemistry*, 2nd ed. New York: Saunders College Publishing, 1999.

Glicksman J. Food applications of gums. In: Lineback DR, Inglett GE, eds. *Food Carbohydrates*. Westport, CT: AVI, 1982.

McWilliams M. *Foods: Experimental Perspectives*, 4th ed. New York: Prentice-Hall, 2001.

Penfield MP, Campbell AM. *Experimental Food Science*, 3rd ed. San Diego, CA: Academic Press, 1990.

Potter N, Hotchkiss J. *Food Science*, 5th ed. New York: Chapman & Hall, 1995.

Vieira ER. *Elementary Food Science*, 4th ed. New York: Chapman & Hall, 1996.

CHAPTER 4

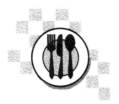

Starches in Food

INTRODUCTION

Starch is a plant polysaccharide stored in roots, tubers, and seeds of plants, and it is in the endosperm of all grains. Starch may be hydrolyzed to glucose and provide humans with energy and the glucose that is necessary for brain and central nervous system functioning. When consumed in the human diet, it yields 4 cal/g.

Starch grains, or **granules**, contain long-chain glucose polymers and are *insoluble* in water. Unlike the *small* molecules of salt and sugar, the larger starch polymers do *not* form a true solution. Rather, starch granules form a temporary suspension when stirred in water. The uncooked granules may swell slightly as they absorb water. However, once starch is cooked, the swelling becomes significant and the granule leaches out starch, enabling starch to be used as a thickener.

Overall, the characteristics of a finished food product are determined by the source of starch, the temperature of heating, concentration of starch used in a formulation, and the other components used with the starch, such as acid and sugar. There are many types of starch and modified starches created for special dietary needs and food applications.

Intermediate, shorter-chain products from starch breakdown may be used to simulate fat in salad dressings and frozen desserts. For example, wheat, potato, and tapioca maltodextrins may be used as fat replacers. They provide the viscosity and mouthfeel of fat in a food product, but with reduced calories compared to fat.

STARCH SOURCES

Starch may come from a variety of sources with different crystalline structures. *Cereal grains* such as corn, wheat, or rice are sources of starch, as are *roots* and *tubers*. Starch is also derived from *legumes* such as soybeans or garbanzo beans. Sago is a powdery starch obtained from the trunks of the sago palm in tropical Asia, used both as a food thickener and fabric stiffener.

If the starch source is root or tuber starch, or a waxy version of starch, a *clear* thick mixture may be achieved. Whereas a *cloudy* thick mixture is typically produced by cereal starches, especially wheat flour more so than *cornstarch* because wheat contains additional nonstarch ingredients. (Approximately twice as much flour as cornstarch is required to thicken a mixture.)

STARCH STRUCTURE AND COMPOSITION

The various starch granules differ in *size*, ranging from 2 to 150 μm, and *shape*, which may be round or polygonal, as seen in photomicrographs of corn, wheat, and waxy maize in Figures 4.1–4.3.

Starch is composed of two molecules, amylose and amylopectin, whose parts are connected by glycosidic linkages (Chapter 3). **Amylose** molecules make up approximately one-quarter of all starch (although some varieties contain no amylose). The structure is a long linear chain composed of thousands of glucose units with α-1,4-glycosidic linkages of the molecules.

It forms a three-dimensional network when molecules associate upon cooling, and is responsible for the gelation of cooked, cooled starch pastes. Therefore, starches high in amylose hold their shape when molded; they gel. Examples of the amylose

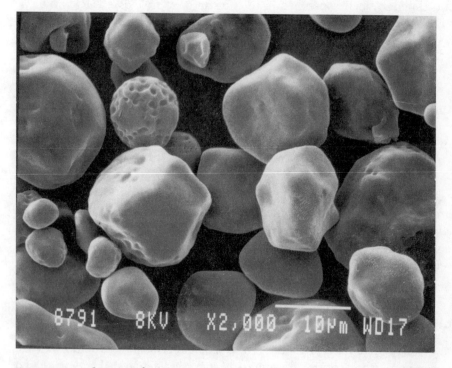

FIGURE 4.1 Scanning electron micrograph of common corn cereal grains magnified 2000 times (*Source*: Purdue University—Whistler Center for Carbohydrate Research).

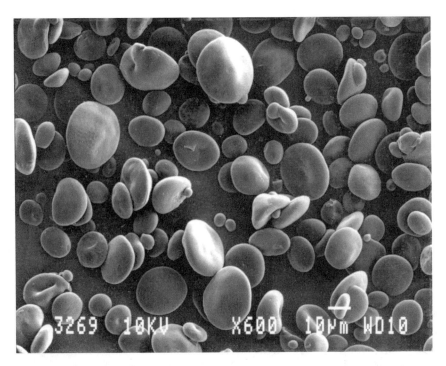

FIGURE 4.2 Scanning electron micrograph of wheat magnified 600 times (*Source*: Purdue University—Whistler Center for Carbohydrate Research).

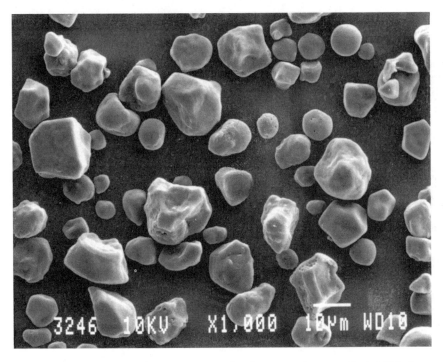

FIGURE 4.3 Scanning electron micrograph of waxy maize magnified 1000 times (*Source*: Purdue University—Whistler Center for Carbohydrate Research).

content of various starch sources include the following: *cereal grains*—26–28% amylose, *roots and tubers*—17–23%, and *waxy varieties of starch*—0%.

Amylopectin molecules (Chapter 3) constitute approximately three-quarters of the polymers in a starch granule. The glucose chain of amylopectin contains α-1,4 linkages with α-1,6 branching at every 15–30 glucose units of the chain. There is a linkage between the carbon-1 of the glucose and carbon-6 of the branch glucose. The chains are highly branched and bushy (but less branched than the animal storage form of carbohydrate, glycogen).

Starches with a high percentage of amylopectin will *thicken* a mixture but will *not* form a gel because, unlike amylose, amylopectin molecules do *not* associate and form chemical linkages in the same manner upon cooling.

GELATINIZATION PROCESS

Starch in its *uncooked* stage is *insoluble* in water. It forms a temporary **suspension** of large particles, which are undissolved in the surrounding medium, and will settle to the bottom of a container of liquid unless agitated. The particles may imbibe a small amount of water, but, generally, a suspension offers minimal change to the starch. The uncooked starch molecule is a highly ordered crystalline structure that refracts light in two directions exhibiting a Maltese cross formation, or **birefringence**, on the granule when it is viewed under polarized light with a microscope (Figure 4.4).

Then, when starch is *heated* in water, **imbibition** or intake of water into the granules occurs. This occurs first in less-dense areas, and subsequently in the more crystalline regions of the starch molecule. Initially, it is a *reversible* step in

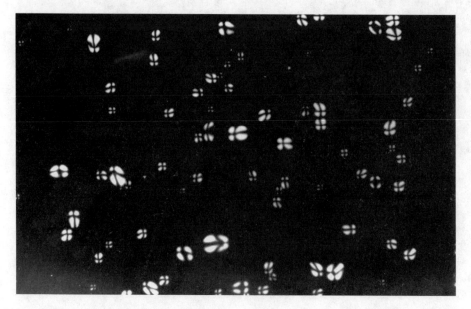

FIGURE 4.4 Photomicrograph of ungelatinized potato starch taken through cross-polarizers (*Source*: Purdue University—Whistler Center for Carbohydrate Research).

the gelatinization process. Then, as heating *continues*, starch granules take up more water *irreversibly* and swell, losing their ordered crystalline structure (thus losing birefringence) and becoming opaque and more fragile. Some short chains of amylose come out of the granules. This process, called **gelatinization**, is responsible for the thickening of food systems.

As starch leaches out of swollen granules in gelatinization, the water–starch mixture becomes a *sol*. A sol is a colloidal two-phase system containing a liquid continuous phase and a solid dispersed phase. This solid-in-a-liquid is pourable and has a low **viscosity** or resistance to flow.

$$\text{SUSPENSION} \xrightarrow[\text{heat}]{} \text{SOL}$$

This gelatinization process may be synonymous with *pasting*, although gelatinization and pasting may be reported as *sequential* occurrences (1). Whether a separate process or the continuation of gelatinization, pasting occurs with the continued heating of gelatinized starch grains.

The temperature at which various starches gelatinize is actually *range* of temperatures specific to a starch. The granules within a starch will swell and thicken mixtures at slightly different temperatures, with the larger granules swelling earlier than smaller granules.

The **steps** in the gelatinization process are as follows:

- The gelatinization temperature is reached—approximately 140–160°F (60–71°C)—depending on the starch type, and is completed at 190–194°F (88–92°C).

- The kinetic energy of the hot water molecules breaks the hydrogen bonds between the starch molecules. Hydrogen-bond interchange occurs as starch forms hydrogen bonds with *water* molecules instead of other *starch* molecules. As hydrogen bonds are formed, water is able to penetrate further into the starch granule and swelling takes place. Sufficient water must be present to enter and enlarge the starch granule.

- Diffusion of some amylose chains occurs as they leach out of the starch granules.

- Birefringence and the ordered crystalline structure of the uncooked granule is lost. Increased translucency is apparent because the refractive index of the expanded granule is close to that of water.

- Granule swelling increases as the temperature increases. The larger starch granules are the first to swell.

- Swollen granules take up more space and the mixture thickens as the enlarged granules leach amylose and possibly amylopectin.

- The starch paste continues to become thicker, more viscous, and resistant to flow as it gelatinizes.

- Cooking the gelatinized starch for 5 minutes longer develops flavor. Overstirring thins the cooked starch mixture as the swollen starch granules implode and rupture and lose some of the liquid held inside the enlarged granule.

FACTORS REQUIRING CONTROL IN GELATINIZATION

Several factors must be controlled during gelatinization in order to produce a high-quality gelatinized starch. These factors include the following:

Acid: Acid hydrolysis during cooking of starch granules results in the formation of **dextrins** or short-chain glucose polymers. As acid fragments the starch molecule, the result is a *thinner hot paste* and *less firm cooled product*. This may be evident when acid is added to sauces in the form of vinegar, tomatoes, or fruit juice, including citrus juice (lemon juice may be added to pie fillings). Hydrolysis of the starch molecules subsequently results in less water absorption by the starch granule, and therefore, the late addition of acid to a mixture is best, after starch has been gelatinized and begun to thicken.

Agitation: Agitation or stirring, both initially and throughout the gelatinization process, enables granules of starch to swell independently and creates a more uniform mixture, without lumps. However, excessive agitation after gelatinization is complete may rupture granules and, consequently, thin starch mixtures.

Enzymes: Starch may be hydrolyzed by the starch-splitting enzymes α-amylase, β-amylase, and β-glucoamylase. *Endoenzymes* such as α-amylase act anywhere on the starch chain and undamaged starch grains to degrade starch into glucose, maltose, and dextrins. The *exoenzyme* β-amylase acts on α-1,4-glycosidic linkages from the nonreducing end and on damaged amylose or amylopectin chains, further hydrolyzing starch two glucose units at a time, thus producing maltose. Beta-amylase cannot hydrolyze starch beyond the branch points of amylopectin. The enzyme β-glucoamylase hydrolyses α-1,4 links, producing glucose, and slowly hydrolyzes α-1,6 linkages in starch.

Fat and proteins: The presence of fat and protein initially coats or **adsorbs** to the surface the starch granules, causing a delay in hydration and viscosity. For example, the high level of fat in pie crusts limits dough swelling by preventing water absorption, and the use of fat acts as a separating agent to prevent starch granules from clumping together in sauces. (See Separating Agents and Lump Formation in this chapter.)

Sugar: The addition of moderate amounts of sugar, especially the disaccharides sucrose and lactose, decreases the firmness of the cooked and cooled starch product. Sugar acts by absorbing water that the granule would absorb. It competes for imbibition and thus delays the absorption of water by starch granules, preventing a speedy or complete swelling of the starch granule.

It follows then that the *partial* addition of sugar to a recipe, before the starch mixture has completed cooking, allows starch to absorb more water and thicken. If *all* of the sugar is added to a starch-thickened formulation at the beginning of cooking, a thinner mixture, with less swelling, is the result. Sugar also elevates the temperature required for gelatinization to occur, and it increases translucency of the finished product.

If both *acid* and *sugar* are added to a starch mixture (as in lemon pie filling), there is less swelling due to the presence of sugar, which competes with starch for water absorption, and there is less hydrolysis from acid.

Temperature: 190–194°F (88–90°C) and up to 203°F (95°C) represents the completion of starch gelatinization, although starches vary in their unique gelatinization temperature.

> **Length of heating**: As the heating time is lengthened, the finished mixture may be thinner due to rupturing of enlarged granules. Alternatively, cooking for a longer time in an uncovered double boiler may evaporate the water that would otherwise thin the mixture.

> **Type of heat**: *Moist* heat is necessary for gelatinization to occur. *Dry heat* causes the starch to hydrolyze, forming shorter-chain dextrins and becoming more soluble in cooking water. When dry heat is applied to flour (and, thus, its starch component), a "browned" flour, with a slightly toasted flavor and brown color is obtained. This effect may be desired in many recipes.

Times and temperatures of when various starches thicken or gel may be observed by reading data (Figure 4.5) from a recording instrument or recording viscometer (Figure 4.6).

The viscosity of a starch and water mixture may be recorded on a moving graph as the mixture is tested and stirred. The recording instrument portrays the thickness

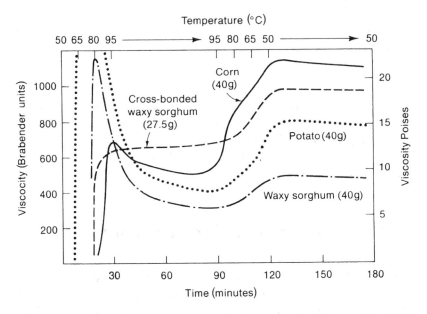

FIGURE 4.5 Graph of the thickening of various starches (*Source*: Schoch TJ. Starches in foods. In: *Carbohydrates Their Roles*, Schultz HW, Cain RF, Wrolstad RW, eds. Westport, CT: AVI Publishing Company, 1969. With permission).

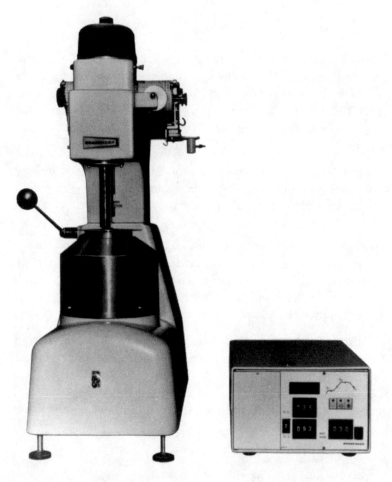

FIGURE 4.6 Brabender amylograph (*Source*: C.W. Brabender Instruments, Inc.).

of starch mixtures during heating, gelatinization, and cooling. It may show the effects of α-amylase on starch mixtures or the thickness of various starches at different times and temperatures. As illustrated in the graph in Figure 4.5, root starches, such as potato and tapioca, and *waxy* cereal starches thicken earlier and at lower temperatures than cereal starches.

GELATION OR SETTING OF GELATINIZED STARCH PASTES DURING COOLING

Beyond gelatinization there may be a further change in the starch granule. For, upon cooling of the sol, or gelatinized starch paste, a starch containing amylose may undergo gelation, or formation of a *gel*. Starch gels are elastic, colloidal, two-phase systems—where the *solid* continuous phase of amylose polymers forms a three-dimensional network that holds a *liquid* dispersed phase (in contrast to a sol).

$$\text{SUSPENSION} \xrightarrow[\text{heat}]{\text{imbibition}} \underset{\text{SOL}}{\overset{\text{maximum gelatinization}}{}} \xrightarrow[\text{cool}]{\text{gelation}} \text{GEL (or a thick sol)}$$

When cooling occurs, energy is reduced. As a result of this reduction, intermittent hydrogen cross-bonds form among *amylose,* reassociating at random intervals, and *forming a gel.* Perhaps, as shown in the above equation, a thick sol, as opposed to a gel, may be formed. Recall that such is the case with molecules of *amylopectin* because the granule exhibits lesser tendency to reassociate or revert to a more crystalline structure than amylose. Amylopectin is a highly branched molecule that *does not* readily form bonds or gels.

If gels are formed they are nonpourable with high viscosity and may cloud depending on the starch source. If cooled undisturbed, the gels remain strong, yet this reassociation may be accompanied by an unacceptable water loss or syneresis (see **Syneresis**). Some starches and their gelling potential are identified in the following listing:

Forms Gel	Does Not Form Gel
Cornstarch	Waxy cereals
Wheat starch	Tapioca
Wheat flour	

In addition to the gelling potential of a particular starch, as shown above, the *concentration* of starch used in a formulation also influences consistency. For example, a white sauce of flour, fat and milk may be thickened to various concentrations by varying the amount of flours shown as follows:

thin—1 tablespoon of flour/cup of liquid
medium—2 tablespoons of flour/cup of liquid
thick—3 tablespoons of flour/cup of liquid

While both amylose and amylopectin molecules, the latter to a minor extent, may participate in a textural change (somewhat more gritty) with time, "waxy" starches maintain the property of high water-binding capacity and show significantly less change. Thus, in addition to their resistance to gel formation, starches without amylose resist retrogradation. **Retrogradation** is the process in which the gelatinized starch reverts or retrogrades to a more crystalline structure upon cooling. Due to this process, a gritty-textured gel may be observed in pudding allowed to age for a few days in the refrigerator. Stale bread also evidences starch retrograding, or amylose realigning. With brief reheating, the hydrogen bonds formed among the amylose components of the starch are broken, and the bread become softer.

SYNERESIS

As a cooked, cooled starch gel ages, it contracts causing water loss and shrinkage. This water loss from the cooked, cooled gel is water of **syneresis** or "weeping." It may occur either when amylose undergoes *retrogradation* (previously discussed), when the gel has been *formed improperly*, and especially, when the gel has been exposed to the effects of *freeze–thaw cycles*. It is noted that as water in a starch gel (such as cream fillings in frozen baked products) is frozen and thawed, the water created from melted ice crystals is not able to reassociate with the starch, and the resulting amylose structures become fragile, readily losing entrapped water. Therefore, the use of modified starches (see Modified Starch) or starches containing only the non-gelling amylopectin are used to control this unwanted effect in a commercial product. Food packaging material that is resistant to moisture–vapor transfer is also important in protecting quality.

SEPARATING AGENTS AND LUMP FORMATION

A problem in the preparation of starch-thickened mixtures is the undesirable formation of lumps. This is due to the unequal swelling, or "clumping" together of individual starch granules. Therefore, **separating agents** such as fat, cold water, and sugar may be added to just the starch/flour ingredients of a recipe, to physically separate starch grains, and allow their individual swelling. Use of these separating agents produces a smooth-textured mixture without undesirable lumps!

Fat: Fat forms a film around individual starch granules, allowing each granule to swell independently of other granules. A *lump-free* sauce or gravy may be obtained by initially combining dry flour with liquid fat prior to addition to a recipe. Then, with adequate agitation, the mixture is thick and free from lumps. The addition of cornstarch or flour to a hot fat such as meat drippings or oil also destroys the α-amylase in flour, which would otherwise thin the mixture. A *roux* commonly prepared by numerous chefs, is prepared by blending fat, such as hot pan drippings, and flour.

Cold water: *Cold* water may be used to physically separate starch granules. When mixed with insoluble starch, water puts starch granules in a suspension called a *"slurry."* The cold water–starch suspension is then slowly mixed into the hot liquid for thickening. Cold water is useful as a separating agent if the product is *fat-free or sugar-free* (the other two separating agents). *Hot* water is not an effective separating agent as it partially gelatinizes the starch.

Sugar: Sugar is a common separating agent. When mixed with starch, prior to incorporation into the liquid, it physically separates starch granules to allow individual swelling. Sugar is useful as a separating agent if sweetening is also a desirable characteristic of a starch mixture.

Once starch granules are successfully separated, so that the granules do not "clump together" forming lumps, the separated starch is then added to a formulation heated slowly, and *stirred constantly*. Extensive or harsh stirring after maximum gelatinization has occurred will rupture starch granules causing the mixture to be thin.

MODIFIED STARCHES

Naturally existing starches may be **modified** chemically to produce physical changes that contribute to shelf stability, appearance, convenience, and performance in food preparation. Some examples of modified starches used in food manufacturing are described as follows:

Pregelatinized starch is an instant starch that has been gelatinized and then dried. It subsequently swells without the application of heat. Pregelatinized starch appears in many foods, such as instant pudding mixes. Some properties of a pregelatinized starch include the following:

- The starch is dispersible in cold water; it can thicken without heat being applied.
- The starch granule can be cooked and dried, yet reabsorb a lot of water without having to be heated again.
- The starch granule undergoes irreversible change and cannot return to its original ungelatinized condition after treatment.
- A greater weight of starch is required to thicken a liquid because *rupturing* of the starch granule has occurred during the process of gelatinization and drying.

Cold water-swelling (CWS) starch is an instant starch that remains as an *intact granule*. It offers convenience, stability, clarity, and texture. Cold water-swelling starches may be either gelling or nongelling. They may be used in no-cook or cold-process salad dressings, and may provide the thick, creamy mouthfeel in no-fat salad dressings.

Cross-linked starches are used in many foods, especially acid food products such as pizza sauce or barbecue sauce, because the modified starch is more acid resistant than an unmodified starch. Cross-linked starch is manufactured by a molecular reaction that occurs at *selected hydroxyl* (–OH) *groups* of two adjoining, intact, starch molecules.

The purpose of cross-linking is to enable the starch to withstand such conditions as low pH, high shear, or *high* temperatures. As a result of cross-linking, a starch swells less and thickens less. The starch becomes less fragile and is more resistant to rupture. Although it is more tolerant to high temperatures, it is not to *cold* temperatures.

Stabilized starches are used in frozen foods and other foods stored at cold temperatures in order to prevent gelling or syneresis. They may also be termed *substituted* starches. These starches are stabilized by addition of bulky groups to the starch molecules, which block molecular association of the starch molecules due to steric hindrance. The added groups are often negatively charged, and so molecular interaction is also inhibited due to ionic repulsion. The result is a stabilized starch that produces pastes that are able to withstand several freeze–thaw cycles before syneresis occurs. Freeze–thaw stabilized starches are essential to the frozen food industry, and are also useful to maintain the quality of processed foods such as sauces and gravies that are stored at cold temperatures.

Stabilized starches are not appropriate in foods that require prolonged heating. However, starches may be modified by a combination of both cross-linking and stabilization. This produces modified starches that are acid, heat and freeze–thaw stable, and have a wide range of uses in food products.

Acid-modified starch is starch that is subjected to treatment in an acid slurry. Raw starch and dilute acid are heated to temperatures less than the gelatinization temperature. Once the starch is mixed into a food product, it appears less viscous when hot but forms a strong gel on cooling.

Waxy Starches

As mentioned earlier in this chapter, waxy starches do *not* contain amylose, *solely* amylopectin. They are highly branched and are derived from some natural strains of barley, corn, rice, and sorghum. They may also be cross-linked for better function. Waxy starches begin to thicken at lower temperatures, but become less thick and undergo less retrogradation than nonwaxy varieties. *Waxy* cornstarch, for example, does not have the same gel-forming properties as cornstarch since it contains none of the gel-producing amylose and is composed of amylopectin.

- *Waxy* cornstarch contains NO amylose, is all amylopectin, and does NOT gel.
- *Ordinary* cornstarch contains 27% amylose and forms a gel.
- *High-amylose* cornstarch contains 55% amylose and forms a gel.

Waxy varieties of starch are commonly used in the preparation of pie fillings that should thicken but not gel. They are noted for their paste clarity.

Starch Uses in Food Systems

Starches may be introduced into foods primarily because of their *thickening* ability, but they also function as *stabilizers*. For example, a white sauce may be added during the preparation of a tomato-and-milk-based soup, in order to control milk protein precipitation due to the tomato acid.

Another use of starch is as a *fat replacer* in food systems. Intermediate-length polymers of D-glucose, **maltodextrins**, are formed from hydrolysis of starches such as tapioca, potato, and wheat. Maltodextrins simulate the viscosity and mouthfeel of oils and are used to reduce the fat content of some foods.

With the use of ordinary cross-breeding procedures, new starches are being discovered that have various applications in food systems. Baking, microwave cakes, frozen sauces, fat replacers, breadings, snacks, and gelled candies are some of the uses of starch (2). Pea starch, for example, may offer an alternative to other modified starches used in the food industry, as it provides a very high viscosity immediately upon agitation. It is available in pregelatinized form for use in cold-processed products such as dessert creams, dressings, instant soups, and sauces (3).

New food starches and their uses are continually being developed. Food starches are commercially manufactured and available for use in products such as baked foods, beverages, canned, frozen, and glassed foods, confections, dairy products, dry goods, meat products, and snack foods (4).

Another example of a new food application of starch granules is their use as flavor carriers. Using normal processing methods, small starch granules may be mixed with gelatin or water-soluble polysaccharides and then spray-dried forming a sphere. *Spherical aggregates* of starch granules contain open porous spaces that can be filled and used to transport material such as flavors, essences, and other compounds. Spherical aggregate carriers potentially offer time-release and protection of these flavors from oxidation (5).

COOKING WITH STARCH

Cooking over boiling water (such as with a double boiler for household preparation) promotes temperature control and even gelatinization. A disadvantage of this cooking method is that it requires cooking for a longer time to reach the thickening stage than a direct-heat cooking method. Of course, cooking with the appropriate starch in the proper concentration is crucial for the success of any starch-thickened product.

If incorporated into a recipe containing raw eggs, a hot starch-thickened mixture should be added gradually (to temper) the eggs, so that the eggs do not coagulate and produce an unacceptable consistency.

NUTRITIVE VALUE OF STARCH

Starch is a complex carbohydrate containing 4 calories/gram. Short-chain maltodextrins derived from the hydrolysis starch may be used in foods to simulate the taste and texture of fat, and they offer 4 cal/g instead of 9 cal/g in fat.

Special nutritional needs may require a dietary restriction of wheat and may lead to use of non-wheat starches in those individuals following gluten-free diets. Some alternatives to wheat are corn, potato, or rice starch. Packages of potato "flour" indicate that the contents are solely potato *starch* (6).

CONCLUSION

Starch is a plant polysaccharide that is the storage form of carbohydrate in roots, seeds, and tubers. It may be derived from cereals such as corn, wheat, rice, oats, or legumes such as soybean. In its uncooked stage, starch is insoluble in water. As it is heated and undergoes gelatinization, factors such as acid, agitation, use of enzymes, fat, proteins, sugar, and temperature require control. A separating agent prevents lumps in a starch mixture.

The source of starch and its concentration determine the thickening, gelling, and clarity of the finished product. Flour and cornstarch may be used to form gels; waxy varieties of starch do not gel. Syneresis may occur as the cooked, cooled starch mixture ages. Modification of starch granules allows starches to be used successfully for various food applications. Starch may be added to foods in order to provide thickening, product stability, or potentially to carry flavors.

GLOSSARY

Adsorb: Surface adherence of gas, liquids, or solids onto a solid.

Amylose: Long, linear chain composed of thousands of glucose molecules joined by an α-1,4-gycosidic linkage.

Amylopectin: Branched chains of glucose units joined by α-1,4 linkages, with α-1,6 branching occurring every 15–30 units.

Birefringence: A Maltese cross appearance on each uncooked crystalline starch granule when viewed under a polarizing microscope due to light refraction in two directions.

Dextrin: Glucose polymers; a product of the early stages of starch hydrolysis.

Gel: Elastic solid formed upon cooling of a gelatinized starch paste; a two-phase system that contains a solid continuous phase and a liquid dispersed phase.

Gelatinization: Starch granules take up water and swell irreversibly upon heating, and the organized granular pattern is disrupted.

Gelation: Formation of a gel upon cooling of a gelatinized starch paste.

Granule: Starch grain of long-chain glucose polymers in an organized pattern; granule shape is particular to each starch type.

Imbibition: Starch granules taking up water and swelling as it is exposed to moist heat.

Maltodextrin: Starch hydrolysis derivative that may be used to simulate fat in formulations.

Modified starch: Specific chemical modification of natural starches to physically create properties that contribute to shelf stability, appearance, convenience, and performance in food preparation.

Retrogradation: Reverting back, or reassociation of amylose as the gelatinized starch once again forms a more crystalline structure upon cooling.

Separating agent: Prevents lump formation in a starch mixture. Physically separates starch grains and allows their individual swelling.

Sol: A two-phase system with a solid dispersed in a liquid continuous phase.

Spherical aggregate: Open, porous starch granules with spaces that can be filled and used to transport materials such as flavor, essences, and other compounds.

Starch: Carbohydrate made up of two molecules—amylose and amylopectin.

Suspension: Large particles undissolved in the surrounding medium. Particles are too large to form a solution or a sol upon heating.

Syneresis: "Weeping" or water loss from a cooked, cooled gel due to excessive retrogradation or improper gel formation.

Viscosity: Resistance to flow of a liquid when force is applied. A measure of how easily a liquid will flow. Thin liquids have a low viscosity. Thick liquids or gels have a high viscosity and flow slowly.

REFERENCES

1. Freeland-Graves JH, Peckham GC. *Foundations of Food Preparation*, New York: Macmillian, 1987.
2. American Maize-Products Company. Hammond, IN.
3. Feinkost Ingredient Company. Lodi, OH.
4. National Starch and Chemical Company—Food Products Division. Bridgewater, NJ.
5. Zhao J, Whistler RL. Spherical aggregates of starch granules as flavor carriers. *Food Technology.* 1994; 48(7): 104–105.
6. Ener-G Foods, Inc. Seattle, WA.

BIBLIOGRAPHY

A. E. Staley Manufacturing Co. Decatur, IL
Bennion M. *The Science of Food.* New York: Harper and Row Publishers, 1980.
Cargill Foods. Eddyville, IA.
Luallen, TE. Starch as a functional ingredient. *Food Technology.* 1985; 39(1): 59–63.
Whistler RL, BeMiller JN, Paschall EF. *Starch: Chemistry and Technology*, 2nd ed. Orlando, FL: Academic Press, 1984.

CHAPTER 5

Pectins and Gums

INTRODUCTION

Pectins and gums are important polysaccharides in foods because of their functional properties. They are widely used as gelling agents, thickeners, and stabilizers. They are constituents of plant tissue and are large, complex molecules whose exact nature is not certain. However, enough is known to understand some of their properties and to make use of their functional properties to produce convenience and special texture foods.

PECTIC SUBSTANCES

Pectic substances including protopectin, pectinic acid, and pectic acid are an important constituent of plant tissue and are found mainly in the primary cell wall. They also occur between cell walls, where they act as intercellular cement. Although their exact nature is not clear, they can be considered as linear polymers of D-galacturonic acid joined by α-1,4-glycosidic linkages, as shown in Figure 5.1. Some of the acid or carboxyl (COOH) groups along the chain are esterified with methanol (CH_3OH) as shown.

Each glycosidic linkage is a *cross-planar* bond, because it is formed by reaction of one hydroxyl group located above the plane of the first ring with another hydroxyl group located below the plane of the second ring. The configuration of these bonds causes twisting of the molecule, and the resulting polymer can be likened to a twisted ribbon. Cross-planar bonds are not readily digested in the human digestive tract, and so pectins are classified as soluble fiber.

Pectic substances may be grouped into one of the three categories depending on the number of methyl ester groups attached to the polymer. *Protopectin* is found in immature fruits, and is a high molecular weight methylated galacturonic acid polymer.

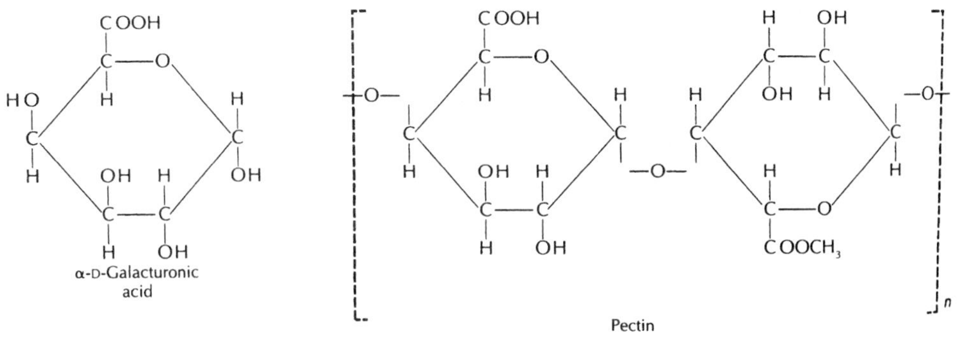

FIGURE 5.1 Basic structure of pectic substances.

It is insoluble in water but can be converted to water-dispersible pectin by heating in boiling water. It cannot form gels. *Pectinic acid* is a methylated form of galacturonic acid that is formed by enzymatic hydrolysis of protopectin as a fruit ripens. High-molecular weight pectinic acids are known as pectins. Pectinic acids are dispersible in water and can form gels. *Pectic acid* is a shorter-chain derivative of pectinic acid that is formed as fruit overripens. Enzymes, such as polygalacturonase and pectinesterase, cause depolymerization and demethylation of the pectinic acid, respectively. Complete demethylation yields pectic acid, which is incapable of gel formation.

PECTIC SUBSTANCES

Protopectin—methylated galacturonic acid polymer found in immature fruits.
Pectinic acid—methylated galacturonic acid polymer; includes pectins.
Pectic acid—short-chain demethylated derivative of pectinic acid found in overripe fruits.

Pectins

Pectins are high-molecular weight pectinic acids and are dispersible in water. Some of the carboxyl groups along the galacturonic acid chain are esterified with methanol. The degree of esterification in unmodified pectins ranges from about 60% in apple pulp to about 10% in strawberries. (Pectins can be deliberately deesterified during extraction or processing.) According to the degree of esterification, pectins are classified as **high methoxyl** or **low methoxyl** pectins. The two groups have different properties and gel under different conditions.

Low-methoxyl pectins. Low-methoxyl pectins contain mostly free carboxyl groups. In fact, only 20–40% of the carboxyl groups are esterified. Therefore, most of them are available to form cross-links with divalent ions such as calcium, as shown in Figure 5.2.

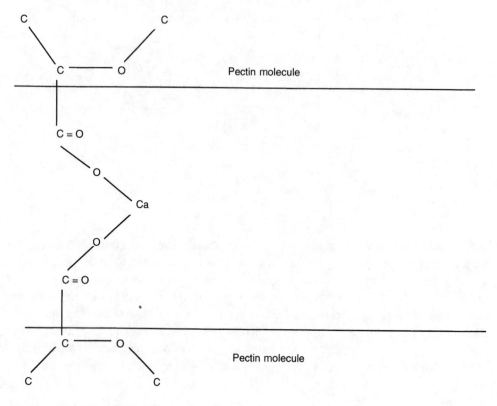

FIGURE 5.2 Cross-links in low-methoxyl pectin.

If sufficient cross-links are formed, a three-dimensional network can be obtained that traps liquid, forming a gel. Low-methoxyl pectins can, thus, form gels in the presence of divalent ions without the need for sugar or acid.

High-methoxyl pectins. High-methoxyl pectins contain a high proportion (usually 50–58%) of esterified carboxyl groups. Most of the acid groups are, therefore, not available to form cross-links with divalent ions, so these pectins do not form gels. However, they can be made to gel with the addition of sugar and acid. It is the high-methoxyl pectins that are commonly used to form pectin jellies.

Pectin Gel Formation

A pectin gel consists mainly of water held in a three-dimensional network of pectin molecules. Pectin is dispersible in water and forms a *sol* (solid dispersed in liquid continuous phase), but under the right conditions, it can be converted into a *gel* (liquid dispersed in solid continuous phase). This occurs when the pectin molecules interact with each other at specific points. It is not easy to form pectin gels; it requires a delicate balance of pectin, water, sugar, and acid.

Pectin is hydrophilic (water loving) due to the large number of polar hydroxyl groups and charged carboxyl groups on the molecule. When pectin is dispersed in *water*, some of the acid groups ionize, and water binds to both the charged and polar groups on the molecules. The negative charge on the pectin molecules, coupled with their attraction for water, keeps them apart so that they form a stable sol.

To form a gel, the forces keeping the pectin molecules apart must be reduced so that they can interact with each other at specific points, trapping water within the resulting three-dimensional network. In other words, the attraction of the pectin molecules for water must be **decreased** and the attraction of the pectin molecules for each other must be **increased**. This can be achieved by addition of sugar and acid.

Sugar competes for water, thus making less water available to associate with the pectin molecules. This reduces the attractive forces between the pectin and water molecules.

Acid adds hydrogen ions, reducing the pH. (The pH must be below 3.5 for a gel to form.) Carboxylic acids contain a **carboxyl group** (COOH), are weak acids and, are not fully ionized in solution; the un-ionized form of the acid exists in equilibrium with the ionized form.

$$-COOH + H_2O \rightleftharpoons -COO^- + H_3O^+$$

When hydrogen ions are added, they react with some of the ionized carboxyl groups to form undissociated acid groups. In other words, the equilibrium is shifted to the left, and more of the carboxylic acid is present in the un-ionized form. Thus, when hydrogen ions are added to pectin, the ionization of the acid groups is depressed and the charge on the pectin molecules is reduced. As a result, the pectin molecules no longer repel each other.

In fact, there is an attractive force between the molecules and they align and interact at specific regions along each polymer chain to form a three-dimensional network. These regions of interaction are called **junction zones,** shown diagrammatically in Figure 5.3. However, there are also regions of the pectin chains that are not involved in junction zones because they are unable to interact with each other. These regions form pockets or spaces between the junction zones that are able to entrap water. Hence, a gel is formed, with water trapped in the pockets of the three-dimensional pectin network.

Exactly how the junction zones form is not certain, but hydrogen bonds are thought to play an important role. The **steric fit** of the molecules (in other words, their ability to fit together in space) is also important. Pectin molecules contain minor components such as rhamnose and other neutral sugars that are bound to the main galacturonic acid chain by 1-2-glycosidic links. These sugars cause branches or kinks in the molecules and make it difficult for them to align and interact to form junction zones. However, there are regions of the pectin chains that do not contain these neutral sugars and it is these regions that are thought to form the junction zones.

High-methoxyl pectins form gels in this way. Low-methoxyl pectins require divalent ions to gel, and intermediate pectins require sugar, acid, and divalent ions to gel.

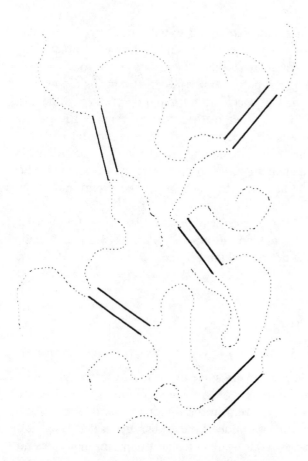

FIGURE 5.3   Junction zones in a pectin gel. Generalized two-dimensional view. Regions of the polymer chain involved in junction zones are shown as —. The other regions of the chain are shown as - - -. Water is entrapped in the spaces between the chains. Adapted from Coultate, 1989 (4).

Pectin Sources

Pectins with a high-molecular weight and a high proportion of methyl ester groups have the best jelly-forming ability. The pectin content of fruits is variable and depends not only on the type of fruit but also on its maturity or ripeness. If jellies or jams are made at home, it is best to add commercial pectin to ensure that there is sufficient pectin to form a gel. Purified pectin is made from apple cores and skins (apple pomace) and from the white inner skin (albedo) of citrus fruits. It is available in either liquid or granular form. The granular products have a longer shelf life than the liquids. Low-methoxyl pectin can be obtained by demethylating pectin with enzymes, acid, or alkali until it is 20–40% esterified (1). Because these pectins gel with divalent ions and need no sugar, they can be used commercially for the production of low-calorie jams, jellies, or desserts. They have also been introduced to the retail market so that such low-calorie products may be made at home.

PECTIN GEL FORMATION

In a pectin sol

- **water** binds to ionic and polar groups on pectin.

- **pectin** molecules are negatively charged and hydrated, therefore they do not interact with each other.

To form a pectin gel

- Attraction of pectin molecules for water must be decreased.

- Attraction of pectin molecules for each other must be increased.

This is achieved with

- **sugar**
  - competes for water,
  - decreases pectin–water attraction.
- **acid**
  - adds hydrogen ions,
  - depresses ionization of pectin,
  - reduces the charge on the pectin molecules,
  - increases pectin–pectin attraction.
- **pectin**
  - interacts at junction zones forming a three-dimensional network,
  - pectin becomes the continuous phase.
- **water**
  - is trapped in pockets within the gel network,
  - water becomes the disperse phase.

Some Principles of Making Jelly

This book does not attempt to describe the practical aspect of making jellies. For such information, the reader is referred to consumer information publications, or to books by authors such as Charley (2) or Penfield and Campbell (3). The intention is to highlight some of the more important scientific principles of jelly-making.

To make jelly, fruit juice (which is a source of water and acid), pectin, and sucrose are combined in a suitable pan and heated until the mixture boils. The temperature and boiling time are monitored, and boiling is continued until the desired temperature is reached.

As boiling continues, water evaporates, the concentration of sucrose increases, and the boiling point of the jelly also increases. Therefore, the boiling point can be used as an index of sucrose concentration. By measuring the temperature of the boiling jelly, it can be determined when sufficient water has been removed to give the desired sucrose concentration in the final jelly. However, all solutes increase the boiling point of water, so it is important to allow for the effect of any additional ingredients on the boiling point; a pure sucrose solution may boil at a lower temperature than a jelly mix containing the same concentration of sucrose. In other words, a boiling jelly may contain less sucrose than expected if the effects of the additional ingredients on the boiling point are not taken into account. This could result in a runny or weak gel.

It is important to control the boiling time, not just the temperature of the boiling jelly, because chemical reactions occur in the presence of heat and acid that need to be controlled to maintain gel quality. Glycosidic links are hydrolyzed in the presence of heat and acid. Therefore, depolymerization of pectin will occur if the boiling time is too long. This will result in loss of gelling power and the gel may not set.

During the boiling process, sucrose is converted to invert sugar, and the presence of invert sugar in the jelly prevents crystallization of sucrose on storage over a long period. A short boiling time may not allow formation of sufficient invert sugar to inhibit sucrose crystallization over time, especially if the jelly is stored at refrigeration temperatures.

IF THE BOILING TIME IS

- too long—depolymerization of pectin occurs, and the gel may not set.
- too short—insufficient invert sugar may be formed, and crystallization of sucrose may occur.

It has already been mentioned that a commercial pectin should be used in addition to the fruit, because the quality of pectin in the fruit varies. An overripe fruit is deficient in pectin, because demethylation and depolymerization occur as the fruit ages. Hydrolysis of only a few glycosidic bonds causes a marked drop in viscosity and gelling power and will produce a weak gel.

GUMS

Gums are a group of complex hydrophilic carbohydrates containing thousands of monosaccharide units. Galactose is the most common monosaccharide found in

---

MAIN CHARACTERISTICS OF GUMS

- Larger highly-branched hydrophilic polymers
- Rich in galactose.
- Hydrocolloids
- Form viscous solutions
- Most do not gel

gums; glucose is usually absent. Gums are often referred to as **hydrocolloids**, because of their affinity for water, and their size; when added to water, they form stable aqueous colloidal dispersions or sols. The molecules are highly branched, and as a result most gums are unable to form gels. However, they are able to trap or bind large amounts of water within their branches. Aqueous dispersions therefore tend to be very viscous, because it is difficult for the molecules to move around freely without becoming entangled with each other.

Gums are classified as soluble fiber because they undergo little digestion and absorption in the body. Therefore, they supply relatively few calories to the diet, as compared with digestible carbohydrates such as starch.

Gums are common in a wide range of food products, including salad dressings, sauces, soups, yogurt, canned evaporated milk, ice cream and other dairy products, baked goods, meat products, and fried foods. They are used as thickening agents in food products, replacing starch. They are also used to assist in the stabilization of emulsions and to maintain the smooth texture of ice cream and other frozen desserts. They are common in reduced fat products, because they are able to increase viscosity and help to replace the texture and mouthfeel that was contributed by the fat.

Gums are obtained from plants, and can be separated into five categories: seed gums, plant exudates, microbial exudates, seaweed extracts, and synthetic gums derived from cellulose.

Seed Gums

The seed gums include guar and locust bean gums. These gums are branched polymers containing only mannose and galactose. Guar gum contains a mannose/galactose ratio of 2:1, whereas the ratio is 4:1 in locust bean gum. Guar gum is soluble in cold water, whereas locust bean gum must be dispersed in hot water. Neither gum forms a gel when used alone. However, they may be used synergistically with other gums to form gels.

Guar gum forms gels with carrageenan and guar gum. It is used to stabilize ice cream, and it is also found in sauces, soups, and salad dressings.

The presence of guar gum in the intestine seems to retard the digestion and absorption of carbohydrates and slow absorption of glucose into the bloodstream. Use of guar gum in foods may, therefore, be useful in treating mild cases of diabetes (4).

Locust bean gum is typically used as a stabilizer in dairy and processed meat products. It may also be used synergistically with xanthan gum to form gels.

Plant Exudates

The plant exudates include gum arabic, which comes from the acacia tree, and gum tragacanth. These are complex, highly branched polysaccharides. Gum arabic is highly soluble in cold water, and is used to stabilize emulsions and to control crystal size in ices and glazes. Gum tragacanth forms very viscous sols, and is used to impart a creamy texture to food products. It is also used to suspend particles, and acts as a stabilizer in products such as salad dressings, ice cream, and confections.

CATEGORIES OF GUMS

- **Seed gums:** guar gum, locust bean gum
- **Plant exudates:** gum arabic, gum tragacanth
- **Microbial exudates:** xanthan, gellan, dextran
- **Seaweed polysaccharides:** alginates, carrageenan, agar
- **Synthetic gums:** microcrystalline cellulose, carboxymethyl cellulose, methyl cellulose

---

Microbial Exudates

Xanthan gum, gellan gum, dextran, and curdlan are all gums produced using fermentation by microorganisms. Of these, *xanthan* is the most common. Xanthan forms viscous sols that are stable over a wide range of pH and temperature. It does not form a gel, except when used in combination with locust bean gum. It is used in a wide range of products as a thickener and stabilizer and suspending agent. Most salad dressings contain xanthan gum.

Seaweed Polysaccharides

The **seaweed polysaccharides** include the agars, alginates, and carrageenans. Unlike most other gums, they are able to form gels under certain conditions.

Carrageenan is obtained from red seaweeds, and especially from Irish moss. It occurs as three main fractions, known as kappa, iota, and lambda carrageenan. Each is a galactose polymer containing varying amounts of negatively-charged sulfate esters. Kappa-carrageenan contains the smallest number of sulfate esters, and is therefore the least negatively charged. It is able to form strong gels with potassium ions. Lambda-carrageenan contains the largest number of sulfate groups, and is too highly charged to form a gel. Iota-carrageenan forms gels with calcium ions.

The carrageenan fractions are generally used in combination. Several different formulations are available, containing different amounts of the individual fractions, and food processors are able to choose formulations that best fit their needs.

The carrageenans are used to stabilize milk products such as ice cream, processed cheese, canned evaporated milk, and chocolate milk, because of their ability to interact with proteins. The carrageenans may also be used with other gums, because of their ability to cross-link with them.

Agar is also obtained from red seaweeds. It is noted for its strong, transparent, heat-reversible gels; that is, agar gels melt on heating and re-form when cooled again.

Agar contains two fractions—agarose and agaropectin, both of which are polymers of β-D- and α-L-galactose. Agaropectin also contains sulfate esters.

The **alginates** are obtained from brown seaweeds. They contain mainly D-mannuronic acid and L-guluronic acid, and they form gels in the presence of calcium ions. Calcium alginate gels do not melt below the boiling point of water; thus, they can be used to make specialized food products. Fruit purees can be mixed with sodium alginate and then treated with a calcium-containing solution to make reconstituted fruit. For example, if large drops of cherry/alginate puree are added to a calcium solution, convincing synthetic cherries are formed. Reconstituted apple and apricot pieces for pie fillings can also be made by rapidly mixing the sodium alginate/ fruit puree with a calcium solution and molding the gel into suitable shapes.

FUNCTIONAL ROLES OF GUMS

Gums my be used to perform one or more of the roles in food peoducts.

- **Thickeners**—salad dressings, sauces, soups, beverages
- **Stabilizers**—ice creams, icings, emulsified products
- **Control crystal size**—candies
- **Suspending agents**—salad dressings
- **Gelling agents**—fruit pieces, cheese analogs
- **Coating agents**—batters for deep-fried foods
- **Fat replacers**—low-fat salad dressings, ice creams, desserts
- **Starch replacers**—baked goods, soups, sauces
- **Bulking agents**—low fat foods
- **Source of fiber**—beverages, soups, baked goods

Synthetic Gums

Cellulose is an essential component of all plant cell walls. It is insoluble in water and cannot be digested by man, and so it is not a source of energy for the body. It is classified as insoluble fiber.

The polymer contains at least 3000 glucose molecules joined by β-1,4-glycosidic linkages. Long cellulose chains may be held together in bundles forming fibers, as in the stringy parts of celery.

Synthetic derivatives of cellulose are used in foods as *nonmetabolizable* bulking agents, binders, and thickeners. *Microcrystalline cellulose*, known commercially as Avicel (FMC Corp.), is used as a bulking agent in low-calorie foods. It is produced by hydrolysis of cellulose with acid. ***Carboxymethyl cellulose*** (CMC) and *methyl cellulose*(MC) are alkali-modified forms of cellulose. The former is the most common, and it is often called simply *cellulose gum*. It functions mainly to increase the viscosity of foods. It is used as a binder and thickener in pie fillings and puddings; it also retards ice crystal growth in ice cream and the growth of sugar crystals in confections and syrups. In dietetic foods, it can be used to provide the bulk, body, and mouthfeel that would normally be supplied by sucrose. *Methyl cellulose* forms gels when cold dispersions are heated. It is used to coat foods prior to deep fat frying, in order to limit absorption of fat. Two other forms of modified cellulose include *hydroxypropyl cellulose* and *hydroxypropylmethyl cellulose*. These are also used as batters for coating fried foods.

CONCLUSION

Pectins and seaweed polysaccharides are useful for various food products because of their gelling ability. In general, gums are important because they form very viscous solutions, but most do not gel. All these carbohydrates are important to the food industry because of their functional properties and their ability to produce foods with special textures. Used in a wide range of food products, as gelling agents, thickeners, and stabilizers, their availability has increased the choice and quality of many convenience foods. Synthetic derivatives of cellulose are important as nonmetabolizable bulking agents, thickeners, and stabilizers in a wide range of calorie-reduced foods.

GLOSSARY

Carboxyl group: COOH group; weak acid group that is partially ionized in solution.

Carboxymethyl cellulose (CMC): Synthetic derivative of cellulose used as a bulking agent in foods. Also known as cellulose gum.

Cellulose: Glucose polymer joined by β-1,4-glycosidic linkages; cannot be digested by humans, and so provides dietary fiber.

Cross-planar bond: Formed when the hydroxyl groups on the carbon atoms involved in the formation of a glycosidic bond are oriented on opposite faces of the sugar rings. Cross-planar bonds occur in pectin and cellulose. They are not digested in the human digestive system.

Gel: Two-phase system with a solid continuous phase and a liquid dispersed phase.

Gums: Complex, hydrophilic carbohydrates that are highly branched and form very viscous solutions; most gums do not gel.

High-methoxyl pectin: Pectin with 50–58% of the carboxyl groups esterified with methanol.

Hydrocolloid: Large molecule with a high affinity for water that forms a stable aqueous colloidal dispersion or sol. Starches, pectins, and gums are all hydrocolloids.

Junction zone: Specific region where two molecules such as pectin align and interact, probably by hydrogen bonds; important in gel formation.

Low-methoxyl pectin: Pectin with 20–40% of the carboxyl groups esterified with methanol.

Pectic acid: Shorter-chain derivative of pectinic acid found in overripe fruits; demethylated; incapable of forming a gel.

Pectic substances: Include protopectin, pectinic acids, and pectic acids.

Pectin: High-molecular-weight pectinic acid; methylated α-D-galacturonic acid polymer.

Pectinic acid: Methylated α-D-galacturonic acid polymer; includes pectins; can form a gel.

Protopectin: Insoluble material found in immature fruits; high molecular weight methylated galacturonic acid polymer; cannot form a gel.

Seaweed polysaccharides: Complex polysaccharides that are capable of forming gels; examples include alginates, carrageenan, and agar; used as thickeners and stabilizers in food.

Sol or dispersion: Two-phase system with a solid dispersed phase and a liquid continuous phase.

Steric fit: Ability of molecules to come close enough to each other in space to interact (or fit together).

REFERENCES

1. Glicksman J. *Food applications of gums*. In: Lineback DR, Inglett GE, eds. *Food Carbohydrates*. Westport, CT: AVI, 1982.
2. Charley H, Weaver C. *Foods. A Scientific Approach*, 3rd ed. New York: Merrill/Prentice-Hall, 1998.
3. Coultate TP. *Food. The Chemistry of Its Components*, 2nd ed. Cambridge: RSC, 1989.
4. Penfield MP, Campbell AM. *Experimental Food Science*, 3rd ed. San Diego, CA: Academic Press, 1990.

BIBLIOGRAPHY

McWilliams M. *Foods: Experimental Perspectives*, 4th ed. New York: Prentice-Hall, 2001.

Potter N, Hotchkiss J. *Food Science*, 5th ed. New York: Chapman & Hall, 1995.

Vieira ER. *Elementary Food Science*, 4th ed. New York: Chapman & Hall, 1996.

BeMiller JN, Whistler RL. Carbohydrates. In: Fennema OR, ed. *Food Chemistry*, 3rd ed. New York: Marcel Dekker, 1996.

CHAPTER 6

Bread, Cereal, Rice, and Pasta

INTRODUCTION

Bread, cereal, rice, and pasta products are important foods consumed throughout the world. The United States Department of Agriculture (USDA) and the World Health Organization (WHO) have placed these foods at the base of their Food Guide Pyramid. It is recommended that 6–11 daily servings from the Bread, Cereal, Rice, and Pasta Group compose the basis of food chosen in the diet.

In this chapter, the *flours* used in breadmaking, as well as *cereals, rice, and pasta products* are discussed. A further study of quick breads, yeast breads, the functions of various added ingredients, and wheat gluten appear in the chapter on Baked products (Chapter 15).

From the nutritional point of view, these foods form the base of the Food Guide Pyramid. Observing from the culinary point of view, these items are included in many menu offerings and have risen substantially in popularity, due in part to a committed number of Americans making more nutritious food selections (1,2).

STRUCTURE OF CEREAL GRAINS

All grains are *structurally* similar to one another. The kernel of grain is composed of three parts: the germ, endosperm, and bran. "Whole grains," such as whole wheat, contain all three parts of the seed, including the bran and germ. The parts of the seed are separated in milling, and if part is removed, the product is "refined" rather than "whole" (Figure 6.1).

The **germ**, or embryo, is the inner portion of the kernel-located on the lower end of the kernel, as it grows. It composes approximately 2.5% of the seed and is where sprouting begins as the new plant begins growth. The germ is the kernel component with the highest percent lipid, containing 6–10% lipid, and it may cause rancidity by

a Kernel of Wheat

The Kernel of Wheat

...sometimes called the wheat berry, the kernel is the seed from which the wheat plant grows. Each tiny seed contains three distinct parts that are separated during the milling process to produce flour.

Endosperm

...about 83 percent of the kernel weight and the source of white flour. The endosperm contains the greatest share of protein, carbohydrates and iron, as well as the major B-vitamins, such as riboflavin, niacin, and thiamine. It is also a source of soluble fiber.

Bran

...about $14^{1}/_{2}$ percent of the kernel weight. Bran is included in whole wheat flour and can also be bought separately. The bran contains a small amount of protein, large quantities of the three major B-vitamins, trace minerals, and dietary fiber — primarily insoluble.

Germ

...about $2^{1}/_{2}$ percent of the kernel weight. The germ is the embryo or sprouting section of the seed, often separated from flour in milling because the fat content (10 percent) limits flour's shelf-life. The germ contains minimal quantities of high quality protein and a greater share of B-complex vitamins and trace minerals. Wheat germ can be purchased separately and is part of whole wheat flour.

Longitudinal Section of Grain of Wheat (enlarged approximately 35 times)

U.S. dietary guidelines recommend 6 to 11 servings of the bread, cereal, rice and pasta group each day. Grain-based foods provide complex carbohydrates, the best source of time-released energy for our bodies. These foods are usually low-fat and provide fiber. Grain foods provide vitamins – especially the three key B vitamins (thiamine, riboflavin and niacin) and iron.

WHEAT FOODS COUNCIL, SUITE 111, 5500 S. QUEBEC, ENGLEWOOD, CO 80111, (303) 694-5828

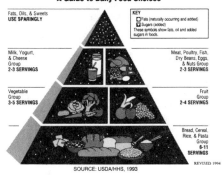

Food Guide Pyramid
A Guide to Daily Food Choices

Fats, Oils, & Sweets
USE SPARINGLY

KEY
☐ Fats (naturally occurring and added)
☑ Sugars (added)
These symbols show fats, oil and added sugars in foods.

Milk, Yogurt, & Cheese Group
2-3 SERVINGS

Meat, Poultry, Fish, Dry Beans, Eggs, & Nuts Group
2-3 SERVINGS

Vegetable Group
3-5 SERVINGS

Fruit Group
2-4 SERVINGS

Bread, Cereal, Rice, & Pasta Group
6-11 SERVINGS

SOURCE: USDA/HHS, 1993

REVISED 1994

FIGURE 6.1 Structure of a wheat kernel (*Source*: Wheat Foods Council).

the action of the lipoxidase enzyme, or by nonenzymatic oxidative rancidity. Therefore, a whole grain product may either undergo germ removal or include antioxidants to control rancidity. The germ contains approximately 8% of the kernel's protein and most of the thiamin.

The **endosperm** is primarily starch, held as part of a protein matrix. Regardless of the grain type, it is the seed component, lowest in fat, containing up to 1.5% of the lipid of the seed, and is lower in fiber than the bran. The endosperm is the source of white flour, makes up approximately 83% of the seed, and approximately 70–75% of the protein of the kernel. The actual ratio of starch to protein differs among grain varieties; for example, soft wheat contains more starch and less protein than hard wheat.

The **bran** is the layered, outer coat of a kernel, offering protection for the seed, consisting of an outside pericarp layer, and inside layer that includes the seed coat. The bran is often removed by abrasion or polishing in the milling process and used in many foods animal feed. It makes up approximately 14.5% of the seed, and contains 19% of the protein, 3–5% lipid, and minerals such as iron.

Bran is high in its fiber content, providing cellulose and hemicellulose bulk or "roughage" in the diet. Yet, functionally, the bran may differ among grain varieties. *Wheat bran,* is an *insoluble* fiber. It functions as a "stool softener." *Oat bran* is a soluble fiber that functions among other ways, to reduce serum cholesterol.

CHEMICAL COMPOSITION OF CEREAL GRAINS

While grains are *structurally* similar, they vary in their *nutrient* composition, containing carbohydrate, fat, protein, water, vitamins, and minerals (Tables 6.1 and 6.2). The main nutrient component of cereal grains is **carbohydrate**, which makes up 79–83% of the *dry* matter of grain. It exists predominantly as starch, with fiber especially cellulose and hemicellullose, composing approximately 6% of the grain.

Lipid makes up approximately 1–7% of a kernel, depending on the grain. For example, wheat, rice, corn, rye, and barley contain 1–2% lipid; oats contain 4–7%. The lipid is 72–85% unsaturated fatty acids—mainly, oleic acid and linoleic acid.

Protein composes 7–14% of the grain and provides half of the protein consumed worldwide. In comparison to meats or eggs, the protein contribution of

TABLE 6.1 Typical Percent Composition of Common Cereal Grains (100 g)

Grain	Carbohydrate	Fat	Protein	Fiber	Water
Wheat flour	71.0	2.0	13.3	2.3	12.0
Rice	80.4	0.4	6.7	0.3	12.0
Corn meal	78.4	1.2	7.9	0.6	12.0
Oats, rolled	68.2	7.4	14.2	1.2	8.3
Rye flour	74.8	1.7	11.4	1.0	11.1
Barley	78.9	Trace	10.4	0.4	10.0
Noncereal flours					
Buckwheat flour	72.1	2.5	11.8	1.4	12.1
Soybean flour, defatted	38.1	0.9	47.0	2.3	8.0

Source: Wheat Flour Institute.

TABLE 6.2 Vitamin, Mineral, and Fiber Content of Wheat Flours (100 g)

Flour	Thiamin B_1 (mg)	Riboflavin B_2 (mg)	Niacin B_3 (mg)	Iron (mg)	Fiber (g)
Whole wheat flour (whole grain)	0.66	0.14	5.2	4.3	2.8
Enriched flour (enriched)	0.67	0.43	5.9	3.6	0.3
White flour (refined)	0.07	0.06	1.0	0.9	0.3

Source: Wheat Flour Institute.

grains is not high, and cereal grains do not include all the essential amino acids contained in animal protein. Protein from plant foods is of low biological value, and less efficient in supporting body needs, because a smaller percentage of protein nitrogen is digested and absorbed. Although potential breeding may produce cereals higher in lysine, it is the limiting amino acid in cereals. Cereals are low in the amino acids tryptophan and methionine.

In cultures throughout the world, the preparation of traditional dishes combine grains with legumes or nuts and seeds to provide the needed amino acids to yield a complete protein. (Note: Botanically, all grains, legumes, nuts, and seeds are *fruits* of a plant.)

Gliadin and *glutenin* are two important proteins present in wheat, especially hard wheat, oats, rye, and barley. To the extent that these two proteins are present, flour has "gluten-forming potential." Then, with hydration and manipulation, a gummy, elastic structure, the **gluten** (Chapter 15) structure, is created, contributing strength and extensibility to the dough. Various flours but, especially wheat, may be utilized in breadmaking to form sufficient levels of gluten for structure.

The enzyme (protein) α-amylase is naturally present in grains and promotes dextrinization of starch molecules to shorter-chain polymers, and the sugar maltose and glucose. The action of α-amylase may thin starch mixtures or be detrimental to the breadmaking industry (Chapter 4).

Water is present in cereal grains at levels of 10–14% of the grain. Soaking and cooking adds water to cereal grains, and the grain size expands as additional water is absorbed.

Vitamins present in cereals are predominantly the B vitamins—thiamin (B_1), riboflavin (B_2), and niacin (B_3). These vitamins may be lost in the milling process and so, are added back through the process of **enrichment**. Today, there is less prevalence of the once deadly diseases beriberi and pellagra, due to cereal enrichment with thiamin and niacin, respectively (Table 6.2). Whole grain products contain some fat-soluble vitamins in the germ.

Minerals are naturally present at higher levels in whole grains (with the bran layer) than in refined grains, although **fortification** of refined flour with iron

(Table 6.2) is common. Zinc and calcium as well as vitamins, may also be added at levels beyond those present in the original grain.

Fiber content is determined by different analysis, and includes crude fiber (CF) and total dietary fiber (TDF). These two measurements are not correlated. CF is composed of cellulose and the noncarbohydrate *lignin*. TDF includes cellulose and lignin, *plus* hemicellulose, pectic substances, gums, and mucilages.

CEREALS

Cereal is a cultivated grass, such as wheat, corn, rice, and oats, which produces an edible grain (fruit or seed). *Cereal* comprises all the cereal products prepared from grain, including milled flour and pasta. Depending on the composition, cereal crops may be processed into various items such as the following:

- bread, using flour or meal from various grains (Chapter 15);
- cereal, ready-to-eat, or cooked breakfast cereal varieties;
- pasta, a dried paste made of various flours (and perhaps legumes, herbs, and spices);
- starch, from the starchy component of endosperm (Chapter 4);
- oil, from germ processing (Chapter 12).

When stored properly, grains are extremely resistant to deterioration during storage, especially when compared to the perishable dairy or meats, or fruit and vegetable crops. Grains are utilized extensively in developing and less affluent countries where animal products are either not available or not used. In more affluent countries, many varieties of processed cereals (i.e., ready-to-eat breakfast cereals) may be consumed.

COMMON CEREAL GRAINS AND THEIR USES

There is a great variety of cereal grains and their uses throughout the world. The most important and the largest cereal grain consumed by man in the United States diet is *wheat*.

Wheat

Wheat is used as whole, cracked (bulgur, couscous), made into flour, breads (quickbreads, pastries, etc.), cereals, and pasta, and is the basis of numerous products that are recognized in diets throughout the world. Some individuals (gluten sensitive, as discussed in a later section of this chapter) exhibit an intolerance of wheat.

The wheat kernel (wheat berry) is the most common cereal milled into flour in the United States. There are over 30,000 varieties of wheat grown in the United States, grouped into the following major classifications: hard red winter, hard red

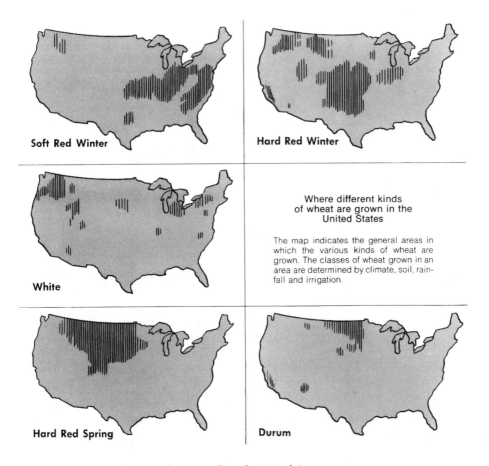

Soft Red Winter

Hard Red Winter

White

Where different kinds of wheat are grown in the United States

The map indicates the general areas in which the various kinds of wheat are grown. The classes of wheat grown in an area are determined by climate, soil, rainfall and irrigation.

Hard Red Spring

Durum

FIGURE 6.2 Map showing wheat growth in the United States (*Source*: Wheat Flour Institute).

spring, soft red winter, hard white wheat, soft white wheat, and durum wheat. Figures 6.2 and 6.3 show where various wheats are grown.

Wheat is named for the *season* (Winter or Spring) in which it is planted, its *texture* (hard or soft) and the *color* (red, white, and amber). Regarding season, *winter* wheat is planted in cold seasons (fall and winter) and harvested in June or July. Examples of winter wheat include—hard red winter, soft red winter, or white winter wheat. The spring planting, or *spring* wheat, is harvested in late summer or fall seasons. It includes hard red spring, white spring, and durum wheat.

Regarding texture wheat is classified hard or soft. *Hard* wheat kernels contain strong protein–starch bonds, the kernel is tightly packed, and there are minimal air spaces. Hard wheat flour forms elastic doughs due to its high gluten-forming protein content, and is the best flour to use for breadmaking. Hard *spring* wheat is 12–18% protein and hard *winter* wheat is 10–15% protein. Conversely, *soft* wheat is lower in protein, i.e., 8–11%, and is desirable for cakes and pastries.

The protein–starch bonds in the kernel break more easily in soft wheat, yet inherent differences in the protein or starch components of hard and soft wheat do

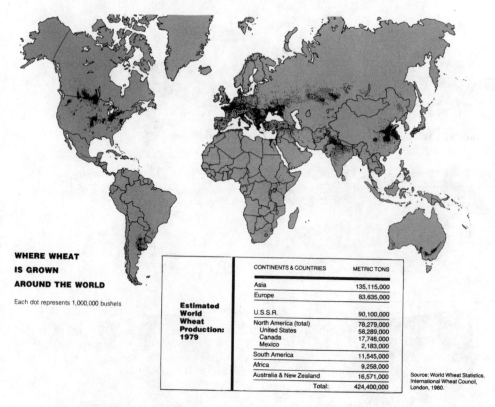

WHERE WHEAT IS GROWN AROUND THE WORLD

Each dot represents 1,000,000 bushels

Estimated World Wheat Production: 1979

CONTINENTS & COUNTRIES	METRIC TONS
Asia	135,115,000
Europe	83,635,000
U.S.S.R.	90,100,000
North America (total)	78,279,000
United States	58,289,000
Canada	17,746,000
Mexico	2,183,000
South America	11,545,000
Africa	9,258,000
Australia & New Zealand	16,571,000
Total:	424,400,000

Source: World Wheat Statistics, International Wheat Council, London, 1980.

FIGURE 6.3   Map showing where wheat is grown around the world (*Source:* Wheat Flour Institute).

not sufficiently explain the differences in hardness. Hard and soft wheat may be blended to create all-purpose flour that contains about 10.5% protein.

In addition to the season and the texture, wheat is classified according to its color, either red or white, depending on the presence of pigment, such as carotenoid. Durum wheat is a hard wheat, i.e., a highly pigmented, gold-toned wheat. The endosperm is milled into **semolina** for pasta, and then the coarse semolina may be ground into durum *flour*.

Milling Process of Wheat. Specific milling tolerances must be met to call the product "flour." Flour is produced when the wheat kernel or berry is ground. The Food and Drug Administration (FDA) then grades, according to the flour composition. When milled, each 100 pounds of wheat yields approximately 72 pounds of white flour and 28 pounds of other product, including animal feed.

The conventional milling process (Figure 6.4) of wheat first involves washing to remove foreign substances such as dirt or rocks. Conditioning or tempering by the addition or removal of water is necessary in the milling process in order to obtain the appropriate water content and to facilitate the easy separation of the kernel components. Next, wheat is subject to coarse breaking of the kernels into middlings. The breaking process separates most of the kernels' outside (bran) and inside core (germ) from the endosperm. Once the endosperm is separated, it is subsequently

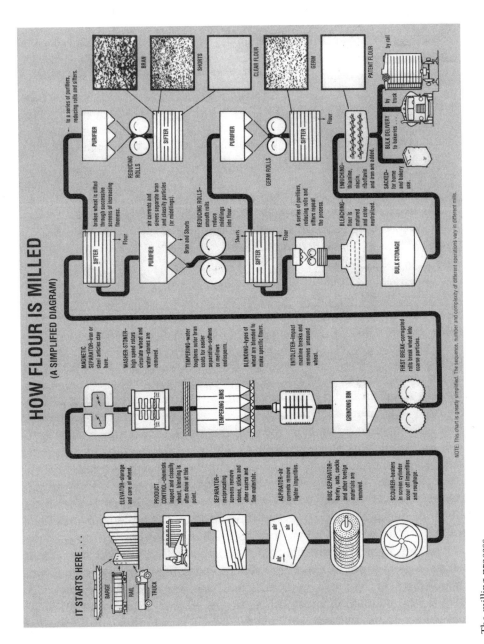

FIGURE 6.4 The milling process (*Source*: Wheat Flour Institute).

Hard wheat: 12–18% protein

- **Bread flour** is typically made of *hard* red spring wheat kernels, with a high protein–starch ratio, and is sold commercially. It has a high gluten-forming potential forming a very strong and elastic structure, and it is not finely milled. Recall that hard *spring* wheat has a greater protein content than hard *winter* wheat. ("Gluten flour," milled from spring wheat, may contain 40–45% protein.)

Hard and soft wheat blend: 10.5% protein

- **All-purpose wheat flour** combines the desirable qualities of both hard and soft wheat flour. It does not contain bran or germ, and is known as white wheat flour, or simply "flour." It forms a less strong and elastic dough than bread flour and it may be enriched or bleached.

Soft wheat: 7–9% protein

- **Cake flour** contains less protein, and more starch than all-purpose flour, has low gluten-forming potential, is highly bleached, and finely milled (7/8 cup all-purpose flour + 2 tablespoons cornstarch = 1 cup cake flour).

- **Pastry flour** maintains intermediate characteristics of all-purpose and cake flour. It contains less starch than cake flour, and less protein than all-purpose flour.

ground in reduction rolls to become finer for flour. As the bran and germ are removed, the flour contains less vitamins and minerals.

Various flours are created if flour streams are blended during the milling process. Although it does not constitute the majority of flour sold on the market, *straight grade* flour is a combination of *all* of the mill streams. Typically, home and bakery operations use **patent flours** that are 85% straight grade flour and the combination of various highly refined mill streams. Patent flour is the highest grade of flour; hence, the highest in value. Short-patent flour, such as cake flour, contains more starch and is produced by combining fewer streams than the higher-protein, long-patent flour. The remainder of flour, not incorporated into patent flours, is *clear flour*. It is used when color is not of importance, as it is slightly gray.

Flours from the same mill vary in composition from one year to the next, and the various flour mills may produce slightly different flours, depending on such factors as geographic location of the crop, rainfall, soil, and temperature. It follows that this variance may produce different baking results depending upon the mill, the geographic location, and so forth. Utilizing the same recipe in different parts of the country may produce slightly different products!

Milling of various textures of wheat produces some of the following flours:

Milling wheat also produces the less common instant-blending, instantized, or "agglomerated" flour (3). Instant-blending flour is all-purpose flour that has been hydrated and dried, forming large "agglomerated" or clustered particles, larger than

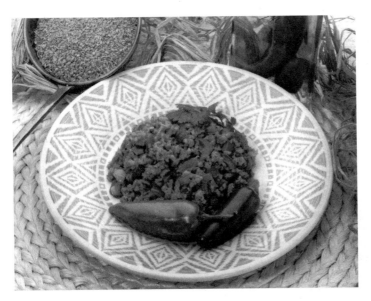

FIGURE 6.5 Bulgur wheat
(*Source:* Wheat Foods Council).

the FDA approves for white wheat flour. It has a more uniform particle size range than white wheat flour and does not readily pack down. Instant-blending flour is easily dispersible in water and is used when dispersibility of flour in liquid is preferred or required. It mixes into a formulation or recipe better than non-instant blending flour and is free-flowing, pouring like salt or sugar.

Other flour treatments include the following:

- **Self-rising flour (phosphated flour)** contains $1\frac{1}{2}$ teaspoons of baking powder and $\frac{1}{2}$ teaspoon of salt per cup of flour and provides convenience.

- *Bleached flour* bleached to a white color naturally by exposure of the yellowish (mainly xanthophyll) pigment to oxygen in the air, or by the chemical addition of either chlorine dioxide gas or benzoyl peroxide. In the process of oxygen addition, the pH is lowered and the bleaching agent evaporates. Not all flour is bleached, and not all bleaching agents necessarily improve the baking qualities of flour (Chapter 18). *Un*bleached flour is aged and bleached naturally.

- *Matured flour* comes naturally with age, or by the addition of maturing agents such as chlorine dioxide (also a bleaching agent which oxidizes wheat flour). Its use improves gluten elasticity and baking properties of doughs by controlling the unwanted effect of excess sulfhydryl groups. These may depolymerize gluten protein molecules, making the dough gummy (Chapter 20).

- *Organic (chemical-free) flour* uses grains that are grown without the application of synthetic herbicides and pesticides.

Wheat foods include bulgur (Figure 6.5), cracked wheat, and farina. *Bulgur* is the whole kernel, i.e., parboiled, dried, and treated to remove a small percentage of

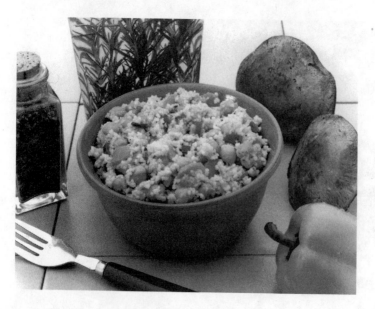

FIGURE 6.6 Couscous
(*Source:* Wheat Foods Council).

the bran. It is then cracked and used as breakfast cereal or pilaf. Bulgur is similar in taste to wild rice. Similarly, *cracked wheat* is the whole kernel broken into small pieces, yet is not subject to parboiling. Because they are whole grains, they should be stored in an airtight container, in a cool, dark place. *Farina* is the pulverized wheat middlings of endosperm used predominantly as a cooked cereal. It is similar in appearance to grits (corn).

A processed form of semolina from wheat is used in the preparation of couscous (Figure 6.6). The WHO places couscous at the bottom of its Food Guide Pyramid. It is popular throughout the world, especially in Northern Africa and Latin America. It is often served as a pilaf or as tabouli.

Rice

Rice is a major cereal grain whose varieties are used as *staple foods* by people throughout the world. It may be the major aspect of a diet, or incorporated into the main dish, side dish, or dessert, and is commonly used in the preparation of ready-to-eat breakfast cereals. Rice is especially important to persons with wheat allergies, and is commonly eaten as a first food by infants, as it offers the least cereal allergy.

Rice may be eaten as the whole grain, or polished, shedding the bran. Generally, rice is polished during milling in order to remove the brown hull, which also removes some of the protein, vitamins, and minerals. [The once-prevalent deadly disease, beriberi resulted from eating polished rice (thiamin removed in the milling process) as a staple food.] Today, most white rice is enriched with vitamins and minerals, to add back nutrients lost in milling. Unpolished, whole rice is more subject to flavor deterioration and insect infestation than polished, white rice.

TABLE 6.3   Primary Nutrients for the Enrichment of Rice

Nutrient	mg/lb
Thiamin	2–4
Riboflavin	1.2–2.4
Niacin	16–32
Vitamin D	250–1000
Iron	13–26
Calcium	500–1000

Enrichment (Table 6.3) of rice is common and may be achieved by two primary methods. One method is to coat the grain with a powder of thiamin and niacin, waterproof it, dry it, and then coat the grain with iron before it is dried again. The another method of enrichment involves parboiling or "converting" rice so that the water-soluble bran and germ nutrients travel to the endosperm by a pressure steam treatment. As a result of this method of enrichment, nutrients are retained when the hull is removed. Following the steaming process, rice is subsequently dried and polished. Optional enrichment may include riboflavin, vitamin D, and calcium.

Rice is grown in a variety of sizes. Extra long grain or long grain rice is higher in amylose content, and therefore less sticky than medium or short grain rice. It follows that in a product such as sushi, e.g., short grain is preferable over long, as it is sticky and holds ingredients together.

AMYLOPECTIN CONTENT OF RICE	
Size variety	*% Amylopectin*
Long grain	74–77%
Medium grain	74–82%
Short grain	80–85%

Rice may be modified to allow *flavor* and aroma variety, very detectable by some palates, or "rice" may even be made from *pasta*, i.e., shaped to resemble rice. It may be processed into flours, starches, cereals, cooking wine, or the Japanese wine, sake. Rice flour (primarily starch), may successfully be made into items such as low-fat tortillas (4) or noodles. (Wild "rice" is actually not rice, but is derived from seeds of another reed-like water plant.)

New rice development shows that rice is used to create many new food and beverage products. Rice-based ingredients are used to reduce the oil content absorbed in the frying process. Genetically modified rice strains have been developed to be high in beta-carotene, have cancer-fighting properties, or be healthy beverage bases. Numerous research studies have focused on shelf-stable cooked rice, ready-to-eat cereal, confectionery applications, rice oils, and flavored rice. Defatted rice bran extracts, aromatic rice, pregelatinized rice flours, starches, and rice syrups are chosen as food ingredients, depending upon the application (5).

While people in Asia may eat as much as 300 pounds of rice per person, in a year, Americans eat less, yet have shown a doubling of rice intake, to eat more than 21 pounds per year (5). Rice use in a wide variety of foods continues to be common.

Corn

The majority of corn is used for animal feed, although corn is a staple cereal food of many people and nations. It is lacking in the two essential amino acids, tryptophan and lysine, but research continues to explore the addition of a protein trait to corn DNA. As well, since corn does not contain the proteins gliadin and glutenin that form gluten, it must be combined with other flour, such as wheat flour, for use in breadmaking.

Sweet corn is a cereal, i.e., commonly eaten as a vegetable, whereas *field corn* has nonvegetable uses, including starch that is of value to growers and consumers alike. The *whole kernels* of special breeds of corn containing 11–16% moisture are desirable for popcorn. The kernel increases in volume as the water escapes as steam.

The *whole* or *partial kernels* may be coarsely ground (perhaps stone-ground) and used to create cornmeal or masa. Cornmeal is popular in cornbread and tamales, corn tortillas, snack foods, and taco shells (Figure 6.7). It may be soaked in alkali, such as lime (calcium hydroxide) for 20–30 minutes, for a better amino acid balance

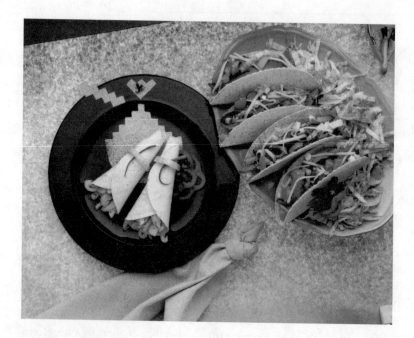

FIGURE 6.7   Corn taco shells and tortillas (*Courtesy of SYSCO® Incorporated*).

and greater protein availability. This soaking process may sacrifice some niacin (vitamin B₃), but it adds calcium.

The *endosperm* of corn may be made into hominy, ground into grits, or used in ready-to-eat breakfast cereals. The starch component may be processed into *cornstarch*. It may be hydrolyzed in hydrochloric acid or treated with enzymes, to produce *corn syrup,* or high-fructose corn syrup (HFCS) (Chapter 14). *Corn oil* is extracted from the *germ*.

OTHER GRAINS

Grains other than wheat, rice, and corn are not abundantly consumed, but they offer great variety (Figure 6.8) and often grow in more adverse environmental conditions, where the more common grains will not grow. The seeds are used both as forage crops and as food cereals in different parts of the world. Some examples of less commonly consumed grains follow.

Barley

Barley is "winter-hardy" and is able to survive in the frost of cold climates. It is used as a cooked cereal, or the hull of the kernel is removed by abrasion to create pearled

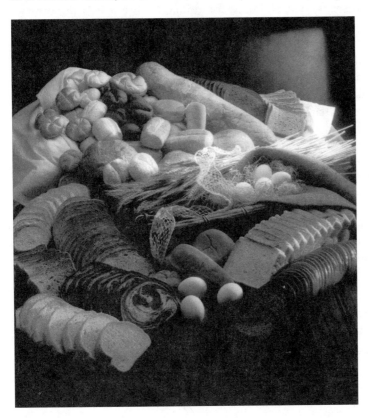

FIGURE 6.8 Breads may be prepared using a variety of grains (*Source:* Wheat Foods Council).

barley, i.e., commonly used in soups. Additionally, barley may be incorporated into breads, pilafs or stuffing, or it may be used for **malt** production.

In order to create malt, the barley grain is soaked in water to sprout the germ and produce an enzyme that hydrolyzes (breaks down) starch to a shorter carbon chain, maltose. Maltose is then used to feed yeast and produce CO_2 and ethyl alcohol, since it is a fermentable carbohydrate. The alcohol and CO_2 are important for brewing alcoholic beverages and for baking. Dried malt is used in a variety of products including brewed beverages, baked products, breakfast cereal, candies, or malted milks. Consumers following a gluten-free diet must *avoid* malt and should read ingredients labels to determine whether malt is an ingredient of a particular food product.

Barley is often used in animal feed—for pigs and cattle (not *poultry* because barley is a grain lower in starch than other grains such as wheat or corn).

Millet

Millet is the general name for small seed grasses. It includes finger (koracan), pearl (cattail), foxtail varieties, and proso (the most common) millet. Sorghum is a special type of millet with large seeds, typically used for animal feed, but it is the primary food grain in many parts of the world, where it is ground and made into porridge and cakes. It is also used to yield oil, sugars, and alcoholic beverages. A common variety of sorghum grown in the United States is milo; there are also waxy varieties that contain very little amylose. Overall, sorghums are resistant to heat and drought, and therefore, are of special value in arid, and hot regions of the world.

A very tiny millet grain that has been used for centuries in the Ethiopian diet is teff or t'ef (*Eragrotis tef*, signifying "love" and "grass"), commonly used in flatbread. Commercial production of teff has been started in the United States (6).

Oats

Oat is an important cereal crop fed to animals such as horses and sheep, and also used by man. It is valued for its high protein content. In milling, the hull is removed and oats are steamed and "rolled" or flattened for use in food, then, oats are incorporated into many ready-to-eat breakfast cereals and snack foods. Oat *bran* is a soluble fiber that has been shown to be effective in reducing serum cholesterol. Due to the fact that oats have a fairly high fat content, as far as grains go, rancidity can rapidly develop. Lipase activity in the grain is destroyed by a few minutes of steam treatment.

Quinoa

Quinoa (keen-wa) is the grain highest in protein. The small, round, light brown kernels are most often used as a cooked cereal (7).

Rye

Rye is richer in lysine than wheat but has a relatively low gluten-forming potential and, therefore, does not contribute a good structure in dough. It is frequently used in combination with wheat flour in breads and quick breads and is made into crackers. There are three types of rye—dark, medium, and light, often baked into bread. Rye may be sprouted, producing malt or malt flour.

Triticale

Triticale is a wheat and rye hybrid, first produced in the United States in the late 1800s (8). As a crop, it offers the disease resistance of wheat and the hardiness of rye. It has more protein than either grain alone, but the overall crop *yield* is not high, so its use is not widespread. Triticale was developed to have the baking property of wheat (good gluten-forming potential) and the nutritional quality of rye (high lysine).

NONCEREAL "FLOURS"

Although they do not have the composition of grains (such as wheat), various legumes and vegetables may be processed into "flour." For example, soy and garbanzo beans (chick peas) are legumes (from the Leguminosae family) that may be ground into "flour" for addition to baked products. Soy stiffens dough and aids in maintaining a soft crumb. Cottonseeds (Malvaceae family), and potatoes (tubers) may also be processed into "flour." Buckwheat (fruit of Fagopyrum esculentum crop) contains approximately 60% carbohydrate, and may also be used in the porridge kasha or animal feed. Cassava (tuber) is the starch-yielding plant that yields tapioca, and is a staple crop in parts of the world, such as Central America.

Pasta

Pasta is the paste of milled grains (alimentary paste), extruded through a die or put through a roller. Figure 6.9 portrays pasta extrusion and Figures 6.10 and 6.11 show some of the diversity, present in pasta. A variety of products including macaroni, noodles, and spaghetti are created by extrusion. [*Macaroni* does not include eggs in its formulation. *Noodles* must contain not less than 5.5% (by weight) of egg solids or yolk (9).]

If pasta is processed to include legumes, as part of the formulation, a complete protein may be formed in a single food. Pasta may be cholesterol-free or made of non-wheat flour, such as rice. "Technological breakthroughs now make it possible to enjoy rice pasta that tastes, looks, and cooks like regular pasta" (10). Pasta may be formulated to include pureed vegetables, herbs, and spices as well as cheeses.

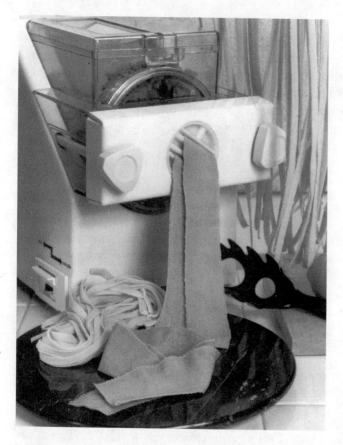

FIGURE 6.9   Pasta extrusion
(*Source*: Wheat Foods Council).

Generally, the crushed (not finely ground) endosperm of milled *durum* spring wheat, known as **semolina,** is used in the preparation of high-quality pasta products. Lower-quality pastas that do not use semolina taste "starchy" and are pasty in texture. Rinsing cooked pasta products prior to service may result in the loss of nutrient enrichment.

Pasta appears at the base of the USDA's Food Guide Pyramid. It frequently appears on restaurant menus and home tables in the form of salads, side dishes, and main dishes.

COOKING CEREALS

Cereal products expand during cooking due to retention of the cooking water. *Finely milled grains* such as cornmeal, corn grits, or wheat farina should be boiled gently and stirred occasionally in order to prevent mushy and lumpy textures. *Whole* or *coarsely milled* grains such as barley, bulgur, rice, and oats (and buckwheat) should be added to boiling water and stirred occasionally. Additional water is added as needed.

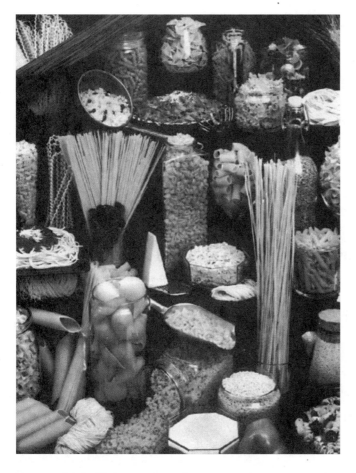

FIGURE 6.10 Various pasta products
(*Source:* Wheat Foods Council).

Excessive stirring of any milled grain results in rupturing of the grain contents and is unpalatable, as the cereal forms a gummy, sticky consistency.

To control heat, cereal products may be cooked in the top of a double boiler over boiling water. A disadvantage of this cooking method is that heating time is lengthened compared to direct heating without a double boiler.

Pasta is added to boiling water and boiled uncovered until the desired tenderness (typically *al dente*) is achieved. The addition of a small amount ($< 1/2$ teaspoon [2.5 ml] household use) of oil prevents boil-over from occurring.

BREAKFAST CEREALS

An American religious group not wanting to consume animal products started the production of ready-to-eat (rte) breakfast cereals. The Western Health Reform Institute in Battle Creek, Michigan produced, baked, and then ground a whole meal product to benefit the healthfulness of its patients. A local townsperson, J.H. Kellogg,

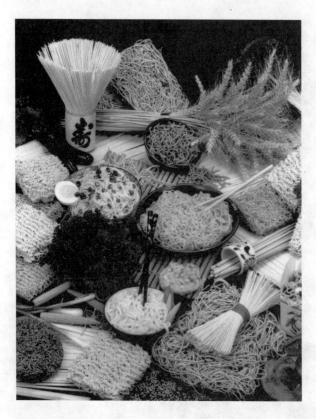

FIGURE 6.11 Various noodles.
(*Source*: Wheat Foods Council)

and his brother *W.K. Kellogg* started a business with this idea, applying it to breakfast food. A patient, *C.W. Post* did the same.

Breakfast cereals in many forms quickly became popular. Flaking, shredding, puffing, etc., and the production of various forms soon expanded although convenient, some criticize the levels of ingredients, including sugar and fiber, in r-t-e breakfast cereals. Enrichment and fortification also became a common practice for breakfast cereals.

NUTRITIVE VALUE OF BREAD, CEREAL, RICE, AND PASTA

Bread, cereal, rice, and pasta make a significant nutritive contribution to the diet (11). Whole grain products and processed cereal products contribute carbohydrates, vitamins such as B vitamins, minerals such as iron, and fiber to the diet in creative ways. Ready-to-eat varieties of breakfast cereals are frequently consumed in the more developed countries. Many are highly fortified with essential vitamins and minerals, including folate (Figure 6.12).

Grains are low in fat, high in fiber, and contain no cholesterol, although cooked or baked breads, cereals, rice and pasta dishes may be prepared with fats, refined

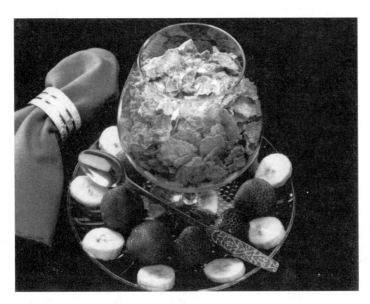

FIGURE 6.12   Ready-to-eat breakfast cereal
(*Source:* Wheat Foods Council).

flours, and eggs, which changes the nutritive value. Many ready-to-eat breakfast cereals are high in sugar and/or low in fiber. The recommend ed number of bread, cereal, rice and pasta servings is 6–11 per day.

CONCLUSION

Cereals are the edible seeds of cultivated grasses and include all the cereal food prepared from grain. A kernel contains bran, endosperm, and germ, but if "refined," cereals contain only endosperm. Common cereal grains include wheat, rice, and corn, although other grains such as barley, millet, oats, quinoa, rye, and triticale may be used as a component in meals. Dried grains have a very long storage life, and much of the world depends on them for food.

Over 30,000 varieties of wheat exist, classified according to season, texture, and color. Hard wheat is used for breadmaking, and soft wheat for cakes and pastries. Semolina flour from hard durum wheat is used for pasta production. Pasta is the paste of milled grains, primarily wheat, and increasingly appears in the American diet. It is a complex carbohydrate and low fat food.

Rice is a staple food of much of the world. It grows as extra long, long, medium, and short grain rice. Rices have a variety of flavors and are used in many entrees, side dishes, even desserts.

Cereals are included as the base of numerous food guides throughout the world, indicating that they are major foods of a nutritious diet. The USDA recommends that 6–11 servings of the Bread, Cereal, Rice, and Pasta group be consumed each day. This recommendation may be met with the great variety of products that are available in the marketplace.

GLOSSARY

All-purpose wheat flour: White flour, not containing the bran or germ. Combining the properties of hard and soft wheat.

Bleached flour: Bleaching the pigment to a whiter color, naturally by exposing pigment to air, or by chemical agents.

Bran: The layered outer coating of the kernel, offering protection for the seed.

Bread flour: Made from a hard wheat kernel, with a high protein–starch ratio; high gluten potential.

Cereal: Any edible grain that comes from cultivated grasses.

Endosperm: The starch-storing portion of the seed that produces white flour and gluten.

Enrichment: Adding back nutrients lost in milling.

Fortification: Adding nutrients at levels beyond that present in the original grain.

Germ: The embryo; the inner portion of the kernel.

Gluten: Protein substances (gliadins, glutenins) left in the flour after the starch has been removed, which when hydrated and manipulated, produce the elastic, cohesive structure of doughs.

Malt: Produced from a sprouting barley germ. Long glucose chains are hydrolyzed by an enzyme to maltose, i.e., involved in both feeding yeast and producing CO_2. May be dried and added to numerous products.

Matured flour: Wheat flour, i.e., aged naturally or by chemical agents to improve gluten elasticity and baking properties of doughs.

Organic flour: Flour from crops grown without the use of chemicals such as herbicides and insecticides.

Patent flour: Highest grade of flour from mill streams at the beginning of the reduction rolls. High starch, less protein than mill streams at the end of reduction rolls.

Pasta: The paste of milled grains, usually the semolina from durum wheat, extruded through a die to produce a diversity of shaped products. They are dried and then cooked in large amounts of water. Included are macaroni, noodles, spaghetti, ravioli, and the like.

Semolina: Flour milled from durum wheat.

REFERENCES

1. National Restaurant Association. Chicago, IL.
2. LeVeille GA. Current attitude and behavior trends regarding consumption of grains. *Food Technology*. 1988; 42(1): 110.
3. Matthews RH, Bechtel EA. Eating quality of some baked products made with instant flour. *Journal of Home Economics*. 1966; 58: 729.
4. Dillon PM. Go with the grain. *Food Engineering*. 1994; 64(5): 96.
5. Pszczola DE. Rice: Not just for throwing. *Food Technology*. 2001: 55(2): 53–59.
6. Arrowhead Mills. Hereford, T.X.
7. Ruales J, Nair BM. Nutritional quality of the protein in quinoa (Chenoposium quinoa). *Plant Foods for Human Nutrition*. 1992; 42(1): 1–11.
8. Lorenz K. Food uses of triticale. *Food Technology*. 1972; 26(11): 66.
9. National Pasta Association. Arlington, VA.

10. Pastariso Products Inc., Scarborough, Ontario, Canada.
11. Sebrell WH. A fiftieth anniversary—cereal enrichment. *Nutrition Today.* January/February, 1992: 20–21.

BIBLIOGRAPHY

American Association of Cereal Chemists. St Paul, MN.

Christensen CM. *Storage of Cereal Grains and Their Products,* 3rd ed. St Paul, MN: American Association of Cereal Chemists, 1982.

ConAgra Specialty Grain. Omaha, NE.

Cooperative Whole Grain Education Association. Ann Arbor, MI.

Ener-G Foods Inc. Seattle, WA.

Farida HA., Rubenthaler GL. Ancient breads and a new science: Understanding flat breads. *Cereal Foods World.* 1983; 28: 627.

Fast RB, Caldwell EF. *Breakfast Cereals and How They Are Made.* St Paul, MN: American Association of Cereal Chemists, 1990.

Grain Processing. Muscatine, I.A.

Innovative Grain Technology. Lincoln, NE.

International Grain Products. Wayzata, MN.

International Wheat Gluten Association. Prairie Village, KS.

National Barley Foods Council. Spokane, WA.

North Dakota Wheat Commission. Bismark, ND.

Rice Council of America. Houston, TX.

The Food Guide Pyramid: A Guide to Daily Food Choices. Washington, DC: US Dept of Agriculture, Human Nutrition Information Service, 1992. Home and Garden Bulletin No. 252.

Wheat Flour Institute. Washington, DC.

Wheat Foods Council. Englewood, CO. www.wheatfoods.org

Wheat Gluten Industry Council. Shawnee Mission, KS.

Wheat Industry Council. Washington, DC.

CHAPTER 7

Vegetables and Fruits

INTRODUCTION

Vegetables are typically the edible portion of plants eaten with or as the main course of lunches or dinners, as salads or in soups. They may be processed into beverages or vegetable starches, eaten fresh or lightly processed, dried, pickled, or frozen. They impart their own characteristic flavor, color, and texture to diets, and undergo changes during storage and cooking. Ranked next to the cereal crops rice, corn, and wheat, potatoes are the most prolific vegetable crop grown for human consumption.

Fruits are defined in several ways. B*otanically*, fruits are the mature ovaries of plants with their seeds. This definition includes all grains, legumes, nuts and seeds, and common "vegetables" such as cucumbers, olives, peppers, and tomatoes. When defined and considered in a *culinary* role, fruit is the fleshy part of a plant, usually eaten alone or served as a dessert. Fruits are high in organic acids and sugar—higher than vegetables.

The nutritive value of vitamins, minerals, fiber, and other compounds contained in fruits and vegetables is extremely important to the diet. Additional dietary and medicinal benefits of fruits and vegetables are being discovered. Three to five servings of vegetables and two to four servings of fruits are recommended for daily consumption on the Food Guide Pyramid (USDA). Examples are shown in Figure 7.1.

STRUCTURE AND COMPOSITION OF CELL TISSUE

Vegetables and fruits are composed of both simple and complex cells. The *simple* cells are similar to one another in function and structure and they make up *dermal* tissue and *parenchyma* tissue. Dermal tissue is the single-layer outside surface of leaves, young stems, roots, and flowers, while **parenchyma tissue** makes up the majority of the plant, and is where basic molecular activity such as the synthesis and storage of carbohydrate by sunlight (photosynthesis) occurs.

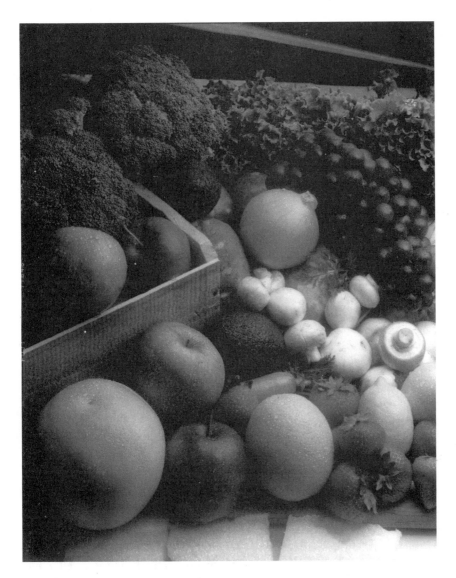

FIGURE 7.1 Fruits and vegetables (*Courtesy of SYSCO® Incorporated*).

Complex tissue includes the *vascular*, collenchyma, and sclerenchyma *supporting tissue*. Major vascular tissue consists of the xylem and phloem; xylem conducts water from the roots to the leaves, and phloem conducts nutrients from the leaves to the roots. These tissues may be located in the center of the vegetable, as is seen in carrots for example.

As mentioned, a plant is made primarily of simple parenchyma tissue (Figure 7.2). Each cell is bounded by a cell wall produced by the protoplast, which serves to support and protect cell contents. It is the cell wall characteristics that determine the shape and contents (content retention, influx, or release) of parenchyma cells. For example, when the wall is firm, the original shape and texture of the cell are

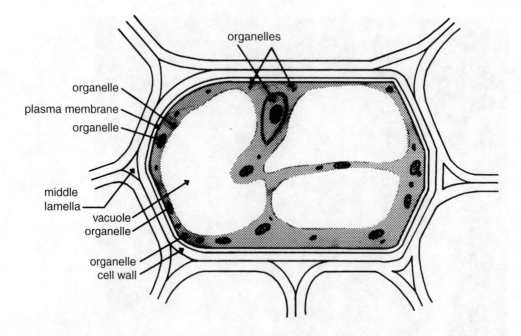

FIGURE 7.2 Components of a parenchyma cell
(*Source:* Division of Nutritional Sciences, New York State College of Human Ecology).

maintained, and when it is destroyed by cutting, dehydration, or cooking, the wall breaks and spills its contents into the surrounding environment. Thus, water, sugars, or water-soluble vitamins of a cell may be lost.

Plants have a *primary* cell wall made of cellulose, hemicellulose, and pectic substances including pectin. Older, more mature plants may also have a *secondary* cell wall composed of lignin (see Chemical Composition of Plant Material), in addition to cellulose, hemicellulose, and pectic substances.

Inside the cell wall is the protoplast, composed of three parts—plasma membrane, cytoplasm, and organelles. The *plasma membrane* surrounds the functional cell, while the **cytoplasm** of the protoplast includes all of the cell contents inside the membrane, yet outside the nucleus. The *organelles* include nucleus, mitochondria, ribosomes, and plastids. It is the plastids that contain *fat-soluble* material such as fat-soluble vitamins, and fat-soluble pigments such as chlorophyll and carotenoids, to be discussed in a subsequent section of this chapter.

Outside the cell wall, between adjacent cells, is the **middle lamella.** This is the "cementing" material between adjacent cells and contains pectic substances, magnesium and calcium, water, and air spaces.

Each cell contains an inside cavity known as a **vacuole.** It may be large in size, holding plentiful water, and comprising the major portion of parenchyma cells, or it may be small in size. In an intact, uncooked cell, vacuoles hold water and provide a desirable crisp texture to the cell. The **cell sap** of the vacuole contains the *water-soluble* materials including vitamins B and C, sugars, inorganic salts, organic acids, sulfur compounds, and the water-soluble pigments. These cell sap components may escape into the surrounding water or water used for cooking.

CHEMICAL COMPOSITION OF PLANT MATERIAL

Carbohydrate

Carbohydrate constitutes the largest percentage of the dry weight of plant material. It is the basic molecule formed during photosynthesis when water (H_2O) and carbon dioxide (CO_2) combine to yield carbohydrate (CHO) and oxygen (O_2). Carbohydrate is present in simple and complex forms. For example, *simple* carbohydrates are the monosaccharides and disaccharides, including the sugars glucose, fructose, and sucrose, that may increase during the fruit ripening process. *Complex* carbohydrates or polysaccharides are synthesized from simple carbohydrates and include cellulose and starch.

Various complex carbohydrates, and the effect of heat on those carbohydrates are discussed as follows (also see Chapter 3):

Starch is the storage component of carbohydrate located in roots, tubers, stems, and seeds of plants. When subjected to heat and water, starch may absorb water and gelatinize (Chapter 4). Vegetables vary in their starch content. Some vegetables such as potatoes are starchy, some moderate in their starch content, and others such as parsley are less starchy. Starch is digestible, as the bonds between the glucose units are α-1,4.

Cellulose is a *water-insoluble* fiber that provides structure to cell walls. The molecular bonds between glucose units that make up cellulose are β-1,4; therefore, cellulose remains indigestible to humans, although it may be softened in cooking.

Hemicellulose fiber provides structure in cell walls, and the majority of it is *insoluble*. It is softened by heating in an alkaline environment (such as, if baking soda is added to cooking water for the purpose of green color retention).

Pectic substances (Chapter 5) are the firm, intercellular "cement" between cell walls, the gel-forming polysaccharides of plant tissue, and are hydrolyzed by cooking. Large, *insoluble* forms of pectin become soluble pectin with ripening of the plant material.

In addition to carbohydrates, a noncarbohydrate material present in the complex vascular and supporting tissue is **lignin**. It is found in older vegetables, remains unchanged by heat and may exhibit an unacceptable "woody" texture.

Protein

Overall, less than 1% of the composition of a fruit is protein. Protein is most prevalent in legumes—peas and beans—but, even then, it is an *incomplete* protein as it lacks the essential amino acid, methionine. Protein, present as enzymes may be extracted and used in other foods. Examples include the proteolytic enzymes that contribute the beneficial tenderizing effects to meats such as papain (derived from papaya), ficin (obtained from figs), and bromelain (extracted from pineapple).

Fat

Fat composes approximately 5% of the dry weight of roots, stems, and leaves of vegetables. It makes up less than 1% of the dry weight of a fruit, except for fruits such as avocados and olives that contain 16 and 14% fat, respectively. Fat is instrumental in development during the early growth of a plant.

Vitamins

The vitamins present in vegetables and fruit are primarily carotene (a vitamin A precursor) and vitamin C. There is also vitamin B_1 or thiamin. Fruits supply more than 90% of the vitamin C and a major percentage of the vitamin A in a diet. Beta-carotene is present in dark orange fruits vegetables and in green vegetables. (It is interesting to note that vitamins A and C are both listed on Nutrient Facts labels as vitamins that Americans may lack although fruits and vegetables are so plentiful.) *Water-soluble* vitamin losses may occur upon soaking and heating, primarily the latter.

Nutritive quality may deteriorate due to enzymatic action. Specifically, the enzymes ascorbic acid oxidase and thiaminase can cause nutritional changes in vitamins C and B_1, respectively, during storage. Therefore, retention of these vitamins is controlled by deactivating the enzymes in blanching prior to freezing (1).

Minerals

Fruits and vegetables, especially the latter, contribute minerals to the diet, notably calcium, magnesium, and iron. Calcium ions may also be added to canned vegetables to promote firmness and lessen softening of pectic substances. The oxalic acid in spinach and the phytates in peas bind calcium, decreasing its bioavailability, therefore, calcium is not added to these vegetables since it does not promote firming.

Water

Water is found in plant cell walls, in cells, and between cells. Some of its functions in plant material are to transport nutrients, to promote chemical reactions, and to provide plants with a crisp texture if cell membranes are intact.

Water constitutes a small percentage (10%) of seeds and is a substantially larger percent of leaves. It makes up 80–90% of a plant, as is evidenced by the drastic size reduction of a measure of vegetables that is subject to dehydration.

Phytochemicals

Phytochemicals are plant chemicals. They are non-nutrient materials that may be especially significant in *disease prevention* and *controlling cancer*. Examples of such plant chemicals include the beta-carotene of carotenoid pigments and the flavonoid group of pigments, as well as the sulfur-containing allyl sulfide and sulforaphane. Additionally, dithiolthiones, indoles, and isothiocyanates in *cruciferous* ("cross-shaped blossom," cabbage family) vegetables, isoflavones, phytosterols, protease inhibitors, and saponins in legumes and limonene and the phenols of citrus fruit are among the plant chemicals that may be effective in disease prevention.

For more in-depth coverage, the reader is referred to other nutrition texts. These chemicals are the focus of much research concerning their importance to human health.

TURGOR PRESSURE

As previously mentioned, the structure of plant material is, to a large degree, dependent on the water content. A *raw* product prior to harvesting is generally crisp because the vegetable or fruit contains a large percentage of water, which provides turgidity to the plant. A plant's **turgor pressure** is the pressure that water-filled vacuoles exert on the cytoplasm and the partially elastic cell wall.

A loss of turgor pressure results in a limp, wilted product, as water is lost to the air, and dehydration occurs. If the parenchyma cell is still intact (not cooked or otherwise destroyed), turgor of the wilted, limp product may be restored. Rehydration or recrisping is possible by soaking in warm, 70–90°F (21–32°C), water. After soaking, plant pores then re-close, and hold the absorbed water if it is drained and refrigerated for 6 hours (2). Yet, soaking raw plant material may be discouraged, as water-soluble nutrients and pigments may, by purely physical means, escape into the soaked water. [To rehydrate *lettuce*, it is suggested that it should not be soaked, but rather, placed in only 2 inches or so of warm water (2).]

Once cooked, osmosis ceases and diffusion occurs, especially changing the texture, flavor and shape of fruits. **Osmosis** represents water movement across a *semi-permeable* membrane. **Diffusion** signifies water *and* solute movement across a *permeable* membrane.

PIGMENTS AND EFFECTS OF ADDITIONAL SUBSTANCES

Plant pigments enhance the aesthetic value of fruits and vegetables for humans, as well as attract insects and birds, which foster pollination. These are subject to change with ripening and processing of the raw vegetables or fruits. The four pigments found in plants are *chlorophyll*, the green pigment; *carotenoids*, a yellow, red, or orange pigment; and the two flavonoids: *anthocyanin*, the red, blue, or purple, and *anthoxanthin*, the white pigment. High-performance liquid chromatography (HPLC) is generally used for plant pigment analysis (3). A discussion of the major pigments and a description of how they may change appears in the following material.

Chlorophyll

Chlorophyll is the green pigment found in the cell chloroplast responsible for photosynthesis (i.e., converting sunlight to chemical energy). It is *fat-soluble* and may appear in vegetable cooking water that contains fat. Chlorophyll is structurally a porphyrin ring containing magnesium at the center of a ring of four pyrrole groups (Figure 7.3). Phytol alcohol is esterified to one of the pyrrole groups, and it confers solubility to fat and fat solvents. Methyl alcohol is attached to another pyrrole group.

If the magnesium in chlorophyll is *displaced* from its central position on the porphyrin ring, an *irreversible* pigment change occurs. A number of factors including prolonged storage, the heat of cooking, changes in hydrogen ion concentration (pH), and the presence of the minerals, zinc and copper, may cause an off-green, unwanted pigment color change.

For example, as vegetables are *heated,* air is removed from the cell and a bright green color becomes apparent. Then, as internal organic acids are released and hydrogen displaces magnesium, pheophytins are produced. Either magnesium-free *pheophytin a,* which is a gray-green pigment, or *pheophytin b,* an olive-green pigment, is formed. These changes to the chlorophyll pigment become more marked with time, so a short cooking time is recommended. Cooking the product *uncovered* for the first 3 minutes is recommended to allow the escape of volatile plant acids that would otherwise remain in the cooking water and react to displace magnesium. In this manner, less change of chlorophyll occurs. Green vegetables that are high in acid content undergo more color change than vegetables low in acid when they are heated.

As mentioned, pigments may change due to heating and release of the plant's internal organic acids. In addition to the *internal* organic acids, an *external* acid environment (i.e., acid added to cooking water) causes the natural green color to change into olive-green pheophytin.

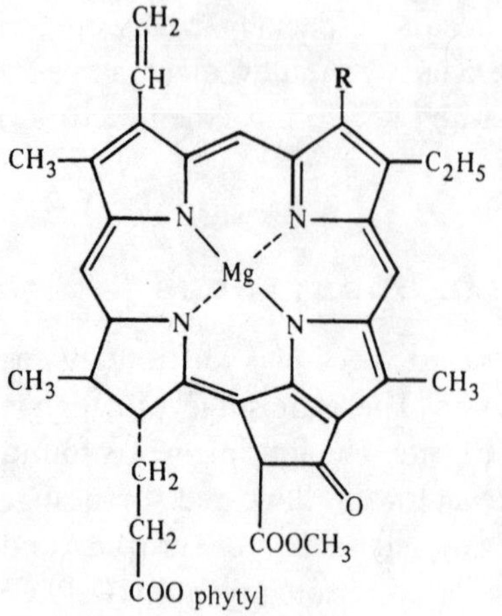

FIGURE 7.3 Chlorophyll.

An *alkaline* environment also affects the green pigment, such as when sodium bicarbonate (baking soda) is added to the vegetable cooking water. The soda reacts with chlorophyll, displacing the phytyl and methyl groups on the molecule, and the green pigment forms a bright-green, water-soluble chlorophyllin. This color change, although producing a desirable appearance, is accompanied by an unacceptable loss of texture, due to softening of hemicellulose and may result in a mushy texture change. It also destroys ascorbic acid (vitamin C) and thiamin (vitamin B_1), and therefore the addition of alkali is *not* recommended.

The minerals, copper and zinc, produce undesirable color changes by displacing magnesium. Regardless of the manner in which chlorophyll is changed, when the chlorophyll is destroyed, a second underlying carotenoid pigment may become apparent.

Carotenoids

The **carotenoids** are red, orange, and yellow *fat-soluble* pigments in fruits and vegetables, including *carotenes* (the hydrocarbon classification) and *xanthophylls* (the oxygenated class). They are found in chloroplasts along with chlorophyll, where the green pigment dominates, and also in chromoplasts without chlorophyll. The carotenoid pigment is seen especially in flowers, fruits, including tomatoes, peppers, and citrus fruits, and roots, including carrots and sweet potatoes.

Carotenes are unsaturated hydrocarbons containing many carbon atoms. They contain conjugated double bonds (i.e., double bonds alternating with single bonds), which are responsible for the color. The greater the number of conjugated double bonds, the deeper the color. For example, *beta-carotene* is *orange* in color and contains a six-membered ring at each end of the chain (Figure 7.4) and *alpha*-carotene has one less conjugated double bond so it is *paler* in color. *Lycopene,* found

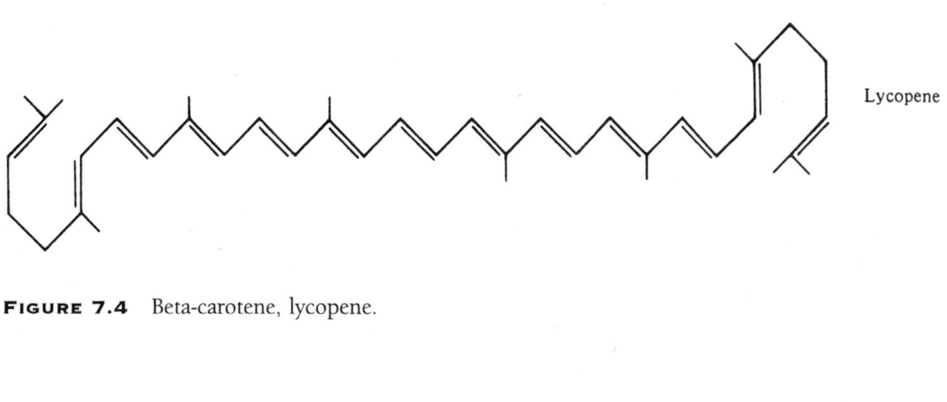

β-carotene

Lycopene

FIGURE 7.4 Beta-carotene, lycopene.

in tomatoes and watermelon, has the *deepest red* color because it has two open rings (Figure 7.4) at each end of the chain and, thus, has two more double bonds than beta-carotene.

There are hundreds of types of carotenes. The most well-known carotene is the aforementioned beta-carotene, cleaved by an enzyme in the intestinal mucosa to yield vitamin A. In all, 40 or more carotenoids are known to be precursors of vitamin A (3).

Xanthophylls are the yellow-orange colored derivatives of carotenes containing carbon, hydrogen, and oxygen. Autumn leaves show evidence of destruction of chlorophyll pigment, as the carotenes, and "autumn xanthophylls" that existed along with the chlorophyll become visible (3). Corn contains the xanthophyll cryptoxanthin, and green leaves contain lutein. Paprika also contains xanthophyll pigment.

The carotenoid pigment may undergo autoxidation due to the large number of double bonds. This oxidation may result in "off-flavor" and color loss, yielding unsatisfactory products. Antioxidants such as butylated hydroxy anisole (BHA), butylated hydroxy toluene (BHT), or tertiary butylated hydroxy quinone (TBHQ) are frequently added to a wide variety of foods containing fruits and vegetables, herbs, or spices to prevent this detrimental oxidation [See food additives (Chapter 18)].

While *oxidation* causes development of a *lighter-color* cooked vegetable, *caramelization* of plant sugar may result in a *darker-color* cooked vegetable. It is recommended that carotene-pigmented vegetables should be either covered during cooking, or cooked quickly, as in stir-frying. Only small amount of table fat such as butter or margarine should be added, while cooking as some carotene may be dissolved in the fat.

Cooking time does not negatively affect carotenoid pigments as it does for chlorophyll, and changes are not as noticeable as changes to the chlorophyll pigments. However, upon *heating,* and in the presence of *acid,* some molecular isomerization occurs. Although the isomer contains the same elements and proportions, the molecule has a different structure with different properties. In carotenoids, the predominant *trans* molecular form, naturally present in plants, is changed to *cis* configuration in a matter of a few minutes, and the pigment becomes less bright. *Alkali* environments do not produce a color change.

Food technologists have developed paprika, annatto, tomato, and carrot extracts to provide color in foods. Herbs and spices also provide coloring. In addition to color and characteristic flavor, they supply advantageous nutrients such as beta-carotene, offering the same nutrients as a diet of yellow, green, and leafy vegetables, although in significantly lesser amounts. Herb and spice addition, albeit in small amounts to foods, contributes to vitamin A values that appear on nutrition labels, and their use is expected to grow (4).

Carotene from vegetables or fruits may prevent oxidation of *body* tissues, and development of cancer, although much remains unknown about possible benefits of *supplements* of this biologically active component of plant material. The American Dietetic Association advocates *foods* in the diet as the best source of good nutrition (see Nutritive Value of Vegetables and Fruit).

The flavonoids are another group of pigmented compounds. They consist of anthocyanins and anthoanthins.

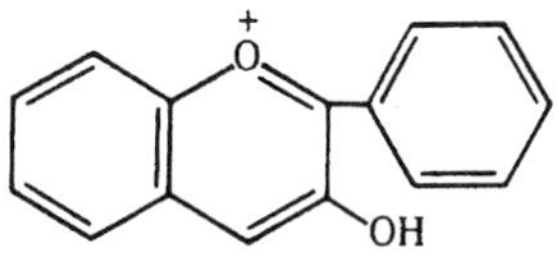

FIGURE 7.5 Anthocyanin.

Anthocyanin

Anthocyanin (Figure 7.5) is red, blue-red, blue, or purple pigment in fruits and vegetables such as blueberries, cherries, raspberries, red cabbage, red plums, and rhubarb (not beets; see Betalaines). The skins of radishes, red apples, red potatoes, grapes, and eggplant also contain anthocyanin pigment. It is prevalent in buds and young shoots, as well as in the purplish area of autumn leaves, visible when chlorophyll decomposes. Anthocyanins contain a positively charged oxygen in the central group of the molecule, and belong to the flavonoid group of chemicals, thus, distinguished from the orange-red found in carotenoids. These pigments are *water-soluble* and are found in the cell sap of plants; thus, they may be released into the cooking water with soaking or prolonged heat exposure.

Care must be taken when working with the anthocyanin pigments of fruit juices, or undesirable color combinations may form in the juice mixtures. The addition of alkali, or an *alkali* cooking medium produces an unwelcome *violet-blue color*, while in an *acidic* environment, the anthocyanin pigment exhibits a *red color*. Therefore, a tart, acidic apple is often added to red cabbage while cooking, in order to produce a more appealing finished product. If acids such as lemon juice or vinegar are added to fruits and vegetables containing the anthocyanin pigment, it should be *after* desired softening has occurred (see Cooking Effect).

Unlike the negative changes to the chlorophyll pigments, covering the cooking utensil containing an anthocyanin pigment is recommended for *better* color because plant acids are then retained in the cooking water. If fruits containing anthocyanins are added to batters and doughs, such as in the preparation of blueberry muffins, acidic buttermilk is also incorporated to assist in preserving color. Color changes that occur are reversible.

Metals, such as iron from non-stainless-steel preparation tools, change the natural purplish pigment to a blue-green color. Therefore, food products containing the anthocyanin pigment are often canned in lacquer-coated (enamel-lined) metal cans to prevent the product acid from interacting with the can metal and causing undesirable color changes.

Anthoxanthin

The fourth major pigment, **anthoxanthin** pigment (Figure 7.6) is also a flavonoid, and is similar to anthocyanin, but it exists in a less oxidized state, as the oxygen on the central group is *uncharged*. This classification represents flavone, flavonol, flavanone, and flavanol pigments, and includes fruits such as apples, or vegetables

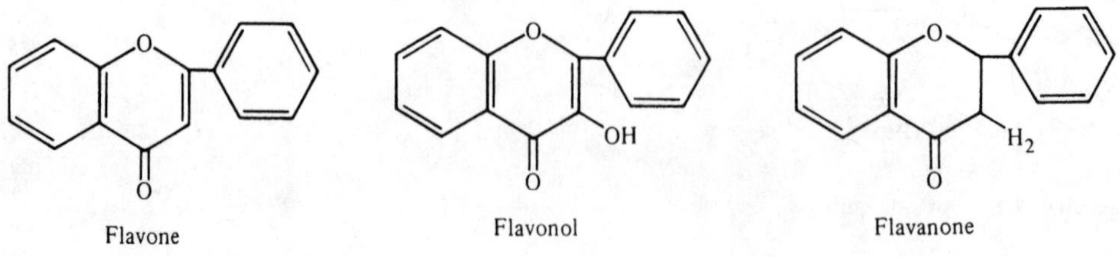

Flavone

Flavonol

Flavanone

FIGURE 7.6 Anthoxanthin.

such as cauliflower, onions, potatoes, and turnips. Anthoxanthins are white, or pale yellowish, *water-soluble* pigments found in a plant's cell sap.

With prolonged *heat,* the pigment turns into brownish gray. White potatoes, with their low orgnic acid content, may become dark colored after prolonged cooking due to formation of an iron–chlorogenic acid complex. Some anthoxanthins may change to anthocyanins and exhibit a pinkish tinge if vegetables are overcooked.

In *acid,* anthoxanthin becomes lighter. (Therefore, in household use, cooking in one teaspoon of cream of tartar per quart of water may be useful in lightening the color.) If cooking water is *alkaline* or contains traces of iron salts, the result may be a yellow or brown discoloration of white cooked vegetables. Cooking in aluminum cookware also causes the same discoloration.

Betalaines

Betalaines are a minor group of pigments that contain a nitrogen group in the molecular structure. They are similar to, but not categorized as anthocyanins or anthoxanthins. These pigments differ in color. For example, the betalaines found in beets, called *betacyanines,* are red-colored like anthocyanins at a pH of 4–7, whereas other betalaines, such as *betaxanthines,* are yellow-colored like anthoxanthins at a pH above 10. Below a pH of 4, the betalaine hue is violet. A lacquered tin (as with anthocyanins) can is used in order to prevent color changes that may result from metals in the can reacting with the betalaine pigment.

Tannins

Tannins (tannic acid) are polyphenolic compounds that add both color and astringent flavor to foods. They may be responsible for the unwanted brown discoloration of fruits and vegetables, as well as for the desirable changes that provide tea leaves with their characteristic color. They range in color from pale-yellow to light brown, and due to their acidic nature, they tend to cause the mouth to pucker. (Astringents shrink mucous membranes, extract water, and dry up secretions.) The term represents a broad group of compounds found in plants—normally in bark, fruit, leaves, and roots. Tannins, such as the brownish pigment found in tea leaves may be used as the brown colored dye in dyeing fabrics or tanning leather. Food tannins found in wines, and teas, contain antioxidant properties correlated with good health.

FLAVOR COMPOUNDS

The flavor of cooked vegetables is greatly influenced by the presence sulfur of both *allium* and *brassica* compounds, although aldehydes, ketones, organic compounds, and alcohols are contributors to flavor. Some of the sulfur compounds, including allyl sulfides may increase carcinogen excretion from the body, according to the American Cancer Society (ACS).

Allium

Vegetables that are of the genus **allium** include chives, garlic, leeks, onions, and shallots, each different members of the lily family. They contain sulfur compounds, and when cut, onions, for example, exhibit enzyme activity causing the eyes to tear (lachrymatory effect). Similarly, garlic undergoes an enzymatic change to sulfur compounds, precursor (+)-S-allyl-L-cysteine sulfoxide, producing the identifiable garlic odor.

Since these flavor compounds in plants are *water soluble*, they may be lost from the vegetable to the water, then volatized as steam during cooking. If a *mild* flavor is desired in cooked onions, a large amount of boiling water and cooking *uncovered* for a long time period is recommended. In that manner, sulfur flavor compounds are degraded and vaporized. Inversely, a sweeter, more *concentrated* flavor is produced if less water and a cover is used. The *most intense* flavor results from cooking in fat.

Brassica

Vegetables of the genus **Brassica** include broccoli, brussels sprouts, cabbage, cauliflower, kale, kohlrabi, mustard, and turnips. They are of the mustard family and are known as *cruciferous* vegetables that have a cross-shaped blossom on the young, growing plant. The naturally mild flavor of the raw vegetables may become quite strong and objectionable with prolonged heat as hydrogen sulfide is produced.

For optimal flavor the use of a *small* amount of briskly boiling cooking water is advised for just a *short* cooking period. In order to allow the volatile organic acids to escape, it is recommended that the vegetables should be *uncovered* at the beginning of the cooking process. Then they may be *covered* to keep the cooking time short.

Some vegetables of the *Brassica* genus, such as cabbage, contain a sulfur compound known as sinigrin. Sinigrin may interact with an enzyme, myrosinase released from the cut or bruised cell and produce potent mustard oil. Another sulfur compound in cabbage, known as (+)-S-methyl-L-cysteine sulfoxide may convert to the more desirable dimethyl disulphide.

Organic Acids

The sour taste of fruits may be attributed to organic acids, such as citric acid, malic acid, or tartaric acid. Vegetables contain a greater variety of organic acids, yet maintain a less acidic pH level than fruits.

Concentrates, Extracts, Oils, Spices, and Herbs

As a flavor alternative to using fresh, frozen, or dehydrated vegetables in a product formulation, concentrates, extracts, oils, herbs, and spices may be incorporated as food is processed. Vegetable *concentrates* may be processed and added in the preparation of numerous items to impart the vegetable's characteristic flavor. The replacement ratio for some vegetables may be 1:30, and for some herbs and spices it may be 1:10 (5). Natural plant *extracts* may be used to yield the flavors and aroma of fresh herbs and spices. Essential *oils* are also removed and concentrated to produce flavoring oils and provide products with a pure, consistent quality of flavor when they are added.

Although there may not be a clear-cut distinction between a herb and spice, a herb is generally from herbaceous plants. According to the American Spice Trade Association (ASTA), a spice is "any dried plant product used primarily for seasoning purposes." (The FDA does not include dehydrated vegetables in its definition of spices, but rather they are "flavors.") Spices may come from fruits, flowers, roots or seeds, as well as from shrubs and vines. They enhance color, flavor, palatability, and they exhibit antimicrobial properties (6).

A tremendous amount of folklore goes along with herbs and spices; they may be used for medicinal as well as culinary purposes. While *traditional medicine* includes the use of herbs and spices, such traditional medicine may be combined today with *Western or modern medicine*. In fact, the National Center for Complementary and Alternative Medicine, established by the National Institutes of Health, has as its mission to seek out effective and alternative medical treatment, to evaluate the outcomes, and report findings to the public.

VEGETABLE CLASSIFICATIONS

The parts of the plant eaten as food by mankind vary throughout the world. The eight most common parts, beginning with underground parts of the plant and progressing to those parts growing above ground, are as follows:

- **Roots**—underground; beet, carrot, jicama, parsnips, radish, rutabaga, sweet potato, turnip, yam (*sweet potatoes* are a yellow to orange color flesh, either dry or moist; *yams* are yellow, white, or purple pigmented flesh root vegetables)

- **Tubers**—underground; enlarged fleshy stem; starch storage area after leaves manufacture carbohydrates; buds or eyes form new plants; Irish potato, Jerusalem artichoke

- **Bulbs**—stems with an underground bulb of food reserve; garlic bulb, leeks, onions, shallots, spring onions (green onions or scallions do not possess a real bulb)

- **Stems**—a plant's vascular system, nutrient pathway; a lot of cellulose; asparagus, celery, kohlrabi, rhubarb

- **Leaves**—the manufacturing organ for carbohydrate that is then stored elsewhere in the plant; brussels sprouts, cabbage, lettuce, parsley, spinach; also seaweed and "greens" such as beet, collards, kale, and mustard greens

- **Flowers**—clusters on the stem; artichoke, broccoli, cauliflower
- **Fruits**—the mature ovaries with seeds, generally sweet, and fleshy; apple, banana, berry, and orange; but including vegetable–fruits such as avocado, cucumber, eggplant, okra, olive, pepper, pumpkin, snap beans, squashes, and tomato that are not sweet, but contain seeds
- **Seeds**—in fruit of a plant; may be in pods; includes legumes such as dried beans, and peas, and peanuts, and, in the United States, sweet corn (although it is a grain, not vegetable); may be sprouted

HARVESTING AND POSTHARVEST CHANGES

Harvesting as well as processing schedules and procedures should be strictly followed to ensure fruits and vegetables with the highest quality. Vegetables and fruits may be harvested at different stages of maturity prior to storage. For example, they are likely to be larger and less tender with age; therefore, it is ideal to harvest less mature fruits and vegetables. The practice of cooling fresh produce in the field, and then canning close to the field, prior to transport is ideal for minimizing negative changes in quality.

After harvest, fruits and vegetables continue to undergo respiration, the metabolic process of taking in oxygen (O_2) and giving off carbon dioxide (CO_2). The maximum rate of respiration occurs just *before* full ripening. *Climacteric* fruits, such as the apple, apricot, avocado, banana, peach, pear, plum, and tomato continue to ripen *after* they are harvested. (Tropical fruits such as the papaya and mango are also climacteric.) Therefore, their maximum level of respiration rate (which occurs just before full ripening) is *after* harvest. On the other hand, *nonclimacteric* fruits, such as the cherry, citrus fruit, grapes, melon, pineapple, and strawberry, demonstrate maximum respiration rate *prior* to harvest.

All fruits are living material that respire and give off *moisture* and *heat*. Thus, proper packaging for shipping is significant (see Chapter 19). Storage conditions that retain this moisture or heat may produce negative changes in the fruit or vegetable, such as mold or rot.

If exposed to natural *postharvest* sunlight, artificial, or fluorescent light, a green chlorophyll pigment and bitter solanine (toxic at high levels) may appear in some vegetables such as onions or potatoes. These compounds are observed as green color spots just below the skin, and small amounts may easily be cut away.

RIPENING

In between the maturity and ripening stages there is a lot of unseen enzymatic activity. Ripening occurs due to internal hormonal and enzyme activity prior to change in the physical appearance. Evidence of ripening can eventually be seen in a physical evaluation. For example, softening of the cell wall, a change from the green color, due to chlorophyll degradation, and more carotenoids are visible in the fruit as it ripens. There is an increase in the sugar and decrease in the acid content.

The odorless and colorless ethylene gas is responsible for noticeable ripening changes. Ethylene gas is a *naturally occurring* hydrocarbon produced by some vegetables and fruits, especially apples, bananas, citrus fruit, melon, and tomatoes. In particular, lettuce and leafy vegetables as well as any bruised fruits are especially susceptible to undesirable respiration due to the presence of ethylene gas. Storage conditions should separate ethylene producers from other fruits that do not require ripening.

In addition to *natural* ethylene gas, there is also *artificially produced* ethylene gas, made by the burning of hydrocarbons. Measured doses of ethylene gas may be introduced into a closed chamber for the purpose of ripening unripened fruits before they are sold to retailers. The effectiveness of ethylene in achieving faster and more uniform ripening is dependent on the pulp temperature and stage of maturity of the fruit, and the relative humidity of the ripening room (7).

To control the unwanted effects of natural ethylene gas, which may result in poor fruit quality, gibberellic acid may be added to the external storage environment of fruits and vegetables. A pre-harvest application of this plant growth regulator delays ripening, and retains firmness in a fruit, both of which are important considerations in postharvest handling and storage. Refrigeration, as well as CO_2 and O_2 manipulation through controlled atmosphere storage, controlled atmosphere packaging, and modified atmosphere packaging (Chapter 19) offers another control of ripening.

Overripe fruits and vegetables become soft or mushy as protopectin develops into pectin in the process of *senescence* or overripening. To control unwanted ripening and extend shelf life, edible waxes and other treatments, including irradiation, may be applied to fruits and vegetables (Chapter 19).

ENZYMATIC OXIDATIVE BROWNING

When bruised or cut during preparation, discoloration of some fruits or vegetables may occur. For example, when some varieties of apples, apricots, bananas, cherries, peaches, pears, or potatoes are cut, and enzymes are exposed to the atmosphere, they are subject to undesirable browning. This is referred to as **enzymatic oxidative browning**—the oxidation of organic, phenolic compounds (that contain an unsaturated molecular ring with multiple –OH groups) in cut fruits and vegetables as enzymes are exposed to oxygen, and the product is subsequently discolored.

Enzymatic oxidative browning occurs when several factors are present. A *substrate* such as the phenolic compound in fruits, *oxygen*, and an *enzyme* (phenol oxidase, phenolase, or polyphenolase) are needed. Control measures to prevent enzymatic oxidative browning may not be easy. For example, more than one substrate may exist in a fruit or vegetable, oxygen may come from intercellular spaces, not solely surface air, and the responsible enzyme must be denatured.

One effective control of browning is to avoid contact between the substrate and oxygen. For example, food may be covered with a syrup to block oxygen, or it may be covered with a film wrap that limits oxygen permeability. Another control is the application of a commercially prepared citric acid powder or ascorbic acid to the cut fruit surface. Lemon juice in a ratio of 3:1 with water may be applied to the surface of the fruit, according to the Produce Marketing Association (2). In this manner, the vitamin C juice is oxidized instead of the pigment, and the acidic pH inhibits enzymatic action.

Pineapple juice, because of its sulfhydryl groups (–SH) that act as antioxidants, is another effective means of protection against browning. (As with lemon juice, the Produce Marketing Association recommends dipping cut fruits in pineapple juice [3:1 ratio, pineapple juice to water] for controlling enzymatic oxidative browning.) Sulfur compounds interfere with the darkening of various foods, such as cut fruit, cut lettuce leaves, and white wine. However, due to health concerns of a small percentage of the population allergic to sulfites, the use of *sulfiting agents* to prevent browning is restricted in *raw* products.

Home gardeners usually blanch fruits or vegetables prior to freezing. Blanching destroys the polyphenol oxidase enzyme and enables the product to withstand many months of freezer storage without degradation. Blanching entails the placement of the fruit or vegetable in boiling water for a precise time (depending on volume and texture of product) prior to freezing.

COOKING EFFECT

Vegetables and fruits are prepared by methods such as baking, boiling, frying, sautéing, steaming, stir-frying (Figure 7.7), and pressure cooking. When short cooking periods and cooking methods such as steaming are selected, there is minimal loss of flavor and nutritive value. Cooking introduces color and texture changes, as well as flavor and nutritive value changes, as shown in the following.

Color

The *natural color* of fruits and vegetables varies, and the color of *cooked* fruits and vegetables is influenced by a number of factors as previously discussed. These factors include the natural plant pigment, duration of cooking, use of a pan lid, and cooking method employed. As well, blanching serves to expel intercellular air and produces a brighter colored vegetable. Cooking in aluminum and cast-iron cookware may discolor cooked products, therefore, the use of stainless steel is recommended for cooking vegetables or fruits. Another color change accompanies the use of sodium bicarbonate, which yields a brighter green color. However, as previously mentioned, it is not recommended, as vitamin and texture loss occurs.

Texture

In addition to color changes, cooking changes the texture of a vegetable. The *texture* of the cooked vegetable depends on the length of cooking, the water composition and temperature, and pH. For example, lengthy cooking in boiling alkaline water drastically softens texture as hemicelluloses break down, cellulose is softened, and pectins dissolve in solution. The addition of acid, such as the addition of a tomato to another vegetable recipe, yields a firm cooked vegetable because tissues do not soften and pectin precipitates. Calcium ions, either naturally present in hard water or those

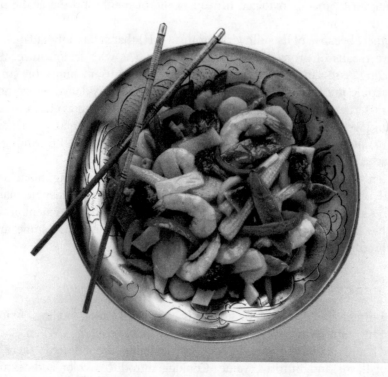

FIGURE 7.7 Various vegetables in Oriental stir-fry (*Courtesy of SYSCO® Incorporated*).

added to canned vegetables in commercial processing, retain the texture of cooked plant tissue forming insoluble salts with pectic substances. Of course, the texture is also related to maturity of the plant, which may become tougher and "woody" due to the presence of lignin.

Flavor

The *flavor* of cooked vegetables is dependent on the vegetable's classification as *Allium* or *Brassica* and loss of water-soluble organic acids and sugars from the vacuole. Additionally, any ingredients in a recipe, such as sugar, fat, herbs, and spices vary the flavor of vegetables.

Nutritive Value

The *nutritive* value of cooked fruits and vegetables is influenced by specific nutrients naturally present in specific products, type of cooking medium, and duration of cooking. Through diffusion, water-soluble nutrients are lost from parenchyma cells and may be oxidized. Minerals are inorganic substances that cannot be destroyed (although they may be discarded in fruit or vegetable trimmings).

In summary, cooking produces changes in the appearance, texture, flavor, and nutritive value. Once cooked, the cell membranes lose their selective permeability, and unlike the simple movement of water or **osmosis** that occurs in *raw* fruits, the *cooked* cell membranes allow the additional movement of sugars and some nutrients. Consequently, simple **diffusion** occurs as substances move from an area of higher concentration to an area of lower concentration and water enters the cell.

FRUITS—UNIQUE COOKING AND PREPARATION PRINCIPLES

In this chapter, special attention must be given to some of the unique aspects of cooking and preparing fruits. Further discussion of "fruits" in this section will be limited to the fleshy fruits with seeds, although it should be kept in mind that bananas and seedless grapes are examples of fruits without seeds.

To repeat a previously mentioned concept, the *botanical* definition of a fruit includes all grains, legumes (beans and peas), nuts, as well as some plant parts commonly eaten as "vegetables" (e.g. tomatoes) and thus is different from the *culinary* definition. According to its culinary role, fruit is the sweet, fleshy part of a plant, usually eaten alone or served as dessert. Grains, legumes, and nuts do not fit into this culinary definition of fruit; neither do avocadoes, cucumbers, eggplant, okra, olives, peppers, pumpkin, snap beans, squash, and tomatoes, which are typically considered as *vegetables*, or vegetable-fruits in dietary regimes.

A 1893 tax dispute led to the ruling by the United States Supreme Court that a tomato was a vegetable. "Botanically, tomatoes are considered a fruit of the vine, just as are cucumbers, squashes, beans, and peas. But in common language of people, whether sellers or consumers of provisions, all these are vegetables which are grown in kitchen gardens, and which, eaten cooked or raw, are, like potatoes, carrots, parsnips, turnips, beets, cauliflower, cabbage, celery, and lettuce, usually served at dinner in, with, or after the soup, fish, or meats which constitute the principal part of the repast, and not like fruits, generally, as dessert" (United States Supreme Court) (8).

As fruits are cooked in plain water, water moves into the tissues, sugar (12–15% level naturally) diffuses out, and the fruit, including dried fruit, becomes plump. Pectins become soluble and diffuse into water; cells become less dense, and the product becomes tenderer. Cellulose is softened, and lignins remain unchanged.

When large amounts of sugar (amounts greater than that found naturally in fruits) are added to the cooking water at the beginning of cooking, tenderization is diminished and the fruit will hold its shape. This is because the water moves out, and the higher concentration of sugar outside of the piece of fruit moves in by diffusion. The sugar interferes with plant pectin solubility. It also dehydrates cellulose and hemicellulose resulting in shrunken, tough walls.

Therefore, if the shape of fruits is to be maintained, sugar is added to the cooking water early in cooking. For example, when cooking berries or apple, pear and peach slices, initial sugar addition is beneficial for retaining the shape. Conversely, when fruits are cooked in plain water, and sugar is added late, after cooked fruit loses its shape and softens, fruit sauces such as applesauce are formed.

There are flavor changes that occur in a cooked fruit perhaps due to the fact that water-soluble sugars and other small molecules, including some vitamins, escape to the surrounding water. Consequently, the cooked fruit tastes blander, unless sugar is added during cooking.

During preparation, cut fruit such as strawberries may be sprinkled with sugar. If so, it loses water through osmosis, as can be seen in the bowl of strawberries that form liquid in the bowl after being sprinkled with sugar. In preparation, fruits may also show brownish-red discoloration due to enzymatic oxidative browning.

Fruit Juices and Juice Drinks

"Juices" are 100% fruit, while "juice drinks" must contain at least 10% real juice. Each may be formulated from a variety of fruits, resulting in various yield percentages. Data on yield and amounts of produce needed to extract juice becomes important in studies on diet and disease (9). The FDA requires pasteurization of commercial juices, and allows ultraviolet (UV) irradiation to reduce the pathogens and other detrimental microorganisms.

GRADING

Grading by the United States government, USDA, is a voluntary function of packers and processors. It is not an indication of safety, nutritive value, or type of packs. Wholesalers, commercial, and institutional food service may purchase according to grade, although consumers may be unaware of grading.

Dried and *frozen* forms of fruits and vegetables are graded, but grading indications appear less commonly than on *canned* or *fresh* products. In the highly competitive wholesale food-service market, *canned* fruits and vegetables receive US Grade A, B, or C. US Grade A is the highest rating and indicates the best appearance and texture, including clarity of liquid, color, shape, size, absence of blemishes or defects, and maturity. US Grade C is the lowest grade. *Fresh* fruits and vegetables are rated US Fancy, US No. 1, and US No. 2.

Private labeling may have specifications that state a narrow range within a grade. *Generic* products may not offer as high of a grade as privately labeled products.

ORGANICALLY GROWN FRUITS AND VEGETABLES

In February 2001, the USDA provided a *federal* definition for "organically grown," and a federal standard for its production, handling, and processing. Rules for implementing The Organic Foods Production Act of 1990 took several years to go into effect and proposals were released several years prior to the final ruling. A tremendous amount of public input was obtained in an attempt to satisfy both the organic farmer and the consumer. An intent of the final comprehensive standard was to ease potential confusion in domestic and export sales, and makes use of just *one* product label, eliminating the need for *individual* state and/or private standards. The USDA Organic Seal was also redesigned for better consumer understanding, and became effective for use in August 2002.

Foods labeled "organic" must be grown without the use of chemical pesticides, herbicides, or fertilizers (10), and have verifiable records of their system of production. Organic products must be 95% organically produced; processed foods may be labeled "made with organic ingredients." If organic production and handling is not followed, yet a product is offered for sale as organic, a large monetary fine may be imposed. Although there is the absence of chemical pesticides, herbicides, and fertilizers used during growth, which would be desirable to some individuals, there is no evidence that organically grown foods are higher in *nutrient content* than conventionally grown foods. A poor nutrient soil may yield a lower crop, but not one of lesser nutritive value (11). Although the *pesticide residue* would certainly be lower, *bacterial counts* of organically grown plant material may be higher than conventionally grown foods. Organically grown is not synonymous with food safety either, therefore, as with all produce, care must be taken to wash contaminants off all fruits and vegetables.

It should be noted in this discussion that the National Organic Program (NOP) applies to more than fruits and vegetables. Crop standards, livestock standards, and handling standards are addressed by the Act.

BIOTECHNOLOGY

Growers have strived to increase *availability* and *yield* of their crops, despite factors such as weather conditions in the growing region, insect infestation, and the lengthy time period of conventional breeding. Modern methods of biotechnology or genetic engineering have addressed these factors, and developments have led to breeding new types of produce, disease-resistant strains, and longer shelf life. **Biotechnology** assists in providing a better, less expensive, safer, and tastier food supply (12). Several years of conventional breeding techniques are immensely shortened by gene manipulation, possibly by 50% for some foods (13).

Genetic engineering, in practice since 1970s, is a biotechnology development that inserts a desired gene into another crop's chromosomes. The resultant cells are grown into plants, and then *conventional* breeding techniques followed to yield crops with specific desirable traits. The individual plants of a crop are unique, and the entire crop is not representative of clones of one original plant.

Genetic engineering of living systems is not restricted to fruits and vegetables. For example, the enzyme rennin, used in cheesemaking, and traditionally obtained from the stomach of calves, may be massproduced by insertion of genetic material into bacteria. Enzymes may be withdrawn from animal or plant cells, or microorganisms, and used to alter or create new products.

A combination of 1) *conventional breeding,* by plant breeders including selection, crossing, and mutation, with 2) *biotechnology,* including recombinant DNA, gene transfer, tissue culture, and plant regeneration (14), produces new germplasm, which increases production potential and resistance to pests, disease, drought, and pollution while developing more nutritious plant products. Close collaboration between scientists using both approaches is needed in order to improve product quality and meet consumers' demands.

To date, many Genetically Modified Organisms, or GMOs, have been approved, and seeds have received approval for planting. For example, genetically modified seeds for crops including soy, maize, and cotton are routinely planted in the U.S. The food industry is responsible for (and is credited by the Institute of Food Technologists) promoting safe and environmentally sound practices in utilizing GMOs. Biotechnology is one agricultural tool that assists in promoting sustainable agriculture, which includes the goals of environmental health and socioeconomic equity.

Areas of research focus on improving the nutritive content of plant foods, such as improving the protein content of plants, increasing their resistance to pests, or improving their storage. In addition to providing the consumer with greater economy, convenience, and improved nutritive value, *safety* is a factor that is important to both the grower and consumer. Safety of biotechnology has been debated and discussed by the public, educators, environmentalists, and scientists. The future may hold more such debate. Many consumers want to have genetically altered food products so-labeled. Several years ago, surveys showed that "biotechnology is not an issue for most American consumers" (15). A comparable 1998 survey with a cross-section of respondents showed the same or even higher support for biotechnology among Japanese and American consumers (16).

The safety of the first genetically engineered food designed for human consumption was demonstrated to the FDA and approval was granted for use of the Flavr-Savr® tomato in May 1994. Its shelf life is 10 days longer than other tomatoes. Polygalacturonase (PG) enzyme allows it to stay on the vine longer, thus it can be vine ripened with enhanced flavor. In 1996, the planting of corn, potato, soybeans, and tomato varieties developed through biotechnology began following FDA decisions on safety (17). Dairy products from cows treated with genetically engineered growth hormones are also on the market in the U.S.

The USDA's Agricultural Research Service (ARS) along with private industry and academic research centers maintain the goal of developing improved genetic engineering. To date, there are some food companies that have ceased using, or announced that they will not use GMOs due to negative consumer reaction. The debate continues.

The FDA ensures the safety of genetically altered foods and food ingredients, in two ways: 1) regulating adulteration, and 2) regulating by the food additive provision of their rules. Neither of these regulating methods is different from safety standards of any other non-bioengineered food product (18). Providing human and environmental safety, as well as high-quality foods is of great significance to public. The FDA requires that all bioengineered foods be labeled if they are significantly different from the conventional food in nutritive value, or in posing food allergies.

The Position Statement of The American Dietetic Association (see additional references) regarding biotechnology is as follows: "It is the position of the American Dietetic Association that the techniques of biotechnology are useful in enhancing the quality, nutritional value, and variety of food available for human consumption and in increasing the efficiency of food production, processing, distribution and waste management" (19). "Dietitians can regard the tumultuous public discussions of biotechnology as a source of stress or as an opportunity to become a more valuable resource to consumers"(20).

For a more in-depth report on biotechnology and foods, see the Institute of Food Technologists three-part series titled IFT Expert Report on Biotechnology and Food (19–21).

IRRADIATION

Much discussion on irradiation is reported elsewhere in this text (see Chapters 17 and 18), and in other writings. For example, seeds may be irradiated to control pathogens. Some fresh fruits, juices, and sprouts have also been treated in this manner. On the horizon are the results of further studies seeking suitable methods to control pathogens in fruit and vegetable products.

VEGETARIAN FOOD CHOICES

Vegetables are increasingly used by a growing number of vegetarians in creating purely vegetarian foods (22). They may also be added to traditional foods for increased nutritional value. In fact, the National Restaurant Association reports that 97% of colleges and universities, and 80% of restaurants incorporate vegetarian main dishes into the menus (NRA). Some processing companies may offer vegetable *flavors* as less costly replacements for vegetables in recipe formulations (see Chapter 9 for vegetarian diets and protein needs).

In order to meet the needs of vegetarian diets, the number of new product introduced that meet the requirement for vegetarian diets continues to increase. Ninety-four new product introductions in a recent year were followed by 124 new products the next year, and 75 for the first half of the following year (21). It is estimated that in the United States, the number of vegetarians may be 24 million people. Yet, only 4% of the general population omits *all* animal food from their diet, including meat, milk, cheese, and eggs (22).

Vegans are vegetarians who omit all animal products from their diet. Since animal products are the only significant source of vitamin B_{12}, vegans need reliable fortified foods or vitamin B_{12} supplementation in order to maintain the myelin sheath surrounding the nerves and prevent permanent nerve damage and paralysis. It becomes important to know that microwave heating inactivates vitamin B_{12} in foods (23, see Chapter 9). If other types of vegetarian cuisines are followed, vegetarians might consume milk, or eggs, white meat, or fish.

NUTRITIVE VALUE OF VEGETABLES AND FRUITS

Due to a worldwide supply and international purchasing potential, vegetables and fruits have year-round availability. Achieving good nutrition is enhanced by availability of the nutrients present in fruits and vegetables. Vitamins, notably vitamins A and C, pro-vitamin A (carotene), minerals (calcium and iron), and dietary fiber, are among the great benefits of a high fruit and vegetable diet, whether canned, frozen, or fresh. Other non-nutrients, such as the ***phytochemicals*** (phyto = plant) in fruits and vegetables, may function in the prevention of human disease. More evaluation and research is needed in order to address the many potential health benefits/disease-preventing properties of plant material. Some nutrition facts are included in Figures 7.8 and 7.9.

Consumption of three to five servings of vegetables per day and two to four of fruit per day are recommended in the Food Guide Pyramid of the USDA. A diet that

VEGETABLES
NUTRI-FACTS
UPDATE

NUTRITION FACTS FOR RAW VEGETABLES[1]

Vegetables, Serving portion (gram weight/ounce weight)	Calories	Calories From Fat	Total Fat (g/%DV)	Sodium (mg/%DV)	Potassium (mg/%DV)	Total Carbohydrate (g/%DV)	Dietary Fiber (g/%DV)	Sugars (g)	Protein (g)	Vitamin A (%DV)	Vitamin C (%DV)	Calcium (%DV)	Iron (%DV)
Asparagus, 5 spears (93 g/3.3 oz)	25	0	0 / 0	0 / 0	230 / 7	4 / 1	2 / 8	2	2	10	15	2	2
Bell Pepper, 1 medium (148 g/5.3 oz)	30	0	0 / 0	0 / 0	270 / 8	7 / 2	2 / 8	4	1	8	190	2	2
Broccoli, 1 medium stalk (148 g/5.3 oz)	45	0	0.5 / 1	55 / 2	540 / 15	8 / 3	5 / 20	3	5	15	220	6	6
Carrot, 7" long, 1 1/4" diameter (78 g/2.8 oz)	35	0	0 / 0	40 / 2	280 / 8	8 / 3	2 / 8	5	1	270	10	2	0
Cauliflower, 1/6 medium head (99 g/3.5 oz)	25	0	0 / 0	30 / 1	270 / 8	5 / 2	2 / 8	2	2	0	100	2	2
Celery, 2 medium stalks (110 g/3.9 oz)	20	0	0 / 0	100 / 4	350 / 10	5 / 2	2 / 8	0	1	2	15	4	2
Cucumber, 1/3 medium (99 g/3.5 oz)	15	0	0 / 0	0 / 0	170 / 5	3 / 1	1 / 4	2	1	4	10	2	2
Green (Snap) Beans, 3/4 cup cut (83 g/3.0 oz)	25	0	0 / 0	0 / 0	200 / 6	5 / 2	3 / 12	2	1	4	10	4	2
Green Cabbage, 1/12 medium head (84 g/3.0 oz)	25	0	0 / 0	20 / 1	190 / 5	5 / 2	2 / 8	3	1	0	70	4	2
Green Onion, 1/4 cup chopped (25 g/0.9 oz)	10	0	0 / 0	5 / 0	70 / 2	2 / 1	1 / 4	1	0	2	8	0	0
Iceberg Lettuce, 1/6 medium head (89 g/3.2 oz)	15	0	0 / 0	10 / 0	120 / 3	3 / 1	1 / 4	2	1	4	6	2	2
Leaf Lettuce, 1 1/2 cups shredded (85 g/3.0 oz)	15	0	0 / 0	30 / 1	230 / 7	4 / 1	2 / 8	2	1	40	6	4	0
Mushrooms, 5 medium (84 g/3.0 oz)	20	0	0 / 0	0 / 0	300 / 9	3 / 1	1 / 4	0	3	0	2	0	4
Onion, 1 medium (148 g/5.3 oz)	60	0	0 / 0	5 / 0	240 / 7	14 / 5	3 / 12	9	2	0	20	4	2
Potato, 1 medium (148 g/5.3 oz)	100	0	0 / 0	0 / 0	720 / 21	26 / 9	3 / 12	3	4	0	45	2	6
Radishes, 7 radishes (85 g/3.0 oz)	15	0	0 / 0	25 / 1	230 / 7	3 / 1	0 / 0	2	1	0	30	2	0
Summer Squash, 1/2 medium (98 g/3.5 oz)	20	0	0 / 0	0 / 0	260 / 7	4 / 1	2 / 8	2	1	6	30	2	2
Sweet Corn, kernels from 1 medium ear (90 g/3.2 oz)	80	10	1 / 2	0 / 0	240 / 7	18 / 6	3 / 12	5	3	2	10	0	2
Sweet Potato, medium, 5" long, 2" diameter (130 g/4.6 oz)	130	0	0 / 0	45 / 2	350 / 10	33 / 11	4 / 16	7	2	440	30	2	2
Tomato, 1 medium (148 g/5.3 oz)	35	0	0.5 / 1	5 / 0	360 / 10	7 / 2	1 / 4	4	1	20	40	2	2

Most fruits and vegetables provide negligible amounts of saturated fat and cholesterol.

[1] Raw, edible weight portion. Percent Daily Values are based on a 2,000 calorie diet.

Developed by: Food Marketing Institute, American Dietetic Association, American Meat Institute, Food Distributors International, National Broiler Council, National Cattlemen's Beef Association, National Fisheries Institute, National Grocers Association, National Turkey Federation, Produce Marketing Association, United Fresh Fruit and Vegetable Association

Data Source: U.S. Food and Drug Administration

(7/96)

FIGURE 7.8 Vegetables Nutri-Facts
(*Data Source:* US Food and Drug Administration *Developed by:* Food Marketing Institute et al.).

includes five servings of fruits and vegetables per day exerts a protective effect against chronic disease. Yet, only 9% of the population is reported to have met the guidelines of three servings of vegetable and two servings of fruits a day in a National Health and Nutrition Examination Survey (NHANES II) (24). According to the American

FRUITS
NUTRI-FACTS
UPDATE

NUTRITION FACTS FOR RAW FRUITS[1]

FRUIT, Serving portion (gram weight/ounce weight)	Calories	Calories From Fat	Total Fat (g/%DV)		Sodium (mg/%DV)		Potassium (mg/%DV)		Total Carbohydrate (g/%DV)		Dietary Fiber (g/%DV)		Sugars (g)	Protein (g)	Vitamin A (%DV)	Vitamin C (%DV)	Calcium (%DV)	Iron (%DV)
Apple, 1 medium (154 g/5.5 oz)	80	0	0	0	0	0	170	5	22	7	5	20	16	0	2	8	0	2
Avocado, California, 1/5 medium (30 g/1.1 oz)	55	45	5	8	0	0	170	5	3	1	3	12	0	1	0	4	0	0
Banana, 1 medium (126 g/4.5 oz)	110	0	0	0	0	0	400	11	29	10	4	16	21	1	0	15	0	2
Cantaloupe, 1/4 medium (134 g/4.8 oz)	50	0	0	0	25	1	280	8	12	4	1	4	11	1	100	80	2	2
Grapefruit, 1/2 medium (154 g/5.3 oz)	60	0	0	0	0	0	230	7	16	5	6	24	10	1	15	110	2	0
Grapes, 1 1/2 cups (138 g/4.9 oz)	90	10	1	2	0	0	270	8	24	8	1	4	23	1	2	25	2	2
Honeydew Melon, 1/10 medium melon (134 g/4.8 oz)	50	0	0	0	35	1	310	9	13	4	1	4	12	1	2	45	0	2
Kiwifruit, 2 medium (148 g/5.3 oz)	100	10	1	2	0	0	480	14	24	8	4	16	16	2	2	240	6	4
Lemon, 1 medium (58 g/2.1 oz)	15	0	0	0	5	0	90	3	5	2	1	4	1	0	0	40	2	0
Lime, 1 medium (67 g/2.4 oz)	20	0	0	0	0	0	75	2	7	2	2	8	0	0	0	35	0	0
Nectarine, 1 medium (140 g/5.0 oz)	70	0	0.5	1	0	0	300	9	16	5	2	8	12	1	4	15	0	2
Orange, 1 medium (154 g/5.5 oz)	70	0	0	0	0	0	260	7	21	7	7	28	14	1	2	130	6	2
Peach, 1 medium (98 g/3.5 oz)	40	0	0	0	0	0	190	5	10	3	2	8	9	1	2	10	0	0
Pear, 1 medium (166 g/5.9 oz)	100	10	1	2	0	0	210	6	25	8	4	16	17	1	0	10	2	0
Pineapple, 2 slices, 3" diameter, 3/4" thick (112 g/4 oz)	60	0	0	0	10	0	115	3	16	5	1	4	13	1	0	25	2	2
Plums, 2 medium (132 g/4.7 oz)	80	10	1	2	0	0	220	6	19	6	2	8	10	1	6	20	0	0
Strawberries, 8 medium (147 g/5.3 oz)	45	0	0	0	0	0	270	8	12	4	4	16	8	1	0	160	2	4
Sweet Cherries, 21 cherries; 1 cup (140 g/5.0 oz)	90	0	0.5	0	0	0	300	9	22	7	3	12	19	2	2	15	2	2
Tangerine, 1 medium (109 g/3.9 oz)	50	0	0.5	1	0	0	180	5	15	5	3	12	12	1	0	50	4	0
Watermelon, 1/18 medium melon; 2 cups diced pieces (280 g/10.0 oz)	80	0	0	0	10	0	230	7	27	9	2	8	25	1	20	25	2	4

Most fruits and vegetables provide negligible amounts of saturated fat and cholesterol; avocados provide 1g of saturated fat per ounce.

[1] Raw, edible weight portion. Percent Daily Values are based on a 2,000 calorie diet.

Developed by: Food Marketing Institute, American Dietetic Association, American Meat Institute, Food Distributors International, National Broiler Council, National Cattlemen's Beef Association, National Fisheries Institute, National Grocers Association, National Turkey Federation, Produce Marketing Association, United Fresh Fruit and Vegetable Association

Data Source: U.S. Food and Drug Administration

(7/96)

FIGURE 7.9   Fruits Nutri-Facts
(*Data Source:* US Food and Drug Administration *Developed by:* Food Marketing Institute et al.)

Diabetic Association Exchange List, one serving of vegetables contains 25 calories and one serving of fruit contains 60 calories.

Americans have made positive dietary changes in the past 20 years, including increasing fruits, vegetables and grains, yet, they still fail to reach the appropriate number of servings of fruits, dark green leafy vegetables, deep yellow vegetables, dried beans and other legumes (25).

The USDA Department of Health and Human Services has noted: "In this land of plenty, millions of Americans aren't eating wisely. Not because they haven't had enough to eat, but because they eat too many of the wrong things or too little of the right." Taste is the most important factor that influences food choices; positive messages about benefits of diets with plenty of fruits and vegetables help with making choices (26). On a regular basis, the American Public eats too little of fruits and vegetables containing nutrients, such as vitamins A and C (on all Nutrition Facts labels), or the antioxidant vitamin E, all of which have an important role in preventing or delaying major degenerative diseases of Americans (27).

Citrus fruits provide protection against cancer, heart disease, and neural tube defects (28). They contain limonene and phenols that block formation of nitrosamines and facilitate carcinogen excretion from the body. In addition, citrus fruits contain antioxidants, vitamin C, and relatively good amounts of folic acid that has been shown to prevent reoccurrence of neural tube defect in pregnant women.

Membranes and juice sacs of fruit contain pectin, unless removed in processing. Several possible dietary benefits of this fiber include glycemic, cholesterol, and cancer control (29). The FDA allows a label claim regarding foods with dietary fiber and a reduction of cancer incidence.

There may be loss of water-soluble vitamins in cooking, for example, ascorbic acid (vitamin C) and thiamin (vitamin B_1) may diffuse out to the water and be oxidized. Sugars and mineral salts may also be lost in soaking or cooking water. Excessive peel removal with the expectation of eliminating pesticide residues, or chopping to create small pieces, results in high nutrient losses. Prolonged or high-temperature storage also results in vitamin loss. Succulents, full of moisture, and leafy fruits and vegetables should be stored covered in the refrigerator. Tubers should be stored in a dark, cool place for quality, including nutrient retention.

Fruits and vegetables provide many nutritional benefits, including the non-nutrient benefits of phytochemicals as mentioned. This further supports the idea that nutrition is obtained from *food* rather than isolated compounds. Isolated compounds of fruits, vegetables, and other foods that are thought to provide health and medicinal benefits to the diet are nutraceuticals. The FDA has not recognized the term **nutraceuticals** or allowed health claims on products beyond those that are supported by the scientific community (Chapter 20).

The American Dental Association recommends eating fruits such as apples and oranges and many uncooked vegetables such as carrots and celery. These act as "detergent" foods, cleaning teeth, and gums of food debris that may otherwise lead to the major nutrition-related problem of tooth decay.

Nutrition information regarding the top 20 commonly eaten fruits and vegetables is available to the consumer at the point of sale as a result of strong encouragement in the Nutrition Education and Labeling Act of 1990. Most supermarkets have nutrition in booklets, posted, or on produce bags. Individual items do not need to be labeled with a nutrition label.

There are numerous compounds in plant material that have antioxidant properties (beta-carotene, vitamin C, and vitamin E), or have been shown to have anticarcinogenic properties. The American Dietetic Association states that eating a wide variety of foods, including an emphasis on grains, vegetables, and fruits is the best way to obtain adequate amounts of beneficial food constituents: "It is the position of The American Dietetic Association that the best nutritional strategy for promoting optimal health and reducing the risk of chronic disease is to obtain adequate nutrients from a variety of foods. Vitamin and mineral supplementation is appropriate when well-accepted, peer-reviewed scientific evidence shows safety and effectiveness" (30).

According to "Shopping for Health 2000" survey by the Food Marketing Institute/Prevention, the following factors motivate purchase decisions: general health (95%), fat (82%), doctor (70%), cholesterol (72%), lower risk (72%), avoid additives/preservatives (68%), manage/treat (58%), food intolerance (49%), and slow aging (48%) (31).

SAFETY OF VEGETABLES AND FRUITS

Fruits and vegetables are not considered "potentially hazardous foods" that allow the "rapid and progressive growth of infectious or toxigenic microorganisms" (Model FDA Food Code). In comparison to animal-based foods, there are few problems with plant-based products, but, unfortunately, they can carry disease. The public is encouraged to eat more fruits and vegetables for health and expects that food to be safe (The USDA's 2000 Dietary Guidelines for Americans encourages individuals to "keep food safe to eat" too!).

Pathogenic microorganisms are found in the environment and can contaminate food, causing illness. Of serious concern are *Salmonella, Escherichia coli, Campylobacter, isteria, Staphylococcus aureus, Shigella, Clostridium botulinum, Bacillus cereus,* and *Hepatitis A*, to name a few (see Chapter 16) (32). *Salmonella* bacteria have been found on cantaloupe, watermelon, and tomatoes, *Listeria* on cabbage, and *Campylobacter* on mushrooms (33). Imports from less-developed regions of the world may be implicated as a contributing factor in the increase in fruit- and vegetable-related foodborne illness.

Regardless of its source, it is recommended that "ready-to-eat" value-added fresh produce be washed prior to consumption, and then refrigerated in order to maintain food safety. Cross-contamination from other foods, such as meats, should be avoided, pull dates should be adhered to, and assembly/preparation areas should be sanitary. Of course personal hygiene is crucial to food safety.

Various antimicrobials are used in industry to improve the safety of fruits and vegetables, especially in the growing market for minimally processed fruits and vegetables. Chlorine has proven to be less than effective in limiting growth of some bacteria, e.g., *Listeria monocytogenes*, and therefore hydrogen peroxide (H_2O_2)

disinfection has been considered. Hydrogen peroxide is a generally recognized as safe (GRAS) substance that has also been used as a bleaching agent (as in milk used for cheese), and as an antimicrobial agent in foods (34).

Chlorine dioxide, hydrogen peroxide (H_2O_2), and ozone may be useful in reducing the microbial load on some fruits and vegetables, the last two leaving no residues following treatment. Peroxyacetic acid may also be used.

Some antimicrobials are effective due to their low pH, but are not usable due to the unacceptable flavor that they impart. Other substances having antimicrobial properties include essential oils from citrus, coriander, mint, parsley, and vanillin juice peels. Overall, it is the use of such antimicrobial chemicals, coupled with good washing, high-intensity pulsed light, irradiation, ultra-violet light, good manufacturing practices, and Hazard Analysis and Critical Control Points (HACCP) principles that contribute to ensure safety in fresh produce (32).

Precautions against contamination and growth of harmful bacteria include the following (33):

- Buying only what is necessary for short-term needs; longer storage allows multiplication of any bacteria that are present.

- Careful washing of hands *before* handling fresh produce (even after holding a public banister or door knob) and *between* cutting and eating fresh produce.

- Rinsing produce to remove harmful bacteria prior to consumption (even uneaten, disposed of rinds) and after removing outer leaves and peels.

- Refrigerate leftovers to slow any bacterial growth.

- Prepare fruits and vegetables on sanitary work surfaces with sanitary utensils.

The FDA recommends that, where feasible, products are to be *cooked* after the addition of spices, in order to destroy microorganisms, although *commercial processing* of herbs, spices, and their extracts reduces bacterial count.

It bears repeating that personal hygiene standards should be high in order to minimize the incidence of food contamination. As well, juices should be pasteurized to eliminate *E. Coli* 0157:H7 that may be carried to the fruit by fecal contamination or improper handling.

LABELING OF VEGETABLES AND FRUITS

Nutrition Facts

Vitamins A and C content of foods are identified on all food labels for products produced in the United States. Most Americans would do well to increase their intake of these two vitamins that are simultaneously so prevalent in fruits and vegetables. The label provides the consumer with information regarding the percentage of Daily Value that they are consuming in each serving. Individual fresh fruits and vegetables do not have labels, yet supermarket brochures, posters, or plastic bags relate the nutrient contribution.

Label Terms

Labeling terms that apply to fruits and vegetables include the following and must appear as a product descriptor after the product name, for example, "green beans, fresh":

- A "**Fresh**" food must be a raw food, alive and respiring. Some skin surface treatment is acceptable, such as application of wax, or pesticides. Treatment with less than one kGy irradiation, to inactivate pathogenic and spoilage microorganisms is allowed. (The FDA is considering use of the term "*fresh*" for alternative nonthermal technologies that function to protect the US food supply, and clearly convey food characteristics to consumers.)

- "**Freshly prepared**" is food that has not been frozen, heat processed, or preserved.

- A "**Good Source of**" must contain 10–19% of the Daily Value of that nutrient per serving.

- If an item states "**Fat-free,**" it must have less than 1/2 g of fat per serving. "**Low-fat**" indicates that the product must contain 3 g of fat or less per serving.

- **Calorie level** is important to many consumers. If an item states "**Low-calorie,**" it must contain less than 40 calories per serving.

- "**Sodium-free**" signifies that a product contains less than 5 mg of sodium (Na) per serving. "**Very-low-sodium**" is used for a product that contains less than 35 mg of Na per serving, and "**Low-sodium**" is less than 140 mg Na per serving.

- "**High-fiber**" is 5 mg or more of fiber per serving.

The 1991 nutrition labeling produce regulations were amended by the Food and Drug Administration (FDA). Regulations exist for labeling nutritive value of the 20 most frequently consumed vegetables and fruits (Figures 7.8, 7.9). In addition to the top 20, other vegetables and fruits must be labeled if nutritional claims are made. Such labeling is voluntary and will continue to be voluntary if there is sufficient compliance noted by the FDA.

CONCLUSION

Plant tissue is composed primarily of parenchyma tissue. The structure and composition of a fresh fruit or vegetable changes as the cell is destroyed. As fruits and vegetables typically contain a very large percentage of water, the maintenance of turgor pressure is an important factor in determining plant material quality.

The desirable pigments and flavor compounds contained in fruits and vegetables may undergo unacceptable changes upon preparation and cooking. Discoloration of some cut vegetables or fruits is known as enzymatic oxidative browning, which must be controlled. Improper storage or cooking can result in quality losses.

Three to five servings of vegetables and two to four servings of fruits are recommended in the USDA. Food Guide Pyramid. As a group, fruit and vegetables are major contributors of pro-vitamin A (carotene) and vitamin C. Many are excellent sources of vitamins and dietary fiber, but are low in fat content. Vegetarian food choices may be met with consumption of a variety of fruits and vegetables.

Biotechnology provides the consumer with greater economy and convenience. Coupled with an understanding of the role of phytochemicals in disease prevention, vegetables and fruits may provide a greater nutrient contribution to the human diet. Irradiation is utilized as a means of ensuring food safety.

A specialty produce supplier has said, "Produce is a living commodity, forever changing, with new items appearing every year" (35). Fruits and vegetables require special handling to maintain high quality. Items of high nutritional value that were once unfamiliar and not used, as well as new items from around the world, are now available on grocery shelves.

GLOSSARY

Allium: Flavor compounds in the genus *Allium* that contain sulfur compounds and offer phytochemical value.

Anthocyanin: Red-blue pigmented vegetables of the Flavone family.

Anthoxanthin: Whitish pigmented fruits and vegetables of the Flavone group of chemicals.

Biotechnology: Biogenetic engineering of animals, microorganisms, and plants to alter or create products that have increased resistance to pests, improved nutritive value, and shelf life.

Brassica: Flavor compound of *Brassica* genus including cruciferous vegetables with sulfur compounds.

Carotenoid: The group of red-orange pigmented fruits and vegetables; some are precursors of vitamin A and also have antioxidant value.

Cellulose: Glucose polymer joined by β-1,4 glycosidic linkages; cannot be digested by human enzymes, thus it provides insoluble dietary fiber.

Cell sap: Found in the plant vacuole; contains water-soluble components such as sugars, salts, and some color and flavor compounds.

Chlorophyll: The green pigment of fruits and vegetables.

Cytoplasm: Plant cell contents inside the cell membrane, but outside the nucleus.

Diffusion: Movement of solute across a permeable membrane from an area of greater concentration to lesser concentration in heated products that do not have an intact cell membrane.

Enzymatic oxidative browning: Browning of cut or bruised fruits and vegetables due to the presence of phenolic compounds, enzymes, and oxygen.

Fresh: Alive and respiring as evidenced by metabolic and biochemical activities.

Fruit: The mature ovaries of plants with their seeds.

Hemicellulose: The indgestible fiber in cell walls that provides bulk in the diet; may be soluble, but primarily insoluble.

Lignin: The noncarbohydrate component of fiber of plant tissue that is insoluble and excreted from the body. It provides the undesirable woody texture of mature plants.

Middle lamella: The cementing material between adjacent plant cells, containing pectic substances, magnesium, calcium, and water.

Nutraceuticals: The name given to a proposed new regulatory category of food components that may be considered a food or part of a food and may supply medical or health benefits including the treatment or prevention of disease. A term not recognized by the FDA.

Osmosis: The movement of water across semipermeable membranes from an area of greater concentration to lesser concentration in products with an intact cell membrane.

Parenchyma tissue: Majority of plant cells containing the cytoplasm and nucleus.

Pectic substances: The intercellular "cement" between cell walls; the gel-forming polysaccharide of plant tissue.

Phytochemicals: Plant chemicals; natural compounds other than nutrients in fresh plant material that help in disease prevention. They protect against oxidative cell damage and may facilitate carcinogen excretion from the body to reduce the risk of cancer.

Turgor pressure: Pressure exerted by water-filled vacuoles on the cytoplasm and the partially elastic cell wall.

Vacuole: Cavity filled with cell sap and air.

REFERENCES

1. Barrett DM, Theerakulkait C. Quality indicators in blanched, frozen, stored vegetables. *Food Technology.* 1995; 49(1): 62–65.
2. Produce Marketing Association, Newark, DE.
3. Gross J. *Pigments in Vegetables–Chlorophylls and Carotenoids.* New York: Chapman & Hall, 1991.
4. Tufts University. Herbs and spices contain beneficial dietary components. *Food Engineering.* 1992; 64(6): 38.
5. Tufts University. Achieving consistency and cost-savings in savory foods. *Food Engineering.* 1993; 65(9): 28.
6. Sherman PW, Flaxman SM. Protecting ourselves from food. *American Scientist.* 2001; 89 (March–April): 142–151.
7. SYSCO Foods. Ethylene Gas and Applications.
8. Cunningham E. Is a tomato a fruit *and* a vegetable? *J Am Diet Assoc.* 2002; 102:817.
9. Newman V, Faerber S, Zoumas-Morse C, and Rock CL. Amount of raw vegetables and fruits needed to yield 1 c juice. *J Am Diet Assoc.* 2002; 102: 975–977.
10. Newsome R. Institute of Food Technologists' Expert Panel on Food Safety and Nutrition. A scientific status summary, organically grown foods. *Food Technology.* 1990; 44(12): 123–130.
11. Wardlaw GM, Insel PM, Seyler MF. *Contemporary Nutrition,* 2nd ed. St Louis, MO: Mosby, 1992.
12. Katz F. Biotechnology—New tools in food technology's toolbox. *Food Technology.* 1996; 50(11): 63–65.
13. Liu K, Brown EA. Enhancing vegetable oil quality through plant breeding and genetic engineering. *Food Technology.* 1996; 50(11): 67–71.
14. Hoban TJ. How Japanese consumers view biotechnology. *Food Technology.* 1996; 50(7): 85–88.
15. Hoban TJ. Consumer acceptance of biotechnology in the United States and Japan. *Food Technology.* 1999; 53(5): 50–53.
16. Giese J. Identifying bioengineered and irradiated foods. *Food Technology.* 1997; 51(11): 88–91.
17. ADA Position of the American Dietetic Association: biotechnology and the future of food. *Journal of the American Dietetic Association.* 1993; 93: 189–192.
18. Greger JL. Biotechnology: Mobilizing dietitians to be a resource. *Journal of the American Dietetic Association.* 2000; 100(11): 1306–1314.

19. IFT Expert Report on Biotechnology and Foods. Inroduction. *Food Technology*. 2000; 54(8): 124–136.
20. IFT Expert Report on Biotechnology and Foods. Inroduction. *Food Technology*. 2000; 54(9): 53–61.
21. IFT Expert Report on Biotechnology and Foods. Inroduction. *Food Technology*. 2000; 54(10): 61–79.
22. Vegetarian introductions sprouting upward. *Food Engineering*. 1994; 66(9): 15.
23. Whitney EN, Rolfes SR. *Understanding Nutrition*, 9th ed. Belmont, CA: West/Wadsworth, 2001.
24. Patterson BH, Block G, Rosenberger WF, Pee D, Kahle LL. Fruit and vegetables in the American diet: Data from the NHANES II survey. *American Journal of Public Health*. 1990; 80: 1443–1449.
25. Kantor LS. A comparison of the U.S. food supply with the Food Guide Pyramid Recommendations. In Frazao E, ed. *America's Eating Habits: Changes and Consequences*, Washington DC: US Department of Agriculture. 1999; 71–95. Agriculture information Bulletin No. 750.
26. ADA Position of the American Dietetic Association: Total diet approach to communicating food and nutrition information. *J Am Diet Assoc*. 2002; 102: 100–108.
27. Block G, Langseth L. Antioxidant vitamins and disease prevention. *Food Technology*. 1994; 48(7): 80–84.
28. Rouseff RL, Nagy S. Health and nutritional benefits of citrus fruit components. *Food Technology*. 1994; 48(11): 125–132.
29. Baker RA. Potential dietary benefits of citrus pectin and fiber. *Food Technology*. 1994; 48(11): 133–139.
30. Position of The American Dietetic Association: Vitamin and mineral supplementation. *Journal of the American Dietetic Association*. 1996; 96: 73–77.
31. Sloan AE. Clean foods. *Food Technology*. 2001; 55(2): 18.
32. Cherry JP. Improving the safety of fresh produce with antimicrobials. *Food Technology*. 1999; 53(11): 54–59.
33. Tufts University. Harmful bacteria grow on fresh produce. *Tufts University Diet & Nutrition Letter*, 1997; 14(11): 1–2.
34. Sapers GM, Simmons GF. Hydrogen peroxide disinfection of minimally processed fruits and vegetables. *Food Technology*. 1998; 52(2): 48–52.
35. Coosemans Worldwide. Coosemans-Denver, Inc.

BIBLIOGRAPHY

Addy ND, Stuart DA. Impact of biotechnology on vegetable processing. *Food Technology*. 1986; 40(10): 64–66.
American Cancer Society. *Nutrition and Cancer: Cause and Prevention*. New York: American Cancer Society, 1984.
American Dietetic Association. Chicago, IL.
American Soybean Association. St. Louis, MO.
Arrowhead Mills. Hereford, TX.

Barrett DM, Theerakulkait C. Quality indicators in blanched, frozen, stored vegetables. *Food Technology.* 1995; 49(1): 62–65.

Basic Vegetable Products. Suisun, CA.

Bourne MC. Physical properties and structure of horticultural crops. In: Peleg M, Bagley E, eds. *Physical Properties of Foods.* Westport, CT: AVI, 1983.

Dwyer JT, Goldin BR, Saul N, Gualtieri L, Barakat S, Adlercreutz H. Tofu and soy drinks contain phytoesterogens. *Journal of the American Dietetic Association.* 1994; 94: 739–742.

Fresh-cut Produce Association. *How to Buy Canned and Frozen Fruits.* Home and Garden Bulletin No. 167. Washington, DC: Consumer and Marketing Service, USDA, 1976.

How to Buy Canned and Frozen Vegetables. Home and Garden Bulletin No. 191. Washington, DC: USDA, 1977.

How to Buy Dry Beans, Peas, and Lentils. Home and Garden Bulletin No. 177. Washington, DC: USDA, 1970.

How to Buy Fresh Fruits. Home and Garden Bulletin No. 141. Washington, DC: USDA, 1977.

How to Buy Fresh Vegetables. Home and Garden Bulletin No. 143. Washington, DC: USDA, 1980.

Liu K. Biotech crops: Products, properties, and prospects. *Food Technology.* 1999; 53 (5): 42–49.

McCormick and Co. Hunt Valley, MD.

Russell M. Value-added fresh produce. *Food Engineering.* 1996; 50(2): 37–42.

Shattuck D. Eat your vegetables: Make them delicious. *J Am Diet Assoc* 2002; 102: 1130–1132.

Spicetec. Carol Stream, IL.

Starchier potatoes make low-fat fries. *Food Engineering.* 1992; 46(11): 24.

The Food Guide Pyramid: A Guide to Daily Food Choices. Home and Garden Bulletin No. 252. Washington, DC: US Dept of Agriculture, Human Nutrition Information Service, 1992.

Tropical Nut and Fruit. Charlotte, NC.

United Soybean Board. St. Louis, MO.

United States Department of Agriculture. *Results from the 1994–96 Continuing Survey of Food Intakes by Individuals.* Washington, DC: United States Department of Agriculture. http://www.barc.usda.gov.bhnrc/foodsurvey/96results.html.

USA Dry Pea & Lentil Industry. Moscow, ID.

Vaclavik, VA, Pimentel, MH, Devine, MM. *Dimensions of Food,* 5th ed. Boca Raton, Florida: CRC Press, 2002.

Van Duyn MAS, Pivonka E. Overview of the health benefits of fruit and vegetable consumption for the dietetics professional. Selected literature. *J Am Diet Assoc* 2000; 100: 1511–1521.

Whitney EN, Rolfes SR. *Understanding Nutrition,* 8th ed. St Paul, MN: West Publishing Co, 2000.

Wilkinson JQ. Biotech plants: From lab bench to supermarket shelf. *Food Technology.* 1997; 51(12): 37–42.

PART III

Proteins in the Food Guide Pyramid

C H A P T E R   8

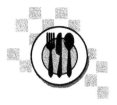

Proteins in Food—An Introduction

INTRODUCTION

Proteins are the most abundant molecules in cells, making up 50% or more of their dry weight. Every protein has a unique structure and conformation or shape, which enables it to carry out a specific function in a living cell. Proteins comprise the complex muscle system and the connective tissue network, and they are important as carriers in the blood system. All enzymes are proteins; enzymes are important as catalysts for many reactions (both desirable and undesirable) in foods.

All proteins contain carbon, hydrogen, nitrogen, and oxygen. Most proteins contain sulfur, and some contain additional elements; for example, milk proteins contain phosphorus, and hemoglobin and myoglobin contain iron. Copper and zinc are also constituents of some proteins.

Proteins are made up of amino acids. There are at least 20 different amino acids found in nature, and they have different properties depending on their structure and composition. When combined to form a protein, the result is a unique and complex molecule with a characteristic structure and conformation and a specific function in the plant or animal where it belongs. Small changes, such as a change in pH, or simply heating a food, can cause dramatic changes in protein molecules. Such changes are seen, for example, when cottage cheese is made by adding acid to milk or when scrambled eggs are made by heating and stirring eggs.

Proteins are very important in foods, both nutritionally and as functional ingredients. They play an important role in determining the texture of a food. They are complex molecules, and it is important to have an understanding of the basics of protein structure to understand the behavior of many foods during processing. This chapter covers the basics of amino acid and protein structure. Individual proteins, such as milk, meat, wheat, and egg proteins, are covered in the chapters relating to these specific foods.

131

AMINO ACIDS

General Structure of Amino Acids

Every *amino acid* contains a central carbon atom, to which is attached a carboxyl group (COOH), an amino group (NH_2), a hydrogen atom, and another group or side chain R specific to the particular amino acid. The general formula for an amino acid is

$$
\begin{array}{c}
H \\
| \\
COOH - C - NH_2 \\
| \\
R
\end{array}
$$

Glycine is the simplest amino acid, with the R group being a hydrogen atom. There are more than 20 different amino acids in proteins. Their properties depend on the nature of their side chains or R groups.

In a solution at pH 7, all amino acids are *zwitterions;* that is, the amino group and carboxyl groups are both ionized and exist as COO^- and NH_3^+, respectively. Therefore, amino acids are *amphoteric* and can behave as an acid or as a base in water depending on the pH. When acting as an acid or proton donor, the positively charged amino group donates a hydrogen ion, and when acting as a base the negatively charged carboxyl group gains a hydrogen ion, as follows:

$$
\text{Acid:} \quad
\begin{array}{c}
H \\
| \\
R - C - COO^- \\
| \\
NH_3^+
\end{array}
\underset{\longleftarrow}{\longrightarrow}
\begin{array}{c}
H \\
| \\
R - C - COO^- + H^+ \\
| \\
NH_2
\end{array}
$$

$$
\text{Base:} \quad
\begin{array}{c}
H \\
| \\
R - C - COO^- + H^+ \\
| \\
NH_3^+
\end{array}
\underset{\longleftarrow}{\longrightarrow}
\begin{array}{c}
H \\
| \\
R - C - COOH \\
| \\
NH_3^+
\end{array}
$$

Categories of Amino Acids

Amino acids can be divided into four categories, according to the nature of their side chains, as shown in Figure 8.1. The first category includes all the amino acids with *hydrophobic* or **nonpolar** side chains. The hydrophobic (water-hating) amino acids contain a hydrocarbon side chain. Alanine is the simplest one, having a methyl group (CH_3) as its side chain. Valine and leucine contain longer, branched, hydrocarbon chains. Proline is an important nonpolar amino acid. It contains a bulky five-membered ring, which interrupts ordered protein structure. Methionine is a sulfur-containing nonpolar amino acid. The nonpolar amino acids are able to form hydrophobic interactions in proteins; that is, they associate with each other to avoid association with water.

The second group of amino acids includes those with **polar uncharged** side chains. This group is *hydrophilic*. Examples of amino acids in this group include serine, glutamine, and cysteine. They either contain a hydroxyl group (OH), an amide

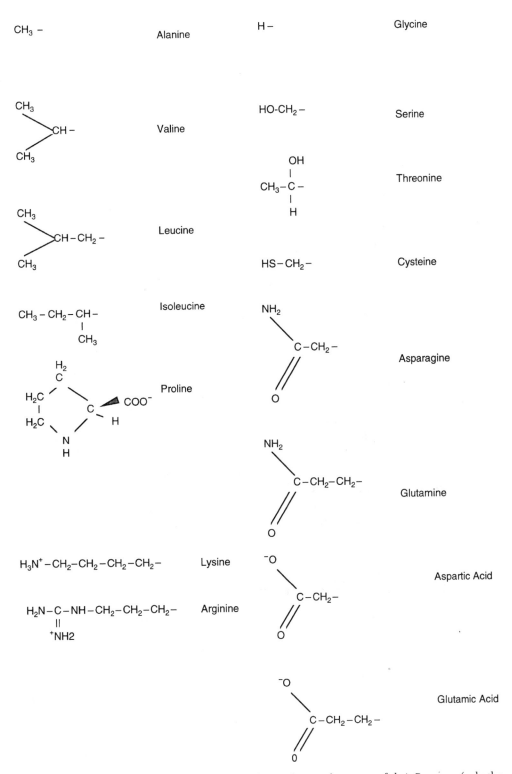

FIGURE 8.1 Examples of amino acids classified according to the nature of their R groups (only the side groups are shown).

group ($CONH_2$), or a thiol group (SH). All polar amino acids can form hydrogen bonds in proteins. Cysteine is unique because it can form **disulfide bonds** (–S–S–), as shown below:

$$X - CH_2 - SH \ + \ HS - CH_2 - X \longrightarrow X - CH_2 - S - S - CH_2 - X \ + \ H_2$$

cysteine   cystine

$$X = NH_2 - \overset{\displaystyle H}{\underset{\displaystyle COOH}{C}} -$$

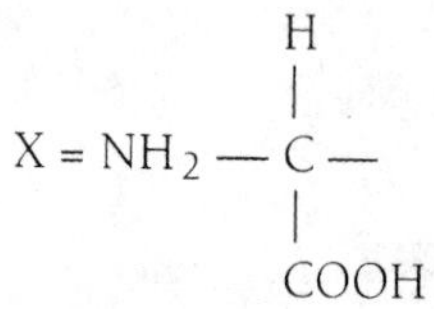

A disulfide bond is a strong covalent bond, unlike hydrogen bonds, which are weak interactions. Two molecules of cysteine can unite in a protein to form a disulfide bond. A few disulfide bonds in a protein have a significant effect on protein structure, because they are strong bonds. Proteins containing disulfide bonds are usually relatively heat stable, and more resistant to unfolding than other proteins. The presence of cysteine in a protein therefore tends to have a significant effect on protein conformation.

The third and fourth categories of amino acids include the charged amino acids. The **positively charged (basic)** amino acids include lysine, arginine, and histidine. These are positively charged at pH 7 because they contain an extra amino group. When a basic amino acid is part of a protein, this extra amino group is free (in other words, not involved in a peptide bond) and, depending on the pH, may be positively charged.

The negatively charged (acidic) amino acids include aspartic acid and glutamic acid. These are negatively charged at pH 7 because they both contain an extra carboxyl group. When an acidic amino acid is contained within a protein, the extra carboxyl group is free and may be charged, depending on the pH.

Oppositely charged groups are able to form ionic interactions with each other. In proteins, acidic and basic amino acid side chains may interact with each other, forming ionic bonds or salt bridges.

PROTEIN STRUCTURE AND CONFORMATION

All proteins are made up of many amino acids, joined by **peptide bonds** as shown below:

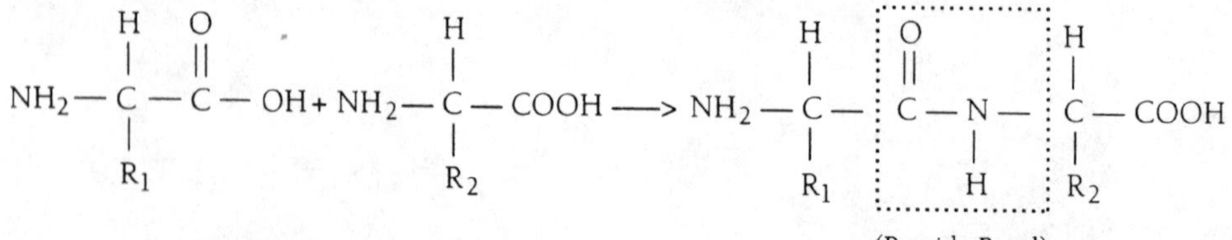

(Peptide Bond)

Peptide bonds are strong bonds and are not easily disrupted. A **dipeptide** contains two amino acids joined by a peptide bond. A **polypeptide** contains several amino acids joined by peptide bonds. Proteins are usually much larger molecules, containing several hundred amino acids. They can be hydrolyzed, yielding smaller polypeptides, by enzymes or by acid digestion.

The sequence of amino acids joined by peptide bonds forms the backbone of a protein, as shown below:

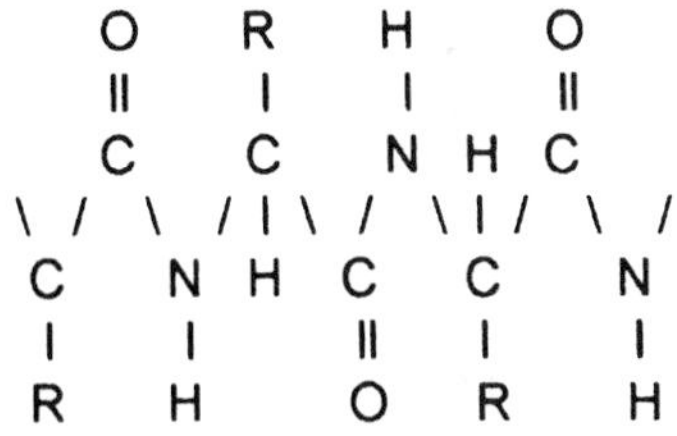

```
    O     R     H        O
    ||    |     |        ||
    C     C     N  H     C
   \ /  \ / | \ /  \ | / \ /
    C    N  H  C     C     N
    |    |     ||    |     |
    R    H     O     R     H
```

- The protein backbone consists of repeating N–C–C units.
- The amino acid side chains (R groups) project alternately from either side of the protein chain.
- The nature of the R groups determines the structure or **conformation** of the chain. (In other words, the shape the protein assumes in space.)

Each protein has a complex and unique conformation, which is determined by the specific amino acids and the sequence in which they occur along the chain. To understand the function of proteins in food systems and the changes that occur in proteins during processing, it is important to understand the basics of protein structure. Proteins are described as having four types of structure—primary, secondary, tertiary, and quaternary structure—and these build on each other. The primary structure determines the secondary structure and so on. The different types of protein structures are outlined below.

Primary Structure

The primary structure (*protein primary structure*) of a protein is the specific sequence of amino acids joined by peptide bonds along the protein chain. This is the simplest way of looking at protein structure. In reality, proteins do not exist simply as straight chains. However, it is the specific sequence of amino acids that determines the form or shape that a protein assumes in space. Therefore, it is essential to know the primary structure if a more detailed understanding of the structure and function of a particular protein is desired.

Secondary Structure

The secondary structure (*protein secondary structure*) of a protein refers to the three-dimensional organization of segments of the polypeptide chain. Important secondary structures include the following:

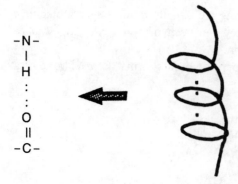

FIGURE 8.2 Schematic three-dimensional structure of an α-helix.

- Alpha helix—ordered structure
- Beta pleated sheet—ordered structure
- Random coil—disordered structure

The **alpha (α) helix** is a corkscrew structure, with 3.6 amino acids per turn. It is shown in Figure 8.2. It is stabilized by intrachain hydrogen bonds; that is, the hydrogen bonds occur within a single protein chain, rather than between adjacent chains. Hydrogen bonds occur between each turn of the helix. The oxygen and hydrogen atoms that comprise the peptide bonds are involved in hydrogen bond formation. The α-helix is a stable, organized structure. It cannot be formed if proline is present, because the bulky five-membered ring prevents formation of the helix.

The **beta (β) pleated sheet** is a more extended conformation than the α-helix. It can be thought of as a zigzag structure rather than a corkscrew. It is shown in Figure 8.3. The stretched protein chains combine to form β-pleated sheets. These sheets are linked together by interchain hydrogen bonds. (Interchain hydrogen bonds occur between adjacent sections of the protein chains rather than within an individual chain.) Again,

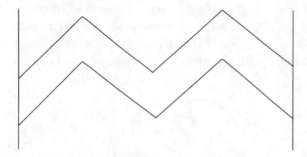

FIGURE 8.3 Schematic three-dimensional structure of β-pleated sheets.

the hydrogen and oxygen atoms that form the peptide bonds are involved in hydrogen bond formation. Like the α-helix, the β-pleated sheet is also an ordered structure.

The **random coil** is a secondary structure with no regular or ordered pattern along the polypeptide chain. This is a much more flexible structure than either the α-helix or β-pleated sheet. It is formed when amino acid side chains prevent formation of the α-helix or β-sheet. This may occur if proline is present or if there are highly charged regions within the protein.

A protein may contain regions of α-helix, β-sheet, and random coil at different places along the chain. How much of each type of secondary structure it contains depends on the sequence of amino acids or, in other words, on the primary structure of the protein.

Tertiary Structure

The **tertiary structure** of a protein refers to the three-dimensional organization of the complete protein chain. In other words, it refers to the spatial arrangement of a protein chain that contains regions of α-helix, β-sheet, and random coil. So, this structure is really an overview of a protein chain, rather than a detailed look at a small section of it. Again, the tertiary structure is built on the secondary structure of a specific protein.

There are two types of protein tertiary structure:

- Fibrous proteins
- Globular proteins

Fibrous proteins include structural proteins such as collagen (connective tissue protein), or actin and myosin, which are the proteins that are responsible for muscle contraction. The protein chains are extended, forming rods or fibers. Proteins with a fibrous tertiary structure contain a large amount of ordered secondary structure (either α-helix or β-sheet).

Globular proteins are compact molecules and are spherical or elliptical in shape, as their name suggests. These include transport proteins, such as myoglobin, which carry oxygen to the muscle. The whey proteins and the caseins, both of which are milk proteins, are also globular proteins. Globular tertiary structure is favored by proteins with a large number of hydrophobic amino acids. These orient toward the center of the molecule and interact with each other by hydrophobic interactions. Hydrophilic amino acids orient toward the outside of the molecule and interact with other molecules; for example, they may form hydrogen bonds with water. The orientation of the hydrophobic amino acids toward the center of the molecule produces the compact globular shape that is characteristic of globular proteins.

Quaternary Structure

Protein quaternary structure, or the quaternary protein structure, involves the noncovalent association of protein chains. The protein chains may or may not be identical. Examples of quaternary structure include the actomyosin system of muscles and the casein micelles of milk. For more information on these structures, the reader is referred to the chapters on meat and milk, respectively.

Interactions Involved in Protein Structure and Conformation

Protein primary structure involves only peptide bonds, which link the amino acids together in a specific and unique sequence. Secondary and tertiary structures may be stabilized by hydrogen bonds, disulfide bonds, hydrophobic interactions, and ionic interactions. *Steric* or spatial effects are also important in determining protein conformation. The space that a protein molecule occupies is determined partially by the size and shape of the individual amino acids along the protein chain. For example, bulky side chains such as proline prevent formation of the α-helix and favor random coil formation. This prevents the protein from assuming certain arrangements in space.

Quaternary structures are stabilized by the same interactions, with the exception of disulfide bonds. As has already been mentioned, disulfide bonds are strong, covalent bonds, and so only a few disulfide bonds will have a dramatic effect on protein conformation and stability. Hydrogen bonds, on the other hand, are weak bonds, but they are important because there are so many of them.

Each protein takes on a unique native conformation in space, which can almost be considered as a "fingerprint." As has already been mentioned, the exact folding of the protein into its natural conformation is governed by the amino acids that are present in the protein and the bonds that the side chains are able to form in a protein. The amino acid sequence is also important, as the location of the amino acids along the chain determines which types of bonds will be formed and where, and thus determines how much α-helix, β-sheet, or random coil will be present in a protein. This, in turn, determines the tertiary and quaternary structure of a protein, all of which combine to define its native conformation. Knowledge of protein conformation and stability is essential to understanding the effects of processing on food proteins.

REACTIONS AND PROPERTIES OF PROTEINS

Amphoteric

Like amino acids, proteins are *amphoteric* (being able to act as an acid or a base) depending on the pH. This enables them to resist small changes in pH. Such molecules are said to have buffering capacity.

Isoelectric Point

The *isoelectric point* of a protein is the pH at which the protein is electrically neutral (It is denoted by pI). At this pH, the global or overall charge on the protein is zero. This does not mean that the protein contains no charged groups. It means that the number of positive charges on the protein is equal to the number of negative charges. At the isoelectric point, the protein molecules usually precipitate because they do not carry a net charge. (Molecules that carry a like charge repel each other, and thus form a stable dispersion in water. Removal of the charge removes the repulsive force and allows the molecules to interact with each other and precipitate, in most cases.)

The pH of the isoelectric point differs for each protein. It depends on the ratio of free ionized carboxyl groups to free ionized amino groups in the protein.

The isoelectric point is important in food processing. For example, cottage cheese is made by adding lactic acid to milk to bring the pH to the isoelectric point of the major milk proteins (the caseins). The proteins precipitate at this pH, forming curds. These are separated from the rest of the milk and may be pressed and/or mildly salted before being packaged as cottage cheese.

Water-Binding Capacity

Water molecules can bind to the backbone and to polar and charged side chains of a protein. Depending on the nature of their side chains, proteins may bind varying amounts of water—they have a *water-binding capacity*. Proteins with many charged and polar groups bind water readily, whereas proteins with many hydrophobic groups do not bind much water. As proteins get closer to their isoelectric point, they tend to bind less water, because reduced charge on the protein molecules results in reduced affinity for water molecules.

The presence of bound water helps to maintain the stability of a protein dispersion. This is due to the fact that the bound water molecules shield the protein molecules from each other. Therefore, they do not associate with each other or precipitate as readily, and so the dispersion tends to be more stable.

Salting-In and Salting-Out

Some proteins cannot be dispersed in pure water but are readily dispersed in dilute salt solutions. When a salt solution increases the dispersibility of a protein, this is termed "**salting-in**." It occurs because charged groups on a protein bind the anions and cations of the salt solution more strongly than water. The ions, in turn, bind water; thus, the protein is dispersed in water more easily.

Salting-in is important in food processing. For example, brine may be injected into ham to increase the dispersibility of the proteins. This has the effect of increasing their water-binding capacity, and so the ham is moister and its weight is increased. The same is true for poultry to which polyphosphates are added.

Salting-out occurs at high salt concentrations, when salts compete with the protein for water. The result is that there is insufficient water available to bind to the protein, and so the protein precipitates. This is not normally a problem in food processing. However, it may be a contributing factor to the deterioration of food quality during freezing of foods; during the freezing process, water is effectively removed as ice crystals, and so the concentration of liquid water decreases and the solute concentration increases dramatically. This is discussed in Chapter 17.

Denaturation

Denaturation is the change in the secondary, tertiary, and or quaternary structure of a protein. There is no change in the primary structure. In other words, denaturation does not involve breaking of peptide bonds. The protein unfolds, but there is no change in its amino acid sequence. Denaturation may occur as a result of the following:

- Heat
- pH change
- Ionic strength change (changes in salt concentration)
- Freezing
- Surface changes (occuring while beating egg whites)

Any of these factors may cause breaking of hydrogen bonds and salt bridges. As a result, the protein unfolds and side chains that were buried in the center of the molecule become exposed. They are then available to react with other chemical groups and, in most cases, the denatured protein precipitates. This reaction is usually irreversible; it is not possible to regain the original conformation of the denatured protein.

The changes that produce denaturation are usually mild changes. In other words, mild heat treatment, such as pasteurization or blanching, or small changes in pH are sufficient to change the conformation of a protein.

Denatured proteins normally lose their functional properties; that is, they are unable to perform their normal function in a food. Enzymes are inactivated and so the reactions that they catalyzed can no longer take place. This has important implications in food processing.

Denaturation may be desirable and can be deliberately brought about by food processing. Examples of desirable denaturation include heating beaten egg white foams to form meringues, adding acid to milk to form cottage cheese, or inactivating enzymes by heat, as occurs when vegetables are blanched before freezing. Blanching is a mild heat treatment that denatures and inactivates enzymes that would cause rancidity or discoloration during frozen storage.

Sometimes denaturation is undesirable. For example, frozen egg yolks are lumpy and unacceptable when thawed because the lipoproteins denature and aggregate. Overheating of foods can also cause unwanted denaturation. Food processors must be careful to utilize processing methods that do not cause unnecessary deterioration of food quality due to protein denaturation.

Hydrolysis of Peptides and Proteins

Hydrolysis of proteins involves breaking peptide bonds to form smaller peptide chains. This can be achieved by acid digestion, using concentrated acid. This may be appropriate in protein research, but it is not an option in food processing. Hydrolysis is also catalyzed by **proteolytic** enzymes. Examples of such enzymes used in foods include ficin, papain, and bromelain, which are used as meat tenderizers. They hydrolyze muscle protein or connective tissue, making meat more tender. It is important to control the duration of time that they are in contact with the meat so that too much hydrolysis does not occur. Too much hydrolysis would make the texture of the meat soft and "mushy" (see Chapter 9).

Another example of a proteolytic enzyme is rennet, which is used to make cheese (see Chapter 11). This enzyme is very specific in its action, hydrolyzing a specific peptide bond in the milk protein. The result of this hydrolysis reaction is aggregation of the milk proteins to form curds, which can then be processed into cheese.

Maillard Browning

Maillard browning is the reaction that is responsible for the brown color of baked products. A free carbonyl group of a reducing sugar reacts with a free amino group on a protein when heated, and the result is a brown color. The reaction is highly complex and has a significant effect on the flavor of foods as well as the color. It is known as nonenzymatic browning, because the reaction is not catalyzed by an enzyme (Maillard browning must be distinguished from enzymatic browning, which is the discoloration of damaged fruits or vegetables and is catalyzed by an enzyme such as phenol oxidase; enzymatic browning is discussed in Chapter 7).

The Maillard reaction is favored by the following:

- High sugar content
- High protein concentration
- High temperatures
- High pH
- Low water content

Maillard browning is responsible for the discoloration of food products such as powdered milk and powdered egg. Before drying, eggs are usually "desugared" enzymatically to remove glucose and prevent Maillard browning (see Chapter 10).

The reaction causes loss of the amino acids lysine, arginine, tryptophan, and histidine, as these are the amino acids with free amino groups that are able to react with reducing sugars. With the exception of arginine, these are essential amino acids. (The body cannot make them, and so they must be included in the diet.) Therefore, it is important to retard the Maillard reaction, particularly in susceptible food products (such as food supplies sent to underdeveloped countries) in which the nutritional quality of the protein is very important.

ENZYMES

All enzymes are proteins. Enzymes are important in foods, because they catalyze various reactions that affect color, flavor, or texture, and hence quality of foods. Some of these reactions may be desirable, whereas others are undesirable, and produce unwanted discoloration or off-flavors in foods.

Each enzyme has a unique structure or conformation, which enables it to attach to its specific substrate and catalyze the reaction. When the reaction is complete, the enzyme is released to act as a catalyst again. All enzymes have an optimal temperature and pH range, within which the reaction will proceed most rapidly. Heat or changes in pH denature the enzymes, making it difficult or impossible for them to attach to their respective substrates, and thus inactivating them.

If an enzymatic reaction is required in food processing, it is important to ensure that the optimal pH and temperature range for that enzyme is achieved. Outside the optimal range, the reaction will proceed more slowly, if at all. Heat treatment must therefore be avoided. If this is not possible, the enzyme must be added after heat treatment and subsequent cooling of the food.

On the other hand, if enzyme action is undesirable, the enzymes must be inactivated. This is usually achieved by heat treatment, but may also be accomplished by adding acid to change the pH.

Examples of desirable enzymatic reactions include the clotting of milk by *rennet*, which is the first step in making cheese (Chapter 11). Ripening of cheese during storage is also due to enzyme activity. Ripening of fruit is also due to enzyme action (Chapter 7). Other desirable enzymatic reactions include tenderizing of meat by proteolytic enzymes such as *papain, bromelain,* and *ficin* (Chapter 9). As was mentioned earlier, these enzymes catalyze hydrolysis of peptide bonds in proteins. They are added to the meat and allowed to work for a period of time. The reaction must be controlled, to prevent too much breakdown of the proteins. The optimum temperature for these enzymes occurs during the early cooking stages. (Hydrolysis proceeds very slowly at refrigeration temperatures.) As meat is cooked, the enzymes promote hydrolysis. However, as the internal temperature continues to rise, the enzymes are inactivated and the reaction is stopped.

Although useful as meat tenderizers, proteolytic enzymes may be undesirable in other circumstances. For example, if a gelatin salad is made with raw pineapple, the jelly may not set, due to action of *bromelain*, which is contained in pineapple. This can be prevented by heating the pineapple to inactivate the enzyme before making the gelatin salad.

Other examples of unwanted enzymatic reactions include enzymatic browning, which occurs when fruits and vegetables are damaged, due to the action of *polyphenol oxidase*, and produces undesirable discoloration (Chapter 7). Development of off-flavors in fats and fat-containing foods may also be a problem in some circumstances, and this may be caused by *lipase* or *lipoxygenase* (Chapter 12).

Enzymes are inactivated in fruits and vegetables prior to freezing by a mild heat process known as blanching (Chapter 17). The fruits or vegetables are placed in boiling water for a short time, in order to inactivate the enzymes that would cause discoloration or development of off-flavors during frozen storage.

FUNCTIONAL ROLES OF PROTEINS IN FOODS

Proteins have many useful **functional properties** in foods. A functional property is a characteristic of the protein that enables it to perform a specific role, or function, in a food. For example, a protein with the ability to form a gel may be used in a food with the specific intention of forming a gel, as in use of gelatin to make jelly.

Functional properties or roles of proteins in foods include solubility and nutritional value. They may also be used as thickening, binding or gelling agents, and as emulsifiers or foaming agents.

The functional properties of a specific protein depend on its amino acid composition and sequence since these determine the conformation and properties of the protein.

Although no single protein exhibits all the functional properties, most proteins may perform several different functions in foods, depending on the processing conditions. Some proteins are well known for specific functional properties in foods.

Whey protein is an example of a protein that is used for its *solubility* (Chapter 11). Whey is soluble at acid pH, because it is relatively hydrophilic and able to bind a lot of water, and so, unlike many proteins, it does not precipitate at its isoelectric point. Because of its solubility, whey protein is used to fortify acidic beverages such as sports drinks. Whey protein may also be used as a *nutritional fortifier* in other products including baked goods.

Egg proteins are used as *thickening* or *binding* agents in many food products (Chapter 10). Meat proteins are also good binding agents.

Gelatin and egg white proteins are examples of *gelling* agents (Chapter 10). When egg whites are heated, they form a firm gel as can be seen in a boiled egg. Gelatin is used to make jelly and other congealed products. Gelatin gels are formed when the protein molecules form a three-dimensional network due to association by hydrogen bonds. Gelatin gels can be melted by heating, and reformed on cooling. Egg white gels, on the other hand, are formed due to association by hydrophobic interactions and disulfide bonds, and they do not melt on heating. The proteins of gluten are another example of proteins that are able to associate to form a three-dimensional network (Chapter 15). The gluten network is formed during kneading of bread dough, and is responsible for the texture and volume of a loaf of bread. Soy protein may also be used to form food gels.

Many proteins are used as either *emulsifiers* or *foaming agents*, as discussed in Chapter 13. Proteins are **amphiphilic**, containing both hydrophobic and hydrophilic sections in the same molecule. This allows them to exist at an interface between oil and water, or between air and water, rather than in either bulk phase. They are able to adsorb at an interface and associate to form a stable film, thus stabilizing emulsions or foams. Egg white proteins are the best foaming agents, whereas egg yolk proteins are the best emulsifying agents. The caseins of milk are also excellent emulsifiers.

Proteins are used in many foods to control texture, due to their ability to thicken, gel or emulsify. Such food products must be processed, handled and stored with care, to ensure that the proteins retain their functional properties. Some protein denaturation is usually necessary to form an emulsion, a foam, or a gel. However, too much denaturation due to incorrect processing conditions or poor handling and storage may result in undesirable textural changes (such as breaking of emulsions, loss of foam volume, or syneresis in gels) and must be avoided.

CONJUGATED PROTEINS

Conjugated proteins are also known as heteroproteins. They are proteins that contain a prosthetic group that may be an organic or an inorganic component. Examples of conjugated proteins include the following:

- Phosphoproteins—for example, casein (milk protein); phosphate groups are esterified to serine residues.

- Glycoproteins—for example, κ-casein; a carbohydrate or sugar is attached to the protein.

- Lipoproteins—for example, lipovitellin, in egg yolk; a lipid is attached to the protein.

- Hemoproteins—for example, hemoglobin and myoglobin; iron is complexed with the protein.

CONCLUSION

Proteins are complex molecules that are widely distributed in all foodstuffs. It is important to understand their conformation and reactions in order to know how they will behave during food processing and to understand how to maximize their functional properties. This is especially true of protein-rich foods, where the quality of the final product depends to a large extent on the treatment of the protein during processing and handling. This chapter has focused on general properties of food proteins. More details of the composition and functional properties of some specific food proteins are given in the ensuing chapters.

GLOSSARY

Amino acid: Building block of proteins; contains an amino group, a carboxyl group, a hydrogen, and a side chain, all attached to a central carbon atom.

Amphiphilic: A molecule that contains both hydrophobic and hydrophilic sections.

Amphoteric: Capable of functioning as either an acid or as a base depending on the pH of the medium.

Alpha helix: Ordered protein secondary structure: corkscrew shape, stabilized by intrachain hydrogen bonds.

Beta-pleated sheet: Ordered protein secondary structure; zigzag shape, stabilized by interchain hydrogen bonds.

Conformation: The specific folding and shape that a protein assumes in space.

Denaturation: Changes in the conformation (secondary, tertiary, or quaternary structure) of a protein caused by changes in temperature, pH or ionic strength, or by surface changes.

Dipeptide: Two amino acids joined by a peptide bond.

Disulfide bond: Strong covalent bond formed by the reaction of two thiol (SH) groups.

Functional property: Characteristic of the molecule that enables it to perform a specific role in a food. Examples of functional properties of proteins include solubility, thickening, binding, gelation, foaming, and emulsifying capacity.

Hydrolysis: Breaking of one or more peptide bonds in a protein to form smaller polypeptide chains.

Hydrophilic: Water-loving; characteristic of polar and charged groups.

Hydrophobic: Water-hating; characteristic of nonpolar groups.

Isoelectric point: pI; the pH at which the overall charge on a protein is zero; the number of positive charges is equal to the number of negative charges; the protein is most susceptible to denaturation and precipitation at this pH.

Maillard browning: The free carbonyl group of a reducing sugar and the free amino group of a protein react to form a brown color; complex nonenzymatic reaction that is favored by high temperatures.

Peptide bond: Bond formed by the reaction of the amino group of one amino acid and the carboxyl group of another.

Polypeptide: Several amino acids joined together by peptide bonds.

Protein primary structure: Specific sequence of amino acids along the protein chain, joined by peptide bonds, the covalently bonded protein backbone.

Protein quaternary structure: The noncovalent association of protein chains to form a discrete unit.

Protein secondary structure: Three-dimensional arrangement of sections of the protein chain; secondary structures include the α-helix, β-pleated sheet, and random coil.

Protein tertiary structure: Three-dimensional arrangement of the whole protein chain; the shape that a protein chain assumes in space; includes fibrous and globular structures.

Proteolytic: Breaks down or hydrolyses proteins.

Random coil: A protein secondary structure that exhibits no regular, ordered pattern.

Salting-in: Addition of a dilute salt solution to improve the dispersibility of a protein.

Salting-out: Addition of a concentrated salt solution to precipitate a protein.

Steric effects: Effects caused by the size and shape of the amino acids comprising the protein chain; spatial effects; for example, bulky amino acids can prevent a protein from folding upon itself in certain ways.

Water-binding capacity: The ability of a protein to bind water; this ability depends on the number of charged and polar groups along the protein chain.

Zwitterion: Contains a positively charged group and a negatively charged group within the molecule.

BIBLIOGRAPHY

Charley H, Weaver, C. *Foods. A Scientific Approach*, 3rd ed. New York: Merrill/Prentice-Hall, 1998.

Coultate TP. *Food. The Chemistry of its Components*, 2nd ed. RSC: Cambridge, 1989.

Damodaran S. Amino acids, peptides and proteins. In: Fennema O, ed. *Food Chemistry*, 3rd ed. New York: Marcel Dekker, 1996.

McWilliams M. *Foods: Experimental Perspectives,* 4th ed. New York: Prentice-Hall, 2001.

Penfield MP, Campbell AM. *Experimental Food Science,* 3rd ed. San Diego, CA: Academic Press, 1990.

Potter N, Hotchkiss J. *Food Science,* 5th ed. New York: Chapman & Hall, 1995.

Vieira ER. *Elementary Food Science,* 4th ed. New York: Chapman & Hall, 1996.

CHAPTER 9

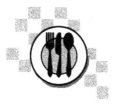

Meat, Poultry, Fish, and Dry Beans

INTRODUCTION

Meat is the edible portion of mammals—the flesh of animals used for food and includes cattle (beef and veal), hogs (pork), and sheep (lamb or mutton). It is also the processed or manufactured products of the tissues. "Meat" may include rabbit, venison, and other game, as well as the nonmammals poultry and fish, and other animal flesh may be used as food in various parts of the world. *Red meat* is the meat from mammals, *white meat* refers to meat from poultry, *seafood* is derived from fish, and *game* is from non-domesticated animals.

Meat is composed of muscle, connective tissue, and adipose tissue (fat). The location of the cut of meat on the animal, muscle contraction, and postmortem changes—all influence the degree of meat tenderness. Some cuts are inherently more tender than others, requiring different cooking methods. Lean meats contain less adipose tissue than well-marbled cuts of meat.

All meat is subject to mandatory inspection by the USDA and voluntary grading. Thereafter, it may be altered by processing methods such as curing, smoking, restructuring, and tenderizing.

Consumption of red meat has declined over the past decades, and intake of poultry has increased. If meat consumption is minimized or omitted from the diet, for any number of reasons, an individual must obtain similar nutrients from a nonmeat source, such as combination of various plant produce (Chapter 7). It becomes important to know that only animal protein is a *complete* protein. It is resynthesized from the *incomplete* plant proteins of animal feed. The USDA recommends consumption of 2–3 daily servings of meat, poultry, or fish (3 ounce servings); dry beans, eggs, or nuts.

CHARACTERISTICS OF MEAT

Physical Composition of Meat

Meat is composed of three tissues: muscle tissue, or the lean part of meat with blood vessels, connective tissue, and adipose or fatty tissue.

Muscle Tissue.   Muscle tissue is referred to as the lean tissue of meat. It includes 1. **cardiac** 2. **skeletal** muscle, both of which are striated muscle that contain transverse striations of the fibers, and 3. **smooth** muscle. *Cardiac* muscle is located in the heart. Skeletal muscle is the primary component of the carcass, and provides support for the weight of the body, and movement, or locomotion for the body. It is usually attached to the bone. Smooth muscle is the visceral muscle, located in the digestive tract, reproduction system, and throughout the blood vessels of the circulatory system.

Inside the muscle cell membrane, (Figure 9.1) there are **myofibrils** containing alternating thin and thick protein filaments, *actin* and *myosin,* which contract and relax in the living animal. The muscle fibers, made up of the myofibrils, are varied in length, perhaps 1 or 2 inches and very small in diameter. Each fiber is cylindrical, with tapered ends, and is covered by a thin connective tissue sheath called **endomysium.** Small bundles of 20–40 fibers make up one primary bundle that represents the "*grain*" of meat. The primary bundle is surrounded by **perimysium** connective tissue.

Several primary bundles form a larger, secondary bundle that contains blood vessels and nerves. Each secondary bundle is surrounded by perimysium connective tissue, and several of the secondary bundles are surrounded by **epimysium**, dividing one skeletal muscle from another.

Between muscle bundles, there are blood vessels (capillaries) and small pockets of fat cells.

Connective Tissue.   Connective tissue is located throughout the muscle (Figure 9.1). It is composed of endomysium, perimysium, and epimysium structures that bind muscle fibers in bundles to form muscle. It extends beyond the muscle fibers to form tendons, which attach the muscle to bones and holds and connects various parts of the body. The tough skin, or hide of an animal, is connected to underlying animal tissue by connective tissue.

Meat that contains a high degree of muscle tissue naturally has a greater amount of connective tissue to hold *myofibrils* and *bundles* in the muscle. The composition of connective tissue is primarily protein, especially **collagen**, held inside mucopolysaccharides. It is the most abundant protein found in the body of intact mammals—found in bone, cartilage, tendons and ligament, enveloping muscle groups, and separating muscle layers. It is in horns, hooves, and skin.

Collagen is a triple-coil protein structure that is white in color and contracts to a thick mass when heated. Yet, it becomes more tender when cooked with *moist* heat, as it is converted (gelatinized) to water-soluble **gelatin** (which may in turn be used for edible gels in the diet.) In *older* animals, the collagen coil may form many cross-linkages that allow less solubilization of collagen to (the more tender) gelatin.

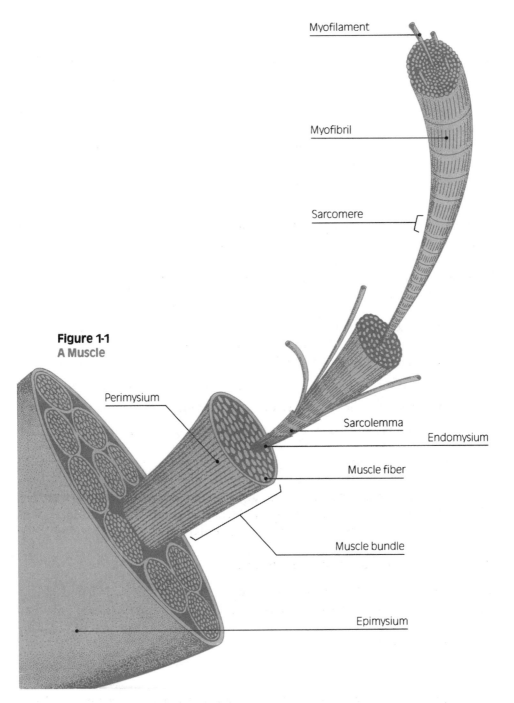

Myofilament

Myofibril

Sarcomere

Figure 1-1
A Muscle

Perimysium

Sarcolemma

Endomysium

Muscle fiber

Muscle bundle

Epimysium

FIGURE 9.1   Diagram of a lean muscle and its connective tissue
(*Source*: National Cattlemen's Beef Association).

A lesser component of connective tissue is the yellow-colored *elastin* protein, which is more elastic than collagen and is found in the walls of the circulatory system and throughout the animal body. It assists in holding bone and cartilage together. Elastin is extensive in muscles used in locomotion, such as legs, and is not softened (solubilized to gelatin) in cooking, as is collagen.

Another minor connective tissue component is *reticulin* connective tissue protein found in younger animals. It may be the precursor of collagen or elastin.

Overall, connective tissue is present to a greater degree in the muscle of *older* animals. Meat high in connective tissue may be ground to break the connective tissue and increase tenderization of the meat.

Fatty Tissue. Cuts of meat may vary substantially in composition and appearance due to the presence of *adipose* or *fatty tissue*. Fat stores energy for animals and its content is dependent on factors such as animal feed, hormone balance, age, and genetics. Fat is held by strands of connective tissue throughout the body and is deposited in several places around organs, under the skin, and between and within muscles. These deposits include the following:

- Adipose tissue—fat is stored around the heart, kidney organs, and in the pelvic canal areas. (Suet refers to the hard fatty tissue around the kidneys and other glandular organs of cattle and sheep.)

- Subcutaneous fat (finish)—fat is visible after the skin is removed.

- Intermuscular fat—the fat between muscles (also known as seam fat).

- Intramuscular fat—the fat within muscles (marbling) (Figure 9.2).

Lean meat is primarily muscle tissue and contains less visible fat than a well-*marbled* meat that contains both intermuscular and intramuscular fatty tissues throughout the muscle. The percentage of fat stores generally increases with age, following the major stage of muscle growth. Melted fat contributes to juiciness, thus the sensation of tenderness, and it contributes to flavor.

CHEMICAL COMPOSITION OF MEAT

Meat contains 45–70% water with the greatest percentage of water found in lean meat and young animals. Meat contains 15–20% protein, and anywhere from 5 to 40% fat, depending on the cut and trim. It contains no carbohydrate (except for the liver, which stores glycogen).

Water

Water is the major constituent of meat. As an animal becomes more mature and fatter, water forms a smaller proportion of the entire makeup compared to young, lean animals. This decrease in the percentage of water is due to the fact that there is an increase in adipose tissue, which contains only a negligible amount of water. Water exists in muscle fibers and, to a lesser degree, in connective tissue. It is released from the protein structure as the muscle coagulates during cooking. The water content is also

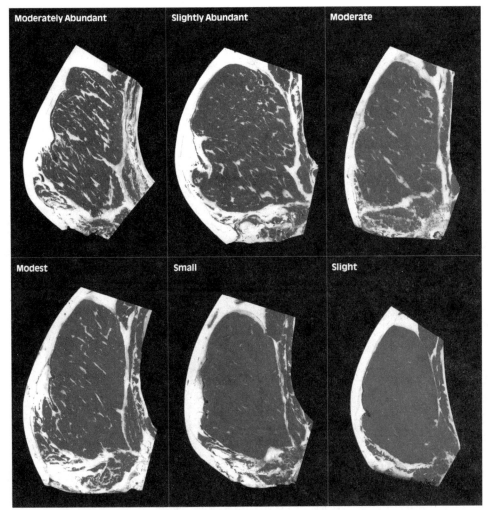

The above illustrations are reduced reproductions of the Official USDA Marbling Photographs prepared for the U.S. Department of Agriculture by and available from the National Live Stock and Meat Board.

FIGURE 9.2   Different levels of fat marbling
(*Source*: National Cattlemen's Beef Association).

decreased as muscle fibers are broken due to chemical, enzymatic, or mechanical tenderization, or salting, or if the pH is changed. Inversely, water may be added to meats such as cured ham.

(A recent repercussion of meeting the government's food safety requirements of raw meats and poultry is water retention. Thus, according to the USDA, processors must list either the maximum percentage of absorbed water, or retained water on applicable food labels.)

Protein

Meat is high in proteins that have a high biological value, that is, they contain all of the essential amino acids in amounts and proportions that can be used in synthesizing body proteins. There are three primary types of proteins in meats: myofibril, stromal proteins, and sarcoplasmic proteins.

Myofibril proteins: Muscle bundles are groups of myofibrils composed of several protein molecules including actin and myosin. During muscle contraction, actin and myosin myofibrils slide together forming an overlap complex called *actomyosin*.

Stromal proteins (connective tissue proteins): The watery connective tissue contains fibrils of stromal proteins: collagen, elastin, and reticulin (discussed earlier).

Sarcoplasmic proteins: A third general classification of meat proteins that includes the pigments and glycolytic enzymes. For example, the *hemoglobin* pigment stores oxygen in the red blood cells bringing it to tissues, including the muscles, while *myoglobin* stores oxygen in the muscle where it is needed for metabolism.

The species, age, sex, and specific muscle show differences in myoglobin concentration. There is more myoglobin in the muscles of cows than pigs, more in older sheep than young lambs, more in bulls (adult males) than cows, and more in frequently exercised portions of the animal, such as muscles of the diaphragm.

There are also numerous *enzymes* in fluid of the muscle cell. Enzymes of the sarcoplasm may be *proteolytic*—degrading protein during the aging of meat, *amylolytic*—degrading carbohydrates or *lypolytic*—degrading fats.

Fat

Fats (in the form of triglycerides) are one of the major components of meat. Triglycerides in the adipose tissue differ in the degree of saturation and number of carbons (see Figure 9.2). Subcutaneous fats are generally more unsaturated than fat deposited first, around glandular organs. While saturation of fats promotes less oxidation, and therefore less rancidity of the meat, and while it contributes to the survival of the living animal at low environmental temperatures, high saturated fat diets are not recommended for health reasons.

Fats in the diet allow the fat-soluble vitamins A, D, E, and K to be carried. As well, fats contain some essential fatty acids that are the precursor material used in the synthesis of phospholipids for every cell membrane.

Cholesterol, a sterol, is present in the animal tissue, as it is in all cell membranes. Typically, lean meats have a lower content. An exception to this is veal (young, lean calf meat), which is low in fat, yet high in cholesterol.

Carbohydrates

Carbohydrates are plentiful in *plant* tissue but are negligible in *animal* tissue. Approximately half of the small percentage of carbohydrates in animals is stored in the *liver* as glycogen. The other half exists throughout the body, especially in *muscles*, and in the blood as glucose. A small amount is found in other glands and organs of animals. If an animal is exercised or not fed prior to slaughter, low glycogen levels in the liver and muscles may occur.

Vitamins and Minerals

Meat contains B-complex vitamins that function as cofactors in many energy-yielding metabolic reactions. The liver contains fat-soluble vitamins A, D, E, and K. The minerals iron (in heme and myoglobin pigments), zinc, and phosphorus are present in meat.

MUSCLE CONTRACTION IN LIVE ANIMALS

Muscle tissue of slaughtered animals undergoes several changes after slaughter. To understand the reactions that occur in meat and their effects on tenderness and quality, it is necessary to have a basic understanding of the structure and function of muscle in a live animal.

Structure of the Myofilaments of Muscle

Muscle fibers contain bundles of myofibrils, which are responsible for contraction in the living animal, as has already been mentioned. The myofibrils themselves are composed of bundles of protein filaments as shown in Figure 9.3. These include *thin* filaments, made mostly of **actin**, and *thick* filaments, which contain **myosin**. They are arranged in a specific pattern within a repeating longitudinal unit called a **sarcomere**. The thin filaments occur at each end of the sarcomere, and they are held in place by **Z-lines**. The Z-lines define the ends of each sarcomere. The thick filaments occur in the center of the sarcomere, and they overlap the thin filaments. The extent of overlap depends on whether the muscle is contracted or relaxed. In a relaxed muscle,

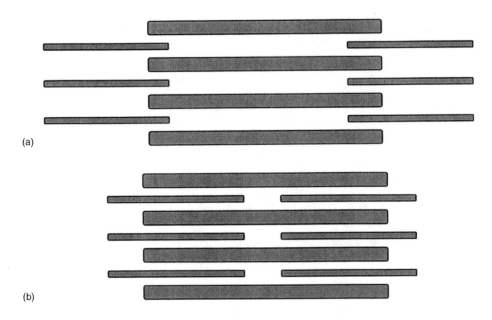

Figure 9.3 Sarcomere and protein filaments (a) relaxed (b) contracted.

the sarcomeres are extended, and there is not much overlap of thick and thin filaments. However, a contracted muscle has a lot of overlap because the sarcomeres shorten as part of the contraction process.

The thin and thick filaments are interspersed between each other in the regions where they overlap. A cross-section of the myofibrils shows that each thick filament is surrounded by six thin filaments, and every thin filament is surrounded by three thick filaments. This facilitates interaction between the thin and thick filaments when contraction occurs.

Muscle Contraction

Muscle contraction starts when a nerve impulse causes release of calcium ions from the sarcoplasmic reticulum into the sarcoplasm, which is a jellylike substance surrounding the thin and thick filaments of the myofibrils. The calcium ions bind to a specific site on the thin filaments, causing the active site on actin to be exposed. Actin molecules are then able to react with myosin, forming actomyosin. Adenosine triphosphate (ATP) is necessary as the energy source for this reaction. The myosin then contracts and pulls the actin-containing filaments further in toward the center of the sarcomere. The actomyosin complex then breaks, and myosin forms another cross-link with a different actin molecule. As the cycle continues, the sarcomere continues to shorten, and contraction occurs.

When the nerve impulse ceases, calcium ions are pumped out of the sarcoplasm and returned to the sarcoplasmic reticulum. Actin and myosin cannot interact without calcium ions, and so the actomyosin complex breaks. The muscle relaxes and returns to its original extended state.

Energy for Contraction

The energy for contraction comes primarily from aerobic respiration, which enables glucose to be broken down completely to yield CO_2 and 36 molecules of ATP. In animals, glucose is stored as glycogen, which is broken down as needed to supply energy. When short bursts of extreme muscle activity are necessary, aerobic respiration does not supply adequate amounts of ATP, and so energy is also obtained by anaerobic glycolysis. This is a more rapid but less efficient way of producing energy, as only two molecules of ATP are produced for every glucose molecule. Glycolysis converts glucose to lactic acid, which builds up in the muscle. (It is the buildup of lactic acid that makes muscles sore and stiff after strenuous exertion. When the strenuous activity ceases, lactic acid is oxidized and removed from the muscle.)

Both aerobic respiration and glycolysis can take place in a live animal. After slaughter, aerobic respiration ceases, but glycolysis continues for a while.

POSTMORTEM CHANGES IN THE MUSCLE

Prior to slaughter, muscle tissue is soft and pliable. Some time after slaughter (from 6 to 24 hours), muscle stiffens and becomes hard and inextensible. This stiffening is due to loss of extensibility by the myofibril proteins, actin and myosin, once energy reserves are nonexistent. The time period for stiffening is species-specific, and it is known as **rigor mortis**, which literally means "the stiffness of death." If meat is cooked at this stage, it is extremely tough. In fact, most meat is aged or conditioned to allow the muscles to become soft and pliable again before it is cooked. This 'resolution of rigor' is due to the enzymatic breakdown of proteins that hold muscle fibers together.

After slaughter, a sequence of events takes place in muscle that leads to the onset of rigor mortis. When the animal is killed, aerobic respiration ceases, blood flow stops, and the muscles are no longer supplied with oxygen. Therefore, anaerobic conditions soon prevail. Glycolysis continues, and glycogen stores are converted to lactic acid with the formation of ATP. The reaction continues until glycogen stores are depleted or until a pH of 5.5 is reached. At this pH, the enzymes that are responsible for glycolysis are denatured, and so the reaction stops. If glycogen is in short supply, glycolysis may stop due to depletion of glycogen, before the pH drops as low as 5.5.

When glycolysis stops, the ATP supply is quickly depleted. Lack of ATP prevents calcium ions from being pumped out of the sarcoplasm, and so the active site on the actin molecules of the thin myofilaments is available to bind with the myosin of the thick filaments. Actin and myosin unite, forming actomyosin cross-links. This cross-link formation is irreversible, as there is no available ATP. (In a live animal, actomyosin cross-links are formed and broken repeatedly, as part of contraction, but the cycle requires ATP.)

Formation of these irreversible actomyosin cross-links causes the muscle to become rigid. This is rigor mortis, and it correlates with the depletion of ATP in the muscle. Once formed, actomyosin cross-links do not break down, even during aging of meat, and their presence makes meat tough [Figure 9.3(b)].

The stiffness of the muscle at rigor depends on the extent of actomyosin formation, which, in turn, depends on the extent of overlap of the thin and thick myofilaments. The greater is the overlap of thin and thick myofilaments, the more extensive the formation of actomyosin, and the stiffer the muscle. This results in tough meat:

- Little overlap—few actomyosin cross-links (tender meat)
- Substantial overlap—many actomyosin cross-links (tough meat)

Because the extent of actomyosin formation affects the toughness of meat, it is important to minimize the number of cross-links formed. This is done in two ways:

1. The meat is hung on the carcass after slaughter to stretch the muscles. This minimizes shortening of the sarcomeres, and results in formation of fewer actomyosin cross-links.

2. Prerigor temperature is controlled to minimize shortening. The optimum temperature is between 59 and 68°F (15–20°C). Above this temperature, increased shortening occurs. Below it, "cold shortening" occurs. At low temperatures, the sarcoplasmic reticulum pump is unable to pump calcium ions out of the sarcoplasm, and so contraction occurs.

The more contraction prerigor, the shorter are the sarcomeres, and the greater the amount of overlap of the thin and thick myofilaments when the muscle goes into rigor. Both hanging the carcass and controlling prerigor temperature minimize contraction before the onset of rigor mortis, resulting in fewer actomyosin cross-links and increasing tenderness.

Ultimate pH

After slaughter, the pH drops due to the buildup of lactic acid, which is normally removed from the blood of the living animal. The ultimate pH is the pH that is reached when glycolysis ceases and is usually around 5.5. As mentioned already, glycolytic enzymes are close to their isoelectric point and are inactivated at this pH, thus preventing glycolysis from continuing. Therefore, a pH of 5.5 is the lowest possible ultimate pH. It is possible to obtain a higher ultimate pH if the animal is starved or stressed before slaughter. This depletes the glycogen reserves, thus glycolysis stops before sufficient lactic acid has been formed to bring the pH to 5.5. Meat with a high ultimate pH has excellent water-holding capacity, because many of the proteins are not as close to their isoelectric point and, therefore, are able to bind more water. However, a low ultimate pH is desirable from a microbiological point of view, because it inhibits microbial growth. A high ultimate pH results in poor resistance to microbial growth.

The rate of change of pH after slaughter also has a significant effect on the quality of meat. A rapid pH change while the temperature is still high causes considerable denaturation of contractile and/or sarcoplasmic proteins and loss of water-holding capacity. Lysozomal enzymes are also released at high temperatures, and these cause hydrolysis of proteins. Such undesirable changes may happen if the carcass is not cooled rapidly after slaughter [e.g., if the pH drops to 6.0 before the temperature of the carcass drops below 95°F (35°C)].

Aging or Conditioning of Meat

Meat *aging* occurs as muscles become more tender due to protein breakdown. The time between slaughter and retail sale is sufficient for natural proteolytic enzymes to tenderize the meat, but controlled (natural) aging is sometimes induced.

Natural aging or conditioning of meat involves holding meat for several days under controlled conditions to allow the muscles to become soft and pliable again and to make the meat tender. Aging is achieved by hanging the carcass in a cold room, at 34–38°F (2°C) for 1–4 weeks. Although the meat regains tenderness after about a week, the best flavor and tenderness develops in about 2–4 weeks. Humidity levels of approximately 70% are controlled, and the meat may be wrapped in vacuum bags to minimize dehydration and weight loss.

Higher temperatures for shorter times, such as 68°F (20°C) for 48 hours, have also been used to age beef, but development of surface bacterial slime tends to be a problem for meat aged by such methods. This can be reduced by exposing the meat to ultraviolet light during aging.

During aging, the actomyosin cross-links that were formed at the onset of rigor mortis are **not** broken down. However, a protease, which is active at around pH 5.5 breaks down the thin myofilaments at the Z-lines. This causes the muscle to become pliable again, and meat to be tender. The sarcoplasmic proteins denature and there is some denaturation of the myofibril proteins, with a resultant loss of water-holding capacity, and so the meat drips. Collagen and elastin do not denature significantly during aging.

Aging methods differ among meat types. Pork and lamb may not require aging, as the animals are slaughtered while they are young and inherently tender. They are usually processed the day following slaughter.

MEAT PIGMENTS AND COLOR CHANGES

Changes in pigment may result from exposure to oxygen, acidity, and light. Major pigments in meat responsible for the red color are myoglobin and hemoglobin. Hemoglobin (with 4 heme groups in its structure) is present at levels of 10–20% of well-bled meat. It functions to transport oxygen and CO_2 in the *bloodstream* of the living animal. Myoglobin (with one heme group as part of its structure) is 80–90% of the total meat pigment. It holds oxygen in the *muscle cells* (see Chemical Composition of Meat).

Myoglobin is the primary pigment contributor of meat, especially dark meat. It is present in heavily exercised portions of the animal that expend greater oxygen (such as leg meat of chicken). The level increases with age and level of muscle exercise. It varies with the species, sex, and muscle of a meat. *Oxymyoglobin* is produced when myoglobin is exposed to oxygen in the air. It is a bright red pigment that remains red due to oxygenation. *Metmyoglobin* is the undesirable, brownish-red colored pigment found in meat. It is due to oxidation of the iron molecule and is found in meat that is not fresh. In raw meat, these pigments exist in dynamic equilibrium, although the reduction of metmyoglobin to myoglobin does not readily occur (Figure 9.4).

MEAT-HANDLING PROCESS

USDA Inspections

The round stamp (Figure 9.5) found on the primal cut of inspected meat carries the abbreviation for "United States Inspected and Passed" and the packaging/processing plant number. The stamp is made of a nontoxic purple vegetable dye. Packaged processed meat must show a somewhat similar stamp, which may be on the carton if the meat is boxed, and it is common for state inspection stamps to display a stamp with the shape of the state. Inspections are a service of the U.S. government and are paid for with tax dollars.

Inspection for meat is *mandatory* (Chapter 20). Meat is inspected for wholesomeness—that it is safe to eat and without adulteration, and the USDA uses the term **wholesome** to mean that examination of the carcass and viscera of the animal did not indicate the presence of disease. It is not meant to imply freedom from all disease-causing microorganisms.

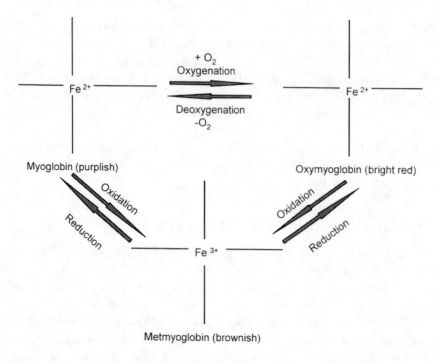

FIGURE 9.4 Pigment change.

The Federal Meat Inspection Act of 1906 requires inspection of all meat packing plants slaughtering and processing meat for *interstate* commerce. The Wholesome Meat Act of 1967 required the same inspection program for *intrastate* transport.

Trained veterinarians and agents of the USDA Food Safety and Inspection Service (FSIS) inspect the health of the animal, as well as the sanitation of the plant, and labeling. Inspections are used before, after, and throughout the meat processing. Diseased and unwholesome animals may not be used; harmful ingredients may not be added; misleading names or labels may not be used, and there must be established sanitation codes for the plant. The Meat Inspection Program also controls and monitors imported meat.

The pathogenic microorganism *E. coli* 0157:H7, found in ground meat, may be undetected if only *visual* inspections are used for inspection, thus the need for bacterial counts in inspections. The Hazard Analysis and Critical Control Point (HACCP) method of food safety (Chapter 16) is the current program for inspecting meat with the inclusion of bacterial count checks.

Wholesomeness and safety of the food supply is of prime importance. Meat is also inspected for accurate labeling.

Kosher Inspection

Kosher inspection indicates that the meat is "fit and proper" or "properly prepared." As applied to food, the word means "fit for consumption." Following Mosaic and Talmudic Laws, a specially trained rabbi slaughters the animal, e.g., beef,

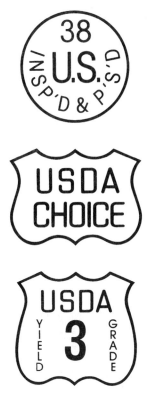

Figure 9.5 The USDA inspection, quality grade and yield grade stamps
(*Source*: USDA).

lamb, goat, meat is well bled, and then salted. All processing is done under the supervision of individuals authorized by the Jewish faith. By Mosaic Law, meat must come from an animal that has split hooves and chews its cud. Therefore, hogs and all pork products cannot be Kosher. The Kosher stamp (Figure 9.6) does not indicate grade or wholesomeness; meat is still subject to federal or state inspection.

Kosher Stamp

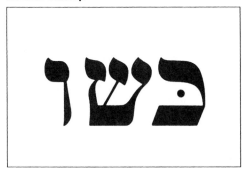

FIGURE 9.6 Kosher Symbol
(*Source*: National Cattlemen's Beef Association).

Overall, there are more that 46,000 kosher-certified products on the market. The market for these foods comprises only 20% Jewish people. Excluding people who are Jewish, Muslims and other religious groups comprise 30% of the kosher market. The lactose-intolerant and vegetarian consumers comprise 25%; 25% are health conscious consumers (1).

It may appear that kosher is considered an acceptable substitute for Muslim religious requirements, but this is not the case. Discussed in the upcoming text is Halal Certification for Muslim requirements.

Halal Certification

The **Halal** certification indicates "proper and permitted." Only foods prepared and processed under Halal standards are to be consumed by Muslims, wherein trained Muslim inspectors assist, participate in, and supervise food production in companies complying with Halal standards. The types of foods permitted, including use of additives, slaughtering, packaging, labeling, shipping, and other aspects of food handling, are regulated. For example, the Halal production does not accept alcohol, gelatin prepared from swine (for use as a food ingredient or packaging ingredient), or meat from animals that was not *individually* blessed. As is true for kosher, the Halal Certification does not indicate grade or whole-someness. It does not employ the same processing as kosher food. A crescent M symbol on the product package indicates that the product meets the halal standards of the Islamic Food and Nutrition Council of America. The Halal stamp of certification (Figure 9.7).

Some products bear certification that they are both kosher and halal (2—My Own Meals). As per the founder and president of a company producing both kosher and halal refrigeration-free meals, "For a product to be kosher or halal means much more than having the product blessed by a religious official" (1).

There exist 13–14 million persons of the Jewish faith, and 1 billion Muslims in the world. Their dietary laws are not interchangeable, but are similar in the two faiths. A look at dietary restrictions of other religions is included in another reference (3).

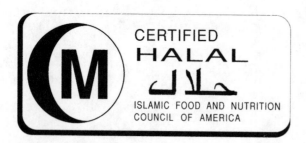

FIGURE 9.7 Halal certification
(*Source*: Islamic Food and Nutrition Council of America).

GRADING OF MEAT

Under another program, established in 1927, *voluntary grading* by the USDA is conducted for **quality** and **yield** (Figure 9.5). Grading is part of the processing cost and is not paid for by tax dollars, as is the inspection. The **quality grades** are based on expected edible quality. As an example, grades standardized for beef are according to the grades listed below, and include an evaluation of *marbling, maturity, texture, and appearance.*

- Prime
- Choice
- Select
- Standard
- Commercial
- Utility
- Cutter
- Canner

Prime grades of beef are very well marbled, followed by Choice, Select, and Standard with less marbling. The younger animal is more likely to be tender and receive a grade of Prime, Choice, Select, or Standard. Older, more mature aged beef can only qualify for Commercial, Utility, Cutter, or Canner grades. Meat is also graded on such factors as the coarseness of muscle fiber bundles (texture, likely to be tough), color, and firmness of the muscle (appearance). For some USDA grade inspections, such as where meat is intended for use as steaks, high levels of marbling provide an expectation of tenderness, and therefore the USDA grade would be high. The inverse is also true, such as when a high grade is assigned to the leanest cut of meat.

Voluntary quality grading characteristics of animals are dependent on factors including age; color of lean, which is pinker in younger animals; external fat quality and distribution, marbling; shape of animal carcass; and firmness and meat texture. Selection of lean, less marbled meat is recommended for low-fat diets.

Meat that is subject to voluntary quality grading is also graded for **yield**, which is useful at the wholesale level. The highest percentage of boneless yield on the carcass is given an assigned yield grade of "1." If yield of a carcass is less, the yield grade may be assigned a value as low as "5." Sales and marketing of meat products are based on grades and yields.

SAFETY

Meat is a potentially hazardous food that supports rapid bacterial growth if stored at improper temperatures (Chapter 16). Because all meat contains bacteria, it should be maintained in a clean and covered condition, at temperatures that retard the growth of microorganisms which may both contaminate and spoil meat, producing changes in the color, odor, and safety. Safe handling instructions appearing on meat packages is shown in Figure 9.8.

Adherence to specific temperatures is necessary for the prevention of growth and the destruction of harmful microorganisms in meat. Adequate refrigeration, cooking, and holding, as well as reheating are all important in controlling bacteria. Personal hygiene and sanitation are also important in preventing the spread of bacteria.

The CDC reports a sustained decline in reported illnesses from several bacteria including Listeria,Campylobacter, and Salmonella over the last few years since 1996. It is attributed in part to "...a change in the way that food safety in meat slaughter, animal slaughter and processing is managed" (CDC). The USDA deputy under-secretary of food safety said "We are strongly encouraging specific interventions for raw meat and poultry in order to further reduce the level and incidence of pathogens such as Salmonella in these products. We feel that there is a whole arsenal of potentially effective interventions that could be utilized" (CDC).

The bacteria, *Clostridium botulinum*, is an anaerobic bacteria that causes the disease botulism. It is a deadly form of food poisoning that may result from consuming improperly processed canned or vacuum-packed meats. To provide control, nitrite is added to processed meat to inhibit the reproduction of spores from this bacteria.

A more common, less deadly bacteria such as *Staphylococcus aureus* may grow in contaminated meat products. This *bacteria* may be destroyed by cooking, but the *toxin* that the bacteria secretes survives cooking and may cause food poisoning. Illness becomes apparent in as little as one hour after consumption of a contaminated meat.

Poultry without sufficient cooking may contain the live, infection-causing *Salmonella* bacteria, which is the most common cause of foodborne infections in

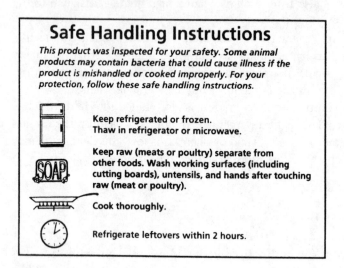

FIGURE 9.8   Safe handling instructions
(*Source*: USDA).

the United States. Most *Salmonella* are destroyed at 161°F (72°C) for 16 seconds, or 143°F (62°C) for 30 minutes. Another *Clostridium*, *Clostridium perfringens*, is found in meats especially those that were allowed to cool slowly following cooking. Undercooked pork may contain the parasite *Trichinella spiralis*, which is killed at temperatures of 155°F (68°C).

Ground beef, the combination of meat from *many* cattle, is more likely to be contaminated with *E. coli 0157:H7* bacteria during processing and handling than a single cut of meat (such as steak) from *one* animal. Cooking temperatures of 155°F (68°C) are necessary to destroy any *E. coli* that might be in the meat. A major challenge to the safety of ready-to-eat (RTE) products includes *Listeria monocytogenes* that may grow under refrigeration, yet is destroyed by thermal processing. A U.S. patent has recently been awarded to a company that uses electricity as the energy source to pasteurize processed and packaged foods, including RTE meats such as hot dogs and luncheon meats (4).

Recently, the USDA has given approval for steam pasteurization as an antimicrobial treatment of beef carcasses (see below). This treatment reduces the risk of *E. coli* 0157:H7 by exposing the entire surface of the carcass to steam that kills the bacteria. Meat processors must avoid subsequent recontamination of the product, and the consumer must handle the meat with care. The use of steam pasteurization for pork and poultry is subject to further research. The use of ozone to disinfect poultry processing water is reviewed on a case-by-case basis.

Other FDA approved treatments include *high-intensity pulsed-light* treatment for the control of microorganisms on the surface of food (61 FR42381-42382). And *irradiation* used to destroy the pathogens that are present in meat and extend refrigerator shelf life. The FDA has approved radiation of fresh, frozen meats such as beef, lamb and pork, to control disease-causing microorganisms (Chapter 16).

The American Meat Institute Foundation (AMIF) speaks for the industry in saying that it sanitizes fresh meat, as well as the RTE meat products, including hams, and hot dogs. This is achieved either by *steam pasteurization*, which exposes the carcass to a steam filled cabinet, or by use of a handheld device in *steam vacuuming*, whereby steam is sprayed directly onto carcass spots where contamination is suspected. With the added food protection provided by the uses of multiple intervention strategies, sprays and organic acid (lactic and acetic acids) and hot water treatment are also used widely (5).

Meat must be kept safe in the defrosting process. The FDA advises thawing below temperatures of 45°F (7°C), under cold, running water, or by microwave, if immediately cooked. Slow thawing, with intact wrappers is the defrosting method that allows the least moisture loss. The USDA recommends refreezing only in the case of properly thawed and cooked meats.

The FDA recommended cooking temperatures to control bacterial growth and prevent foodborne illness are listed in Table 9.1 (check local jurisdiction). For information that can be applied to meat preservation, see Chapter 16.

Current concern exists over Bovine Spongiform Encephalopathy (BSE) or "Mad Cow Disease." Quarantine, slaughter, infection by animal feed made from other infected cattle, as well as hysteria, and false alarms may be issues to many

TABLE 9.1 Minimum Safe Internal Temperature for Selected Meats

Meat	Temperature
Beef steaks (rare)	155°F (68°C) (Upon consumer order)
Roast beef (rare)	130°F (54°C) (Time dependent)
Pork	155°F (68°C) or 170°F (77°C) in a microwave oven
Ground beef	155°F (68°C)
Poultry	165°F (74°C)

Source: FDA.

individuals, groups, and governments as they must manage this disease. Further understanding of the disease, and vigilance is needed to protect the food supply.

More than one million copies of an informational document by NCBA have been financially supported and distributed in the U.S. Foot-and Mouth Disease (FMD) and Bovine Spongiform Encephalopathy (BSE). "FMD & BSE: What Every Producer Needs to Know" addresses, among other issues, prevention, FAQ, as well as the government's emergency response.

HORMONES AND ANTIBIOTICS

Food safety concerns include the use of hormones (growth promotants) and antibiotics in animal feeds. Hormones may be used in animal feeds to promote growth and/or to increase lean tissue growth and reduce fat content. All hormone-use in animal feeding must be discontinued for a specified time period prior to slaughter and must be approved by the FDA. A random sampling of carcasses provides tests for and monitors growth hormone residues.

The FDA also monitors the use of antibiotics in animal feeds to prevent their transfer to man. Antibiotics have been used for over 50 years to treat disease. *Subtherapeutic* doses of antibiotics do more than treating already existing diseases; such doses may be used to prevent disease and promote growth of animals. With this practice, the *therapeutic* administration of antibiotics to humans may be rendered ineffective if antibiotic-resistant strains of bacteria are passed from the livestock to man. A 1989 study by the National Academy of Sciences (NAS) concluded that they were "unable to find data directly implicating the subtherapeutic use of feed antibiotics in human illness."

Although danger to human health has not been shown, the FDA (even recently) has urged that specific antibiotics used to treat animals, be removed from the market, if they have been found to compromise other drugs used in treating animals or humans. "There are many countries [such as Denmark] that do not allow antibiotics as growth promoters in farm animals" (6). Used solely for the purpose of animal growth, antibiotics may be oftentimes debated.

CUTS OF MEAT

Primal or Wholesale Cuts

A *primal cut* is also known as a wholesale cut of an animal. Meat cutting separates cuts into tender and less tender cuts, and lean areas from areas with a greater amount of fat. Cuts differ with species, however, primal cuts of *beef* are identified below and are listed according to tenderness. Less exercised skeletal muscles that provide support (cuts of meat along the backbone, such as the loin) are usually tenderer than other skeletal muscles that are used in locomotion.

Most Tender	Medium Tender	Least Tender
Rib	Chuck	Flank (< brisket)
Short loin	Round	Short plate
Sirloin		Brisket
		Foreshank
		Tip

Subprimal Cuts

Subprimal cuts are divisions of primal cuts. They may be boneless, and if they are vacuum packed, they may be considered as "beef-in-a-bag." The subprimal cuts are boxed (thus the term "boxed meat") and sent to grocery markets for sale. Individual retail cuts such as roasts, steaks, and chops are then made from the subprimal cut as it is further divided.

Retail Cuts

Retail cuts are those available in the retail market, cut from primal or subprimal cuts. They may be named for the primal cut in which they are located or for the bones they contain (Figure 9.9). In general, cuts from the neck, legs, and lower belly are least tender. They are made more palatable when cooked with moist heat to soften connective tissue, although long cooking by dry heat at low temperatures produces a satisfactory product. Tender cuts are cooked with dry heat.

The wholesale and retail cuts of beef are identified in Figure 9.10. In 1970s, The National Livestock and Meat Board (now National Cattlemen's Beef Association) coordinated a committee of retail and meat industry representatives and federal agencies, which standardized names for 314 retail cuts of meat. They published the Uniform Retail Meat Identity Standards (URMIS). URMIS labels include the *kind of meat* (beef, veal, pork, or lamb), the *primal cut* from which the meat originated (chuck, rib, loin, or round of the animal), and the name of the *retail cut*.

Beef (Figure 9.11) is most commonly obtained from carcasses of the following:

- Steer: young, castrated male carcass
- Heifers: young, females before breeding, beyond veal and calf age

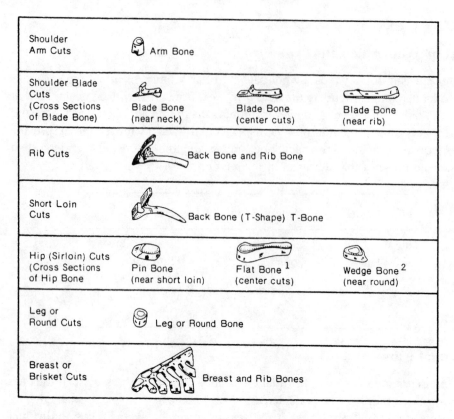

FIGURE 9.9 Bones in retail cuts
(*Source*: USDA).
[1]Formerly part of "double bone" but today the back bone is usually removed leaving only the "flat bone" (sometimes called "pin bone") in the sirloin steak.
[2]On one side of sirloin steak, this bone may be wedge shaped while on the other side, the same bone may be round.

Beef is less frequently obtained from the carcasses of the following:

• Cows: females that have had a calf

• Bulls: adult male

• Baby beef: young cattle, 8–12 months of age

• Calves: young cattle, 3–8 months of age, beyond veal classification

Veal is the flesh of beef calves, generally 3 weeks to 3 months or more. Veal is milk-fed, not grass-fed, thus is low in iron and pale in color. Older calf meat is normally differentiated from veal on the basis of lean color. Calf meat has a grayish red to moderately red lean color, whereas veal is usually grayish pink.

Pork is the flesh of swine (pig).

Lamb is the flesh of young sheep, not more than 14 months old.

Mutton is the flesh of sheep older than two years.

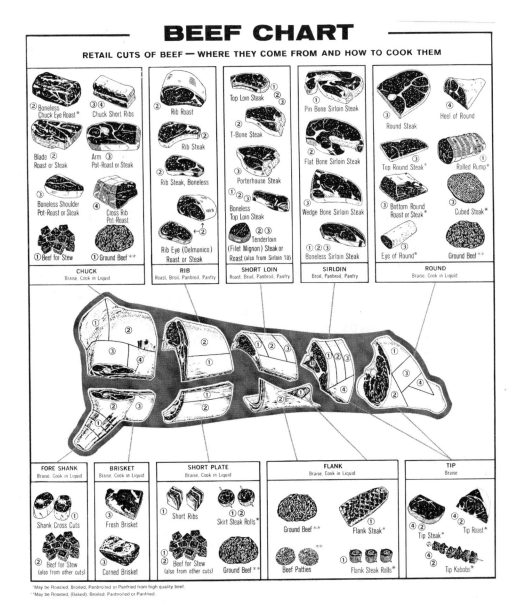

FIGURE 9.10 Wholesale and retail cuts of beef
(*Source*: USDA).

COOKING MEAT

At the turn of this century, beef demand was on the upswing for the first time in two decades (7). Yet, some individuals may have environmental, religious, vegetarian, health, or other concerns related to the consumption of meat, thus they might choose to avoid meat products, or consume meat minimally. Or, consumers may be unfamiliar with types of cuts and cooking methods, or they may be 'short on time.' (It may be a lot to ask, but meat must satisfy the requirements

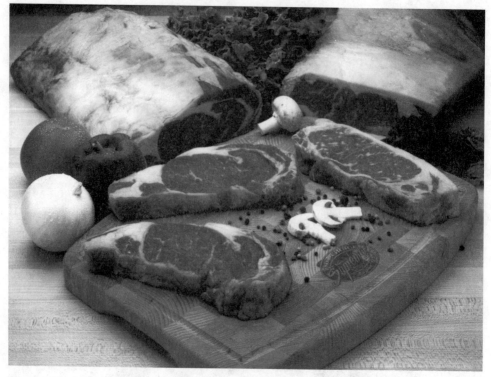

FIGURE 9.11   Beef steak (Courtesy of SYSCO® Incorporated).

of appearance, texture and flavor, as well as nutrition, safety and convenience.) So, it becomes important to know the effects of cooking meat on its various components.

The purpose of cooking is to improve tenderness and flavor while destroying pathogenic microorganisms. In cooking, the peptide chains of amino acid chains uncoil (denature) and reunite or coagulate, releasing water and melted fat (Chapter 8). Consequently, the meat shrinks, and it changes in two ways when heat is applied: muscle fibers toughen and connective tissue becomes more tender. These are opposing effects as far as tenderness of meat is concerned. The overall effect of cooking on meat will depend on the amount of collagen present, the method of cooking, cooking time, and temperature of cooking.

Effects of Cooking on Muscle Proteins

When muscle bundles are physically larger (indicating that they contain a greater number of myofibrils), they produce a coarser grain. Such are the muscles used in locomotion (muscles for physical movement), and muscles of older animals. They contain a greater number of myofibrils in each muscle, causing fibers to be thicker, and meat tougher, when cooked.

Muscle proteins (myofibrils) are sensitive to heat and precipitate, which tends to make the meat tougher. Myosin precipitates at around 131°F (55°C), and actin at 158–176°F (70–80°C). As muscle fibers denature, shortening and toughening because of the shrinkage of the surrounding *connective tissue*, this causes a loss of water-holding capacity. The longer the cooking time, the more serious this effect will be, although at temperature of 170°F (77°C) tenderness may improve.

Tender cuts of meat contain small amounts of connective tissue and should be cooked for a short time at a high temperature with dry heat, or for a longer time at a lower temperature. Such cooking methods minimizes coagulation and shrinkage of muscle fibers and prevent loss of water-holding capacity. Toughening of the muscle fibers is minimized if tender cuts are cooked to rare rather than the well-done stage. This explains why meat that is overcooked tends to be dry and tough.

An increasingly tough, dry product will result from prolonged cooking of tender cuts of meat as the protein coagulates, water is squeezed out, and myofibrils toughen. Greater cooking intensity for a short time is advantageous for tender cuts of meat, and prolonged cooking is recommended for less tender cuts of meat.

Effects of Cooking on Collagen

When collagen, the major component of connective tissue, is heated, hydrogen bonds and some heat-sensitive cross-links are broken. At temperatures between 122°F and 160°F (50–71°C) connective tissue begins shrinking. Some of the tough-structured collagen is then solubilized and converted to gelatin. As the collagen fibers are weakened, and the meat becomes tenderer. When comparing the collagen conversion temperatures with muscle, it is clear that temperatures that solubilize collagen also cause precipitation of muscle proteins, increasing the toughness of meat.

Young animals contain few cross-links in collagen thus, it is readily converted to gelatin and meat tends to be tender. Collagen from *older* animals, on the other hand, contains many more covalent cross-links, most of which are not broken down by cooking; therefore, old animals yield tough meat unless it is heated in a moist atmosphere.

Breakdown (or "melting") of collagen is faster as it reaches higher temperatures. This solubilization of collagen and formation of gelatin requires moist heat (such as stewing or braising), and therefore, the best method of cooking a cut of meat with a lot of collagen is to cook "long and slow" to convert collagen to gelatin without causing too much damage to the muscle proteins.

Cuts of meat low in collagen, such as rib or loin steaks, are inherently tender and do not benefit from slow, moist heat cooking. These cuts are tenderer when cooked quickly, and served rare or medium-rare where the muscle can still remain tender. On the other end of the spectrum, when collagen levels in a cut of meat are high, slow, moist heat cooking, to achieve a well-done stage, gelatinizes the collagen. Some tenderization of the meat surface (1/4 inch) occurs as meats are placed in marinades.

Effect of Cooking on Fat

Fat melts throughout the meat with cooking, and therefore produces a perception of a tenderer product. If a cut is high in fat content, or well marbled, it yields a more tender cooked meat.

Types of Cooking

Generally, cuts of meat that are low in collagen (inherently tender cuts) should be cooked rapidly, with **dry heat**, whereas meat containing more collagen (less tender cuts) benefit from slow, **moist heat** cooking. *Dry heat* methods of cooking include broiling, frying, pan frying, roasting, and stir-frying. Some examples of *moist heat* methods of cooking include braising, pressure cooking, stewing, or using a slow cooking pot to simmer. To some extent, all meat contains moisture, and therefore covering it while cooking provides moist heat cooking. Moist heat cooking reduces surface drying that occurs with dry heat cooking, and gives time for collagen to become gelatin. It results in a less tender, less juicy roast than that obtained by dry heat cooking.

Cooking Application

The myoglobin pigment is denatured with cooking, and therefore meat changes color from a red or purple to pale gray. Although color may be an indication of the degree of doneness, the use of a calibrated thermometer to measure temperature provides the necessary assurance that recommended cooking temperatures are achieved. (Note: a cooking thermometer reads the *average* temperature of foods making contact with the thermometer stem.)

Initial high heat, or "searing" with dry heat imparts flavor, but then, moist heat cooking is used for the continued cooking of less tender cuts of meat, high in collagen-containing connective tissue. As previously mentioned, these cuts become more tender as collagen is gelatinized to the water-soluble gelatin. Elastin-containing connective tissue does not soften.

Large roasts increase in internal temperature for 15–45 minutes or more after removal from the oven. A greater temperature increase following removal from the oven is noted for roasts that are cooked to lesser degrees of doneness before removal from the oven than for roasts removed at the well- done stage. This should be kept in mind when a specific doneness is desired.

Specific temperatures for doneness of meat are as follows:

Doneness	Temperature
Rare	140°F (60°C)
Medium-rare	150°F (65°C)
Medium	160°F (71°C)
Well done	170°F (77°C)

While identical roasts may reach the same end temperature, less water loss and shrinkage is observed by cooking with *moist* heat and slow cooking, than by rapid, *dry* heat application.

ALTERATIONS TO MEAT

Processed Meat

Processed meat is defined as meat that has been changed by any mechanical, chemical, or enzymatic treatment, altering the taste, appearance, and often keeping the quality of the product (National Cattlemen's Beef Association). It may be cured, smoked, or cooked, and it includes cold cuts (lunch meats), sausage, ham, and bacon. Some of these products are available in low-fat formulations.

Of all the meat (beef, veal, pork, and lamb) produced in the United States, about 34% is processed. Approximately 75% of processed meat is pork and 25% is beef and a small amount is lamb or mutton. Meat that has been processed is subject to the same USDA inspection as other meat. If formulated with meat trimmings and variety meats, that must be stated on the label.

Processed meats may contain salt, phosphates, nitrate (NO_3), or nitrite, which provide beneficial microbial control. Additionally, these ingredients supply flavor, texture, and protein-binding contributions (see Restructured Meats) to foods. Some foods may contain a reduction or replacement of sodium, and others, such as some hams, may contain curing solutions that account for 10% or more of the weight. The FSIS allows use of a blend of carrageenan, locust bean gum, and xanthan gum at maximum levels of 0.5% to prevent escape of the brine solution added to cured pork products. Nitrite is added to processed meat to preserve the color of meat and control the growth of *C. botulinum*.

A health concern with the addition of nitrites is that they could combine with amines (the by-product of protein breakdown) in the stomach and form the carcinogenic "nitrosamines." This was addressed in a December 1981 report by the NAS that stated that neither sodium nitrate nor nitrite was carcinogenic. Nitrites remain at levels less than 50 ppm in processed meat at the point of consumption. Many processors add *ascorbic acid* (vitamin C) and *erythorbic acid* and their salts, *sodium ascorbate* and *sodium erythorbate,* to cured meat to maintain processed meat color. These additives also inhibit the production of nitrosamines from nitrites.

Curing and Smoking of Meat

Curing is a modification of meat that increases shelf life, forms a pink color, and produces a salty flavor. **Cured meats** contain nitrite which controls the growth of *C. botulinum*. Additional color changes to the cured meat may result as the pigment in cured meat products oxidizes when exposed to oxygen and fades when exposed to fluorescent light. Exposure to fluorescent light may give cured hams a fluorescent sheen and also causes a graying or fading of the color. Therefore, cured meats are packaged so that they are minimally exposed to oxygen and light.

Ham (pork) and corned (cured) beef as well as bacon and pastrami are very popular cured meats. Corned beef was given the name because beef was preserved with "corns" (grains) of salt.

Smoked meats are popular in parts of the United States; they are relatively unheard of in other localities. Commercially or at home, beef, ham, and turkey are smoked (heat processed) to impart flavor. Liquid smoke could also be used to impart flavor. Smoking treats meat by exposure to aromatic smoke of hardwood, and also dehydrates, thus offering microbial control to the meat.

Restructured Meat

Restructured meat contains lean muscle tissue, connective tissue, and adipose tissue of a natural cut of meat, but proportions of each may differ. In the process of restructuring, meat is 1) flaked, ground, or chunked to a small particle size, 2) reformed, and 3) shaped—perhaps into roasts or steaks. Most boneless hams, for example, are restructured meats.

Myosin in the muscle may be instrumental in causing meat particles to bind together. Salts, phosphates, and other nonmeat binders such as egg albumen, gelatin, milk protein, wheat, or textured vegetable protein may be added for the purpose of holding protein particles together. Generally, the restructuring process provides a less expensive menu item that resembles a whole meat portion. It offers consistency in serving size and appearance.

Artificial Tenderizing

Young animals have less muscle and, therefore, less connective tissue than older animals, with (the exception of veal), therefore they are tenderer and do not need artificial tenderizing. Recall that it is the connective tissue of older animals that contains more covalent cross-links, which is less soluble, less readily converted to gelatin, and less tender. The less tender cuts of meat may be artificially tenderized to break down the proteins of muscle or connective tissue by *mechanical, electrical,* or *enzymatic* treatment.

Meat may subject to *mechanical* tenderization by chopping, cubing, and grinding. An example of mechanical tenderizing is the preparation of cubed steak or ground meat that cuts muscle fibers and, especially, connective tissue, into smaller particle size, producing a more tender meat. Meat may be pounded prior to stuffing or rolling for use in a recipe, which breaks the surface muscle fibers and connective tissue. A special instrument that pierces the meat with multiple thin, tenderizing needles is involved in the "needling" or "blade tenderizing" of meat.

Electrical stimulation such as ultrasonic vibration indirectly tenderizes meat by the physical vibrations that stimulates muscles to breakdown ATP to lactic acid and decreases the pH. The electrical stimulation of a carcass tenderizes without degrading the muscle fibers and texture of meats to a mushy state.

Natural enzyme tenderizers derived from tropical plants are available as powders or seasoning compounds that may be applied by dipping or spraying meat. They are more effective in tenderizing than marinades, which only penetrate approximately one-fourth into the interior of the meat. They include *papain* from the papaya plant, *bromelain* from pineapple, and *ficin* from figs. Some enzymes treat the muscle tissue; others, the connective tissue. For example, the enzymes chymopapain, or papain, and ficin exert a greater effect on tenderizing *muscle fibers* than connective tissue, while bromelain degrades *connective tissue* more than the myofibrils. Any overapplication of natural enzyme tenderizers to meat surfaces, or allowing the treated meat to remain at temperatures conducive to enzymatic activity, could produce an overly soft meat consistency.

The natural enzyme tenderizer papain may also be injected into the jugular vein (bloodstream) of an animal a few minutes before slaughter. It is distributed throughout the animal tissue. The enzyme is heat activated [by cooking at 140–160°F (60–71°C)] and eventually denatured in cooking.

With the addition of acid marinades, collagen is softened to gelatin. The collagen fibers exhibit swelling and retain more water. Tomato and vinegar are acids that cause meat to respond in this manner and become tender.

There is a more recent development utilized in tenderizing meat without affecting appearance and taste. A noninvasive process used to tenderize meat employs a three-minute cycle in a high pressure, water-filled, closed tank. A 4-foot diameter stainless steel tank, sealed with a stainless steel domed lid creates a high-pressure wav as a small explosive charge is detonated within the tank. Lower grades of meat, especially cuts that are low in fat content may increase in value as they are made tender for consumer use (8).

In addition to the age, the origin of the cut on the animal is also a factor contributing to tenderness. This will be discussed in a later section of this chapter.

POULTRY

Poultry (bird) sales have increased, while beef sales have declined. All poultry is subject to inspection under the Wholesome Poultry Products Act of 1968 and is graded US Grade A, B, or C quality based on factors including conformation, fat, and freedom from blemishes and broken bones. The inspection, labeling, and handling of poultry products is similar to the meat inspection process (Chapter 19).

Chicken is the primary poultry consumed in the U.S. diet. It is classified according to age and condition of the bird as follows:

- Broilers/fryers—2–2.5 lbs., 3–5 months of age
- Roasters—3–5 lbs., 9–12 weeks of age
- Capons—4–8 lbs., less than 8 months of age
- Hens, stewing hens, or fowls—2.5–5 lbs., less than 1 year
- Rock Cornish game hen—1–2 lbs., 5–7 weeks of age

Turkey is the second most frequently consumed poultry in the United States and is classified as follows:

- Fryers/roasters—10 weeks of age
- Mature roasting birds—20–26 weeks of age
- Tom turkey (male)—greater than 5 months of age

Duck, **geese**, **guinea**, and **pigeon** provide variety to the diet but are consumed less frequently than chicken or turkey. They are inspected by the USDA's Food Safety and Inspection Service (FSIS).

The dark meat of poultry contains more fat, less protein, and more iron and zinc than white meat, but any poultry that does not have the skin on during cooking allows less drippage of fat into meat than poultry cooked with the skin. Poultry may contain slightly more of the lipid cholesterol than an equal portion of lean beef.

In addition to the whole bird, breasts, legs, or thighs that are used as food, there are many processed poultry products on the American market. For example, many lunch meats contain turkey or chicken, and a benefit is that use of turkey in place of beef or pork reduces fat content. Ground turkey may serve as a replacement for ground beef in cooked dishes, and many formed entrees such as nuggets, patties, or rolls are available to the consumer.

Poultry carries *Salmonella* bacteria, and must be adequately cooked to assure destruction of this pathogen (Chapter 16). The FSIS allows the use of trisodium phosphate as an antimicrobial agent on raw, chilled poultry carcasses that have passed for wholesomeness.

Meat and poultry carcasses and their parts are not permitted to retain water unless it is food safety requirements that led to the retention. A final regulation and labeling disclosure on this matter is deemed helpful in assisting consumers making food choices.

FISH

Fish is edible *finfish* and *shellfish* from marine and freshwater sources. The edible fish represents the flesh from the skeletal muscle, as is the case with mammals and birds. Fish is softer, and flakier than either mammals or poultry, because muscle fibers (myomeres) exist as short bundles, which contain thin layers of connective tissue.

Worldwide, there are several thousand species of seafood, and with current processing, preservation, and marketing methods, greater variety of species are consumed. Yet, only a few species are used as edible fish and shellfish to provide a high-quality protein food to the diet (Figure 9.12).

As mentioned, fish are classified as follows:

- *Finfish* (vertebrate with fins): Finfish are fleshy fish with a bony skeleton and are covered with scales. They may be lean or fat. For example:
  - Lean saltwater fish—cod, flounder, haddock, halibut, red snapper, and whiting

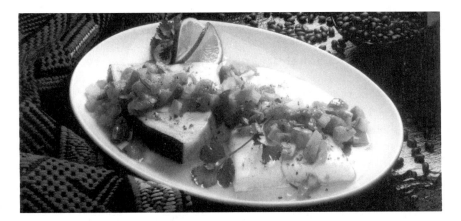

FIGURE 9.12   Fish (Courtesy of SYSCO® Incorporated).

- Lean freshwater fish—brook trout and yellow pike
- Fat saltwater fish—herring, mackerel, and salmon
- Fat freshwater fish—catfish, lake trout, and whitefish

Shellfish (invertebrates): Shellfish are either crustaceans or mollusks—the former with a crustlike shell and segmented bodies, the latter with soft structures in a partial or whole, hard shell. Some examples are as follows:

- Crustacea—crab, crayfish, lobster, and shrimp
- Mollusks—abalone, clams, mussels, oysters, and scallops

The physical components of fish are similar to mammals—for example, neglible carbohydrate content, variable percentages of fat, and high quality protein. Though the fat is primarily liquid (hence, fish *oil*) and not saturated, and fish feed on marine and freshwater plants that contribute to their high content of omega-3 polyunsaturated fatty acids. (Eicosapentaenoic acid—EPA, and docosahexaenoic acid—DHA, both demonstrated to be protective against diseases, such as heart disease.) The proteins are the myofibril proteins—actin and myosin; connective tissue—collagen; and sarcoplasmic proteins—enzymes and myoglobin. The proteins are complete, and are thus, high quality.

As mentioned, basically, all fish may be classified as inherently tender because fish contains less connective tissue than beef, and more of it converts to gelatin during cooking. The flakes that appear in a cooked fish (whole or fillets) are due to a change in connective tissue that occurs with heating and are a sign that cooking is complete. *Restructured* fish of various types that have been minced prior to cooking will not show such flakes.

Minced fish may be produced from less popular varieties of fish, or from the fish-flesh remains of the fillet process. With centuries of production in Japan, and developing technology in this area, the minced fish is used in the production of fish sticks, nuggets, patties, or other unbreaded, "formed" fish items. The washed, minced fish, coupled with heating, produces gel-like properties in the flesh. In the production of *surimi,* for example, minced fish such as pollack is washed first to remove oil, and water-soluble substances such as colors and flavor compounds, leaving only protein fibers as the remains. The washing also removes sarcoplasmic proteins that interfere with the necessary gelling. (Thus, with some oil and sarcoplasmic enzyme residue remaining in the fibers, production requires the addition of cryoprotectants to protect the product from negative oil oxidation and enzyme degradation). Next, the flesh is mixed with salt to solubilize the myofibril proteins—actin and myosin. Other characteristic flavors and pigments, as well as ingredients that promote the elastic texture and stability of the product, are added to the fish so that it may be incorporated into chowders, resembles crabmeat, lobster meat, or sausage-type products. If surimi is used to create these products, they are called "imitation" (e.g., "imitation crabmeat.").

Care in handling is required of raw fish dishes. For example, sliced and prepared raw fish are used in *sashimi,* and vinegared rice, rolled with raw fish, and covered with seaweed is popularly served as *sushi.*

MEAT ALTERNATIVES

Quorn (pronounced "kworn") is a meat alternative that became available to American consumers in January 2002 after being sold in Europe for over a decade. It is a fungus made into many meat-type products including patties and nuggets, and casseroles. A former FDA food safety chief (Sanford Miller, PhD.), senior fellow at the Center for Food and Nutrition Policy states that "This product meets what the nutrition community thinks a product should be and in addition, it tastes good! Modern science can fabricate anything. We can imitate anything, but we always run into problems on how to have it taste good. Not taste *alright*, but taste *good*. This product does that."

The myocoprotein was approved after undergoing a five-year approval process with extensive animal and human testing. This process included a close look at possible allergens, which showed less than the allergens of mushrooms or soy (9).

DRY BEANS AND PEAS (LEGUMES)

Legumes are *incomplete* proteins. Complete proteins containing all of the essential amino acids are present at superior levels in *animal* products such as meat, poultry, fish, or milk and eggs. In order to obtain the same essential amino acids from incomplete *plant* proteins, two or more plant protein foods are typically combined to yield a greater amino acid balance. For example, a vegetarian diet may frequently combine legumes (beans or peas) with either nuts–seeds or grains.

Combining two or more complementary sources of incomplete proteins in a day in order to provide the essential amino acids is referred to as *mutual supplementation*. Examples include combining beans and rice, tofu and vegetables on rice, black-eyed peas served with cornbread, tofu and cashews stir-fry, or chick peas and sesame seeds (hummus).

Legumes

Legumes (Figure 9.13) are the seeds of a pod of the Leguminosae family. The seed, found inside the pod, splits into two distinct parts attached to each other at the lower edge. They include edible peas that may be green, yellow, white, or variegated, including sugar peas with edible pods, black-eyed peas, and more. Legumes also include beans elongated, flattened, spherical, kidney-shaped. Notable are kidney beans, soybeans or the ediblepodded string beans/snap bean or green bean. Some beans, such as mung beans, are sprouted for culinary use. They also include those foods used for animal fodder—such as alfalfa and clover. Often, legumes may be referred to as the pulse, legume, bean, or pea family.

In addition to beans and peas, carob pods, and lentils are legumes. Peanuts, despite their name, are also legumes not true nuts. They are the high protein seeds of a pod that is contracted between the seeds. Their ripening occurs underground.

Legumes—for example, soybean, black-eyed peas, pinto beans; good source of lysine poor source of (limited) tryptophan and sulfur-containing (S–C) amino acids (soybeans contain tryptophan)

Nuts–Seeds—for example, peanuts, sesame seeds; good source of tryptophan and S–C amino acids; poor source of lysine (peanuts contain less S–C amino acids)

Cereals–Grains (whole grains)—corn, rice, whole grains (Chapter 4); good source of tryptophan and S–C amino acids; poor source of lysine (corn is a poor source of tryptophan and good source of S–C amino acids; wheat germ is poor in tryptophan and S–C amino acids but a good source of lysine)

Noticeable changes occur in cooking legumes such as softening due to gelatinization of starch and flavor improvement. The protein is coagulated and its availability is more following cooking.

Beans and peas [along with cruciferous (cabbage family) vegetables and whole grains in the diet], are wholesome food choices recommended by physicians and dietitians for healthy eating. They are low in fat, contain no cholesterol, and are good sources of fiber. Yet, these may cause intestinal distress and gas in some consumers. Therefore, an enzyme derived from *A. niger* has been processed for addition to foods such as these and is available to consumers.

Typically, soybeans are derived from an autumn harvest, and are processed into oil, tofu, frozen dessert, "flour," or textured vegetable protein.

- **Soybean oil,** pressed from the bean, is the highest volume vegetable oil in the United States and is commonly a constituent of margarine.

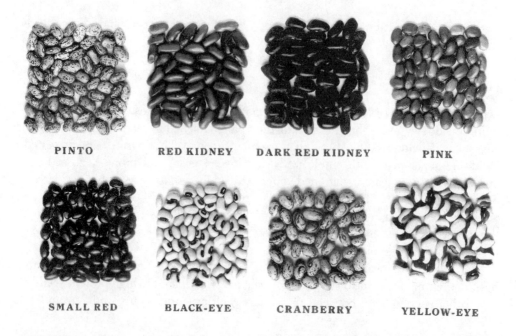

PINTO   RED KIDNEY   DARK RED KIDNEY   PINK

SMALL RED   BLACK-EYE   CRANBERRY   YELLOW-EYE

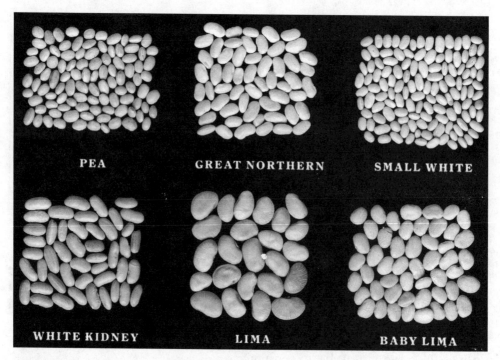

PEA   GREAT NORTHERN   SMALL WHITE

WHITE KIDNEY   LIMA   BABY LIMA

FIGURE 9.13 Examples of some common legumes
(*Source*: USDA).

- **Tofu** is soy milk that has been coagulated to make the gel. Tofu is available in various types, ranging from soft to extra firm, depending on the water content. The *soft* tofu may be an ingredient of "shakes" or frozen, sweetened dessert mixtures. More *firm* tofu may be cut into small pieces and used in stir-fry cooking. If the curd is further processed and sweetened, it may be served as a frozen tofu- based dessert, similar to ice cream or ice milk.

- **Soy flour** is made of dehulled beans with the oil (that was 18%) pressed out. Soy flour is commonly used by consumers who cannot consume wheat or other flour containing gluten-forming proteins. Although a soybean is not a cereal, it may be a source of "flour" in recipes.

- The demand for textured vegetable protein (**TVP**) is noted by many food-service establishments, including school lunch programs that use soy protein on their menus. TVP may simulate ground meat or flakes, it resembles the texture of meat, and is a good source of protein in meatless diets. It is the principal ingredient in artificial bacon sprinkles used for salads and other foods. In combination with colors, flavors, and egg binders (for ease of fabrication), the often unpleasant characteristic flavor of soy beans can be covered.

- **Fermented soybeans** produce soy sauce, miso, and tempeh. Soy sauce is a combination of the fermented soy and wheat; miso is fermented soybean and/or rice used in oriental sauces and soup bases. Tempeh is similar to tofu but is inoculated with different bacteria.

A soy protein *concentrate* is soy that has been defatted, with soluble carbohydrate removed. It is 70% protein. An even higher quality soy ingredient may be manufactured using a soy protein *isolate*. An isolate is 90% protein, with even more of the nonprotein material extracted, and with the addition of flavors and colors, it may be satisfactorily included in numerous foods. Nuts are addressed in the discussion of fruits and vegetables (Chapter 7).

NUTRITIVE VALUE OF MEAT, POULTRY, AND FISH

Some nutritive value aspects of meats (beef, veal, pork, and lamb), chicken and turkey, and fish and shellfish are shown in Figures 9.14–9.17. Nutritive values for calories, calories from fat, total fat, saturated fat, cholesterol, sodium, protein, and iron are reported for beef and veal, pork and lamb, and chicken and turkey. Calories, calories from fat, total fat, saturated fat, cholesterol, sodium, potassium, total carbohydrate, protein, vitamin A, vitamin C, calcium, and iron are also reported for seafood.

Meats are excellent sources of complete protein, many B vitamins, including B_{12} that is only found in animal products, and the minerals iron and zinc. For additional information on the nutritive value of meat and its many vitamins and minerals, the reader is referred to other nutrition textbooks.

Soybeans have antioxidant properties and contain saponins noted for their disease-fighting potential. In 1999, the FDA issued a health claim stating that

BEEF & VEAL
NUTRI-FACTS
UPDATE

BEEF & VEAL NUTRITION FACTS

1/8" fat trim / trimmed of visible fat

BEEF, 3 oz cooked serving	Calories	Calories From Fat	Total Fat (g)	Saturated Fat (g)	Cholesterol (mg)	Sodium (mg)	Protein (g)	Iron (%DV)
Ground Beef, broiled, well done (10% fat*)	210	100	11	4	85	70	27	15
Ground Beef, broiled, well done (17% fat*)	230	120	13	5	85	70	24	15
Ground Beef, broiled, well done (27% fat*)	250	150	17	6	85	80	23	15
Brisket, Whole, braised	290 / 210	190 / 100	21 / 11	8 / 4	80 / 80	55 / 60	22 / 25	10 / 15
Chuck, Arm Pot Roast, braised	260 / 180	160 / 60	18 / 7	7 / 3	85 / 85	50 / 55	24 / 28	15 / 20
Chuck, Blade Roast, braised	290 / 210	190 / 100	21 / 11	9 / 4	90 / 90	55 / 60	23 / 26	15 / 15
Rib Roast, Large End, roasted	300 / 200	220 / 100	24 / 11	10 / 4	70 / 70	55 / 60	20 / 23	10 / 15
Rib Steak, Small End, broiled	280 / 190	190 / 90	21 / 10	9 / 4	70 / 70	55 / 60	20 / 24	10 / 10
Top Loin, Steak, broiled	230 / 180	130 / 70	15 / 8	6 / 3	65 / 65	55 / 60	22 / 24	10 / 10
Loin, Tenderloin Steak, broiled	240 / 180	150 / 80	16 / 9	6 / 3	75 / 70	50 / 55	22 / 24	15 / 15
Loin, Sirloin Steak, broiled	210 / 170	110 / 60	12 / 6	5 / 2	75 / 75	55 / 55	24 / 26	15 / 15
Eye Round, Roast, roasted	170 / 140	60 / 40	7 / 4	3 / 2	60 / 60	50 / 55	24 / 25	10 / 10
Bottom Round, Steak, braised	220 / 180	110 / 60	12 / 7	5 / 2	80 / 80	40 / 45	25 / 27	15 / 15
Round, Tip Roast, roasted	190 / 160	90 / 50	10 / 6	4 / 2	70 / 70	55 / 55	23 / 24	15 / 15
Top Round, Steak, broiled	180 / 150	70 / 40	7 / 4	3 / 1	70 / 70	50 / 50	26 / 27	15 / 15
VEAL, 3 oz cooked serving			(g)	(g)	(mg)	(mg)	(g)	(%DV)
Shoulder, Arm Steak, braised	200 / 170	80 / 40	9 / 5	3 / 1	125 / 130	75 / 75	29 / 30	6 / 6
Shoulder, Blade Steak, braised	190 / 170	80 / 50	9 / 6	3 / 2	130 / 135	85 / 85	27 / 28	6 / 6
Rib Roast, roasted	190 / 150	110 / 60	12 / 6	5 / 2	95 / 95	80 / 80	20 / 22	4 / 4
Loin Chop, roasted	180 / 150	100 / 50	10 / 6	4 / 2	85 / 90	80 / 80	21 / 22	4 / 4
Cutlets, roasted	140 / 130	35 / 25	4 / 3	2 / 1	85 / 90	60 / 60	24 / 24	4 / 4

Not a significant source of total carbohydrate, dietary fiber, sugars, vitamin A, vitamin C, and calcium.

*Before cooking

Serving Size: 3 oz. cooked portion, without added fat, salt or sauces.

Developed By: Food Marketing Institute, American Dietetic Association, American Meat Institute, National-American Wholesale Grocers' Association, National Broiler Council, National Fisheries Institute, National Grocers Association, National Live Stock and Meat Board, National Turkey Federation, United Fresh Fruit and Vegetable Association.

Reviewed By: United States Department of Agriculture

Data Source: USDA Handbook 8–13, revised 1990 and Bulletin Board, 1994 (beef) and USDA Handbook 8–17, 1989 (veal)

3/95

FIGURE 9.14 Nutri-Facts of beef and veal in 3-ounce cooked portions (*Source:* Food Marketing Institute).

PORK & LAMB
NUTRI-FACTS
UPDATE

PORK & LAMB NUTRITION FACTS

The diagonal split cells show two values: upper-left = 1/8" fat trim; lower-right = trimmed of visible fat.

PORK, 3 oz cooked serving	Calories	Calories From Fat	Total Fat (g)	Saturated Fat (g)	Cholesterol (mg)	Sodium (mg)	Protein (g)	Iron (%DV)
Ground Pork, broiled	250	160	18	7	80	60	22	6
Shoulder, Blade Steak, broiled	220 / 190	130 / 100	14 / 11	5 / 4	80 / 80	60 / 65	22 / 23	6 / 8
Loin, Country Style Ribs, roasted	280 / 210	190 / 110	22 / 13	8 / 5	80 / 80	45 / 25	20 / 23	6 / 6
Loin, Rib Chop, broiled	220 / 190	120 / 80	13 / 8	5 / 3	70 / 70	55 / 55	24 / 26	4 / 4
Center Chop, Loin, broiled	200 / 170	100 / 60	11 / 7	4 / 3	70 / 70	50 / 50	24 / 26	4 / 4
Top Loin, Chop, boneless, broiled	200 / 170	90 / 60	10 / 7	3 / 2	70 / 70	55 / 55	25 / 26	4 / 4
Top Loin, Roast, boneless, roasted	190 / 170	90 / 60	10 / 6	4 / 2	65 / 65	40 / 40	24 / 26	4 / 6
Loin, Tenderloin Roast, roasted	150 / 140	45 / 35	5 / 4	2 / 1	65 / 65	45 / 50	24 / 24	6 / 6
Loin, Sirloin Roast, roasted	220 / 180	120 / 80	14 / 9	5 / 3	75 / 75	50 / 55	23 / 25	4 / 6
Spareribs, braised	340	230	26	9	105	80	25	8
LAMB, 3 oz cooked serving			g	g	mg	mg	g	%DV
Shoulder, Arm Chop, broiled	230 / 170	140 / 70	15 / 8	7 / 3	80 / 80	65 / 70	21 / 24	10 / 10
Shoulder, Blade Chop, broiled	230 / 180	140 / 90	16 / 10	6 / 3	80 / 80	70 / 75	20 / 22	8 / 8
Shank, braised	210 / 160	100 / 45	11 / 5	5 / 2	90 / 90	60 / 65	24 / 26	10 / 10
Rib Roast, roasted	290 / 200	210 / 100	23 / 11	10 / 4	80 / 75	65 / 70	19 / 22	8 / 8
Loin Chop, broiled	250 / 180	160 / 80	18 / 8	7 / 3	85 / 80	65 / 70	22 / 25	10 / 10
Leg, Whole, roasted	210 / 160	110 / 60	12 / 7	5 / 2	80 / 75	55 / 60	22 / 24	10 / 10

Not a significant source of total carbohydrate, dietary fiber, sugars, vitamin A, vitamin C, and calcium.

Serving Size: 3 oz. cooked portion, without added fat, salt or sauces.

Developed By: Food Marketing Institute, American Dietetic Association, American Meat Institute, National-American Wholesale Grocers' Association, National Broiler Council, National Fisheries Institute, National Grocers Association, National Live Stock and Meat Board, National Turkey Federation, United Fresh Fruit and Vegetable Association.

Reviewed By: United States Department of Agriculture

Data Source: USDA Handbook 8-10, 1992 (pork) and USDA Handbook 8-17, 1989 and Bulletin Board, 1994 (lamb)

3/95

FIGURE 9.15 Nutri-Facts of pork and lamb in 3-ounce cooked portions (*Source:* Food Marketing Institute).

the consumption of a minimum of 25 g of soy protein per day, coupled with a low-fat, low-cholesterol diet, may reduce risk of coronary heart disease. In 2000, The American Heart Association announced the organization's official recommendation for daily consumption of soy protein.

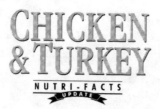

POULTRY NUTRITION FACTS

With skin / Skinless	Calories	Calories From Fat	Total Fat	Saturated Fat	Cholesterol	Sodium	Protein	Iron
Chicken, 3 oz cooked serving			g	g	mg	mg	g	%DV
Whole*, roasted	200 / 130	100 / 35	12 / 4	3 / 1	75 / 75	70 / 75	23 / 23	6 / 6
Breast, baked	170 / 120	60 / 15	7 / 1.5	2 / .5	70 / 70	60 / 65	25 / 24	6 / 4
Wing, baked	250 / 150	150 / 50	17 / 6	5 / 1.5	70 / 70	70 / 80	23 / 23	6 / 6
Drumstick, baked	180 / 130	90 / 35	9 / 4	3 / 1	75 / 80	75 / 80	23 / 23	6 / 6
Thigh, baked	210 / 150	120 / 60	13 / 7	4 / 2	80 / 80	70 / 75	21 / 21	6 / 6
Turkey, 3 oz cooked serving			g	g	mg	mg	g	%DV
Whole*, roasted	180 / 130	70 / 25	8 / 3	2 / 1	70 / 65	60 / 60	24 / 25	8 / 8
Breast, baked	160 / 120	60 / 10	6 / 1	2 / 0	65 / 55	55 / 45	24 / 26	6 / 8
Wing, baked	200 / 140	100 / 25	11 / 3	3 / 1	70 / 60	50 / 75	23 / 26	6 / 8
Drumstick, baked	170 / 140	70 / 40	8 / 4	2 / 1	70 / 65	75 / 80	23 / 24	10 / 15
Thigh, baked	160 / 140	60 / 40	7 / 5	2 / 1.5	70 / 65	70 / 70	22 / 23	10 / 15

*without neck or giblets

Not a significant source of total carbohydrate, dietary fiber, sugars, vitamin A, vitamin C, and calcium.

Serving Size: 3 oz. cooked portion, without added fat, salt or sauces.

Developed By: Food Marketing Institute, American Dietetic Association, American Meat Institute, National-American Wholesale Grocers' Association, National Broiler Council, National Fisheries Institute, National Grocers Association, National Live Stock and Meat Board, National Turkey Federation, United Fresh Fruit and Vegetable Association.

Reviewed By: United States Department of Agriculture

Data Source: USDA Handbook 8-5 and research conducted in cooperation with USDA.

3/95

FIGURE 9.16   Nutri-Facts of chicken and turkey in 3-ounce cooked portions (*Source:* Food Marketing Institute).

CONCLUSION

Meat is the edible portion of mammals, the flesh of animals used for food. Beef, pork, lamb, and veal are included in the definition of meat, and other animal products such as poultry and fish are commonly considered to be "meats." The amount and type of

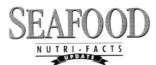

NUTRITION FACTS FOR COOKED SEAFOOD[1]

SEAFOOD (84 g/3 oz)	Calories	Calories From Fat	Total Fat (g/%DV)	Saturated Fat (g/%DV)	Cholesterol (mg/%DV)	Sodium (mg/%DV)	Potassium (mg/%DV)	Total Carbohydrate (g/%DV)	Protein (g)	Vitamin A (%DV)	Vitamin C (%DV)	Calcium (%DV)	Iron (%DV)
Blue Crab	100	10	1 / 2	0 / 0	90 / 30	320 / 13	360 / 10	0 / 0	20	0	0	8	4
Catfish	140	80	9 / 14	2 / 10	50 / 17	40 / 2	230 / 7	0 / 0	17	0	0	0	0
Clams, about 12 small	100	15	1.5 / 2	0 / 0	55 / 18	95 / 4	530 / 15	0 / 0	22	10	0	6	60
Cod	90	0	0.5 / 1	0 / 0	45 / 15	60 / 3	450 / 13	0 / 0	20	0	0	2	2
Flounder/Sole	100	14	1.5 / 2	0.5 / 3	60 / 20	90 / 4	290 / 8	0 / 0	21	0	0	2	2
Haddock	100	10	1 / 2	0 / 0	80 / 27	85 / 4	340 / 10	0 / 0	21	0	0	2	6
Halibut	110	20	2 / 3	0 / 0	35 / 12	60 / 3	490 / 14	0 / 0	23	2	0	4	4
Lobster	80	0	0.5 / 1	0 / 0	60 / 20	320 / 13	300 / 9	1 / 0	17	0	0	4	2
Mackerel, Atlantic/Pacific	210	120	13 / 20	1.5 / 8	60 / 20	100 / 4	400 / 11	0 / 0	21	0	0	0	5
Ocean Perch	110	20	2 / 3	0 / 0	50 / 17	95 / 4	290 / 8	0 / 0	21	0	0	10	6
Orange Roughy	80	10	1 / 2	0 / 0	20 / 7	70 / 3	330 / 9	0 / 0	16	0	0	0	0
Oysters, about 12 medium	100	35	3.5 / 5	1 / 5	115 / 38	190 / 8	390 / 11	4 / 1	10	0	0	6	45
Pollock	90	10	1 / 2	0 / 0	80 / 27	110 / 5	360 / 10	0 / 0	20	0	0	0	2
Rainbow Trout	140	50	6 / 9	2 / 10	60 / 20	35 / 1	370 / 11	0 / 0	21	4	4	6	2
Rockfish	100	20	2 / 3	0 / 0	40 / 13	70 / 3	430 / 12	0 / 0	21	4	0	0	2
Salmon, Atlantic/Coho	160	60	7 / 11	1 / 5	50 / 17	50 / 2	490 / 14	0 / 0	22	0	0	0	4
Salmon, Chum/Pink	130	35	4 / 6	1 / 5	70 / 23	65 / 3	410 / 12	0 / 0	22	2	0	0	2
Salmon, Sockeye	180	80	9 / 14	1.5 / 8	75 / 25	55 / 2	320 / 9	0 / 0	23	4	0	0	2
Scallops, about 6 large or 14 small	120	10	1 / 2	0 / 0	55 / 18	260 / 11	280 / 8	2 / 1	22	0	0	2	2
Shrimp	80	10	1 / 2	0 / 0	165 / 55	190 / 8	140 / 4	0 / 0	18	0	0	2	15
Swordfish	130	35	4.5 / 7	1 / 5	40 / 13	100 / 4	310 / 9	0 / 0	22	2	2	0	4
Whiting	110	25	3 / 5	0.5 / 3	70 / 23	95 / 4	320 / 9	0 / 0	19	2	0	6	0

Seafood provides negligible amounts of dietary fiber and sugars.

[1] Cooked, edible weight portion.
Percent Daily Values are based on a 2,000 calorie diet.

Serving Size: 3 oz. skinless cooked portion, without added fat, salt or sauces.

Developed by: Food Marketing Institute, American Dietetic Association, American Meat Institute, Food Distributors International, National Broiler Council, National Cattlemen's Beef Association, National Fisheries Institute, National Grocers Association, National Turkey Federation, Produce Marketing Association, United Fresh Fruit and Vegetable Association

(7/96)

Data Source: U.S. Food and Drug Administration

FIGURE 9.17 Nutri-Facts of seafood in 3-ounce cooked portions (*Source:* Food Marketing Institute).

meat consumption varies throughout the world. Meat is primarily a muscle tissue and also contains connective tissue with a greater variance in the amount of adipose tissue held inside. Water is present to a greater degree in lean meats and young animals. The protein is a complete protein and contains all the essential amino acids.

Cuts of meat include primal or wholesale, subprimal, and retail cuts, with the latter being more familiar to consumers, as it is what they may purchase at their grocery market. The inherent tenderness of a particular cut depends on such factors as location on the carcass, postmortem changes in the muscle, including the stage of rigor mortis, aging, and the method of cooking. Meat color is dependent on myoglobin and hemoglobin pigments. Changes in the color of meat may result from exposure to oxygen, acidity, and light.

Meat is subject to inspections and grading in order to provide the consumer with safe, more consistent, and reliable meat products. Meat is a potentially hazardous food and adherence to specific temperatures (cold and hot) is necessary for the prevention of growth and the destruction of harmful microorganisms.

Cooking meat causes the uncoiling or denaturation of peptide protein chains to occur. Tender cuts of meat remain tender when cooked by dry heat for a short time at high temperatures. Overcooking tender cuts of meat produces tough, dry meat, because water is released during denaturation. Less tender cuts of meat become more tender as collagen solubilizes during lengthy exposure to moist heat cooking.

Beef, veal, pork, and lamb may be altered by processing, curing and smoking, restructuring, and artificial tenderizing. Ham, corned beef, and bacon are examples of cured meat. Beef, ham, and turkey may be smoked to impart flavor and offer microbial control by dehydration. An alteration to meat occurs as meat is artificially tenderized, and includes mechanical, electrical, and enzymatic treatment.

Poultry makes a significant contribution to the U.S. diet and is classified according to age and condition of the bird. Many processed poultry products, including ground turkey, lunchmeats, and formed entrees are available for use by consumers. Edible fish and shellfish provide high-quality protein food, including restructured fish such as surimi, to the diet.

GLOSSARY

Actin: The protein of muscle that is contained in the thin myofilaments and is active in muscle contraction.

Actomyosin: The compound of actin and myosin that forms in muscle contraction.

Adipose tissue: Fatty tissue; energy storage area in an animal.

Aging: Process in which muscles become more tender due to protein breakdown.

Collagen: Connective tissue protein; the largest component that gives strength to connective tissue; is solubilized to gelatin with cooking.

Connective tissue: The component of animal tissue that extends beyond the muscle fibers to form tendons which attach the muscle to bones; it connects bone to bone; endomysium, perimysium, and epimysium connective tissue surrounds muscle fibers, muscle bundles, and whole muscles, respectively.

Cured meat: Contains nitrite to form the pink color and control the growth of *Clostridium botulinum*.

Dry heat: Method of cooking tender cuts of meat, including broiling, frying, pan frying, and roasting.

Elastin: Connective tissue protein; the yellow component of connective tissue that holds bone and cartilage together.

Endomysium: Connective tissue layer that surrounds individual muscle fibers.

Epimysium: Connective tissue layer that surrounds an entire muscle.

Gelatin: Formed from the tenderization of collagen, used for edible gels in the human diet.

Grain: Primary bundle containing 20–40 muscle fibrils.

Halal: "Proper and permitted" food under jurisdiction of trained Muslim inpection.

Kosher: "Fit and proper" or "properly prepared" food under jurisdiction of the Jewish faith; following the Mosaic or Talmudic Law.

Marbled: Intermuscular and intramuscular fatty tissue distributed in meat.

Moist heat: Method of cooking less tender cuts of meat, including braising, pressure cooking, simmering, or stewing.

Muscle tissue: The lean tissue of meat.

Myofibril: The contractile actin and myosin elements of a muscle cell.

Myosin: Protein of a muscle contained in the thick myofilaments that reacts with actin to form actomyosin.

Perimysium: The connective tissue layer that surrounds muscle bundles.

Primal cut: Wholesale cut of meat; it contains the subprimal and retail cuts.

Retail cut: Cuts of meat available in the retail market; cut from primal cuts.

Reticulin: Minor connective tissue found in younger animals; it may be the precursor of collagen or elastin.

Rigor mortis: Postmortem state 6–24 hours after death in which muscles stiffen and become less extensible; onset of rigor mortis correlates with depletion of ATP in the slaughtered animal.

Sarcomere: Repeating unit of the muscle myofibrils.

Sarcoplasmic protein: The hemoglobin and myoglobin pigments, and enzymes in the cytoplasm of a muscle fiber.

Smoked meat: Meat that has been treated to impart flavor by exposure to aromatic smoke of hardwood; smoking preserves by dehydrating, thus offering microbial control.

Stromal protein: Proteins including collagen, elastin, and reticulin of the connective tissue and supporting framework of an animal organ.

Subprimal cut: Division of a primal cut.

Wholesome: Inspection does not indicate the presence of illness.

Z-lines: Boundaries of the sarcomere; holds thin filaments in place in the myofibril.

REFERENCES

1. Young R. Flexible manufacturing. *Food Engineering*. 2000; 72 (July/August): 49–53.
2. My own meals, *Food Technology*. 2000; 54(7): 60–62.
3. Eliasi J, Dwyer JT. Kosher and Halal: Religious observances affecting dietary intakes. *J Am Diet Assoc*. 2002; 102: 911–913.
4. Portable pasteurization on the way. *Food Engineering*. 2000; 72 (July/August): 18.
5. Mermelstein NH. Sanitizing meat. *Food Technology*. 2000; 55(3): 64–65.
6. Peregrin T. Limiting the use of antibiotics in livestock: Helping your patients understand the science behind this issue. *J Am Diet Assoc*. 2002; 74(6): 768.

7. Sloan, AE. Beefing it up! *Food Technology*. 2000; 54(3): 22.
8. Morris CE. Bigger buck for the bang. *Food Engineering*. 2000; 72(1): 25–26.
9. Peregrin T. Mycoprotein: Is America ready for a meat substitute from fungus? *J Am Diet Assoc*. 2002; 102: 628.

BIBLIOGRAPHY

Bechtel PJ. *Muscle as Food*. Orlando, FL: Academic Press, 1986.

Cargill Incorporated. Minneapolis, MN.

Cargill Protein Products. Cedar Rapids, IA.

Cunningham NA, Cox NA. *The Microbiology of Poultry Meat Products*. Orlando, FL: Academic Press, 1987.

Huxley HE. Molecular basis of contraction. In: Bourne G, ed. *The Structure and Function of Muscle,* 2nd ed. New York: Academic Press, 1972.

Lee CM. Surimi process technology. *Food Technology*. 1984; 38(11): 69.

Meister KA, Grenberg RG. *Antibiotics in Animal Feed: A Threat to Human Health?* Summit, NJ: American Council in Science and Health, 1983.

Nettleton J. *Seafood Nutrition: Facts, Issues and Marketing of Nutrition in Fish and Shellfish*. Huntington, NY: Osprey Books, 1985.

Pearson AM, Dutson TR. *Restructured Meat and Poultry Products*. New York, NY: Chapman & Hall, 1987.

Ritchey SJ, Cover S, Hostetler, RL. Collagen content and its relation to tenderness of connective tissue in two beef muscles. *Food Technology*. 1963; 17(2): 76.

Robinson HE, Goeser PA. Enzymatic tenderization of meat. *Journal of Home Economics*. 1962; 54(3): 195.

Sloan AE. America's Appetite '96: The top ten trends to watch and work on. *Food Technology*. 1996; 50(7): 55–71.

Smith GC, Culp GR, Carpenter ZL. Postmortem aging of beef carcasses. *Journal of Food Science*. 1978; 43(5): 823.

Stanley DW. Relation of structure to physical properties of animal material. In: Peleg M, Bagley E, eds. *Physical Properties of Food*. Westport, CT: AVI, 1983.

Terrel RN. Reducing the sodium content of processed meats. *Food Technology*. 1983; 37(7): 66.

USDA's Meat and Poultry Hotline (1-800-535-4555), Food Safety and Inspection Service, Washington, DC.

ASSOCIATIONS

American Dietetic Association, Chicago, IL.

American Heart Association, Dallas, TX.

National Cattlemen's Beef Association—a merger of the National Livestock and Meat Board, and National Cattlemen's Association, Chicago, IL.

National Cholesterol Education Program (NCEP).

National Heart, Lung and Blood Institute.

National Restaurant Association. The Educational Foundation. *Applied Foodservice Sanitation,* 4th ed. New York, NY: J Wiley, 1992.

CHAPTER 10

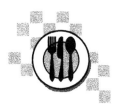

Eggs and Egg Products

INTRODUCTION

The eggs of various birds are consumed throughout the world, but the discussion that follows is regarding hen eggs. Eggs are a natural biological structure offering protection for developing chick embryos. They have numerous functions in food systems and provide nutritive value and culinary variety to the diet, while being an economical source of food throughout the world. Eggs are considered by the World Health Organization to be the reference protein worldwide, to which all other protein is compared.

Two to three servings of the Meat, Poultry, Fish, Dry Beans, *Eggs* and Nuts Group of the Food Guide Pyramid is recommended for daily consumption.

The quality and freshness of eggs is important to regulatory agencies, processors, and consumers. The age, temperature, humidity, and handling of eggs determine freshness. Eggs must be protected against contamination.

PHYSICAL STRUCTURE AND COMPOSITION OF EGGS

The Whole Egg

An average hen egg weighs about 2 ounces (57 g), which includes the weight of the yolk, white, and shell. Each component differs in composition as shown in Tables 10.1 and 10.2.

The Yolk

A cluster of developing yolks, each within its own sac, is present in the hen ovary. Approximately 31% of the weight of an egg, all of the egg's cholesterol, and almost all

TABLE 10.1 Chemical Composition of the Hen's Egg by Percentage

Component	%	Water	Protein	Fat	Ash
Whole egg	100	65.5	11.8	11.0	11.7
Egg white	58	88.0	11.0	0.2	0.8
Egg yolk	31	48.0	17.5	32.5	2.0
Shell	11				

Source: USDA.

of the fat is present in the yolk. Generally, it has a higher nutrient density than the white, containing all of the vitamins known, except vitamin C. Additionally, yolks supply flavor and mouthfeel that consumers find acceptable; they have many culinary uses.

Egg yolks contain all three lipids—triglycerides, phospholipids, and sterols. *Fat*, and a majority of yolk protein are in particles of the aqueous phase of the yolk—in large spheres, granules, and micelles. While the primary phospholipid is phosphatidyl choline, or *lecithin*, the best known sterol is *cholesterol*.

Protein in the yolk is primarily vitellin that is present in a lipoprotein complex as lipovitellin and lipovitellinin. The phosphorus-containing phosvitin and sulfur-containing livetin are also present in yolks.

Concentric rings of slightly different color may appear in the yolk, beginning in the center with a very small white yolk. The pigments (mainly xanthophyll) come from animal feed such as the green plants and yellow corn that the hen eats, and therefore yolks are darker if they have a higher carotenoid content (not necessarily of vitamin A potential). Chickens producing eggs with pale yolks may be fed supplements that darken the yolk.

A colorless sac, the *vitelline membrane* (Figure 10.1), surrounds the yolk and is continuous with the chalazae (kah-lay-za) cord (Figure 10.1). The chalazae is actually found in the albumen, and is a ropelike cord that attaches to the yolk vitelline membrane and holds the yolk in place at the center of the egg, preventing it from hitting the shell.

TABLE 10.2 Protein and Fat Content of Egg Components in Grams

Component	Protein	Fat
Whole egg	6.5	5.8
Egg white	3.6	—
Egg yolk	2.7	5.2

Source: USDA.

COMPOSITION

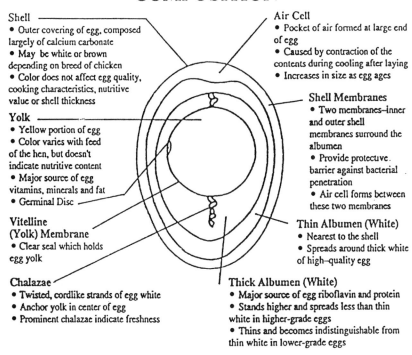

Shell
• Outer covering of egg, composed largely of calcium carbonate
• May be white or brown depending on breed of chicken
• Color does not affect egg quality, cooking characteristics, nutritive value or shell thickness

Yolk
• Yellow portion of egg
• Color varies with feed of the hen, but doesn't indicate nutritive content
• Major source of egg vitamins, minerals and fat
• Germinal Disc

Vitelline (Yolk) Membrane
• Clear seal which holds egg yolk

Chalazae
• Twisted, cordlike strands of egg white
• Anchor yolk in center of egg
• Prominent chalazae indicate freshness

Air Cell
• Pocket of air formed at large end of egg
• Caused by contraction of the contents during cooling after laying
• Increases in size as egg ages

Shell Membranes
• Two membranes–inner and outer shell membranes surround the albumen
• Provide protective barrier against bacterial penetration
• Air cell forms between these two membranes

Thin Albumen (White)
• Nearest to the shell
• Spreads around thick white of high–quality egg

Thick Albumen (White)
• Major source of egg riboflavin and protein
• Stands higher and spreads less than thin white in higher-grade eggs
• Thins and becomes indistinguishable from thin white in lower-grade eggs

FIGURE 10.1   Structure of a hen's egg
(*Source:* California Egg Commission).

As the egg ages, the egg yolks enlarge and become less viscous due to an increase in their water content. This water movement into the yolk occurs because there is a higher concentration of solids in the yolk than in the white.

The White

The egg white, also known as the **albumen** (Figure 10.1), comprises approximately 58% of the weight of an egg. It consists of four concentric layers of white: two thick whites separated by inner and outer thin whites. In lower grade eggs, the thick albumen becomes indistinguishable from the thin whites. As previously mentioned, the chalazae is located within these layers of the albumen.

Eggs contain a very high biological value, or *complete* protein, with all of the essential amino acids in a well-balanced proportion. Over half of the protein in whites is ovalbumin, although conalbumin, ovomucid, and globulins (including lysozyme, which is able to lyse some bacteria) contribute lesser percentages of protein in egg whites. The protein, avidin, is denatured by cooking, but it binds the vitamin biotin in raw egg whites rendering it ineffective when consumed. These proteins attach themselves to the yolk as it descends down the oviduct of the hen.

The egg white contains a negligible amount of fat. It provides more protein than the yolk and is often incorporated into the diet to add protein while limiting fat and cholesterol. Vitamins in the white are riboflavin (which imparts a greenish tint to the white), niacin, and biotin, and minerals contained in the egg white include magnesium and potassium.

The Shell

The shell contributes the remaining 11% weight of the whole egg. The dry shell contains the following:

94% calcium carbonate

1% magnesium carbonate

1% calcium phosphate

4% organic matrix made primarily of protein

Two thin shell membranes (Figure 10.1) are inside of the shell, one of which is attached to the shell. The other is not attached but moves with the egg contents, and the air cell develops as the two membranes separate at the large end of the egg.

The shell itself consists of a *mammillary* or inner layer, a *spongy* layer, and the outer *cuticle* (which may erroneously be referred to as "bloom"). Thousands of pores run throughout these layers of the shell since it is naturally porous for a potentially developing chick inside. As a result of the pores, CO_2 and moisture losses occur while O_2 enters the shell. The shell also functions as a barrier against harmful bacteria and mold entry, as a protein layer of keratin partially seals the shell pores. "Sweating" or moisture condensation on the shell may produce stains.

The presence of animal droppings or simple washing can remove the shell's outer cuticle lining or open its pores resulting in diminished shelf life. Once the outside protection is violated, microorganisms from the outside can travel to the inside contents and contaminate the egg.

Color

Egg *shell color* depends on the *breed* of hen. White Leghorn hens are the chief breed for egg production in the United States. They have white ears under their feathers, and produce *white shells*. *Brown shells* are popular in some regions of the United States, and are produced from hens with reddish-brown ears, such as Rhode Island Red hens, Plymouth Rock hens, and New Hampshire breeds. The shell pigment has no effect on egg flavor or quality, including the nutritive quality of the egg contents. Brown eggs are more difficult to classify as to interior quality than are white eggs (USDA).

Yolk color depends on the *feed* given to the hen. The yellow pigment may be carotene, xanthophyll, or lycopene but does not necessarily have vitamin A potential. Pale yolk may be high in vitamin A value if the chicken received vitamin A supplements.

Changes Due to Aging

Numerous changes to the egg occur as contents inside the shell shrink and the air cell (Figure 10.1) enlarges due to water loss (1). For example, the *yolk* flattens as the vitelline membrane thins, and the surrounding thick white becomes thinner, no longer holding the yolk centered in the egg. The thick *white* thins as sulfide bonds break, and it loses CO_2 with age, subsequently changing the pH from 7.6 to 9.6, which allows bacterial growth. With age, the chalazae cord appears less prominent.

Abnormalities of an Egg Structure and Composition

The USDA cites several abnormalities that may be apparent in the structure and composition of eggs:

- Double-yolked egg—results when two yolks are released from the ovary about the same time or when one yolk is lost into the body cavity and then picked up when the ovary releases the next day's yolk.
- Yolkless eggs—usually formed around a bit of the tissue that is sloughed off the ovary or oviduct. This tissue stimulates the secreting glands of the oviduct and a yolkless egg results.
- Egg within an egg—one day's egg is reversed in direction by the wall of the oviduct and is added to the next day's egg. A shell is formed around both.
- Blood spots—rupture of one or more small blood vessels in the yolk follicle at the time of ovulation, although chemically and nutritionally they are fit to eat.
- Meat spots—either blood spots that have changed in color due to chemical action, or tissue sloughed off from the reproductive organs of the hen.
- Soft-shelled eggs—generally occur when an egg is prematurely laid and insufficient time in the uterus prevents the deposit of the shell (e.g. minerals).
- Thin-shelled eggs—may be caused by dietary deficiencies, heredity, or disease.
- Glassy- and chalky-shelled eggs—caused by malfunctions of the uterus of the laying bird. Glassy eggs are less porous and will not hatch but may retain their quality.
- Off-colored yolks—due to substances in feed that cause off-color.
- Off-flavored eggs—may be due to certain feed flavors, such as fish oil or garlic. Eggs stored near some fruits and vegetables or chemicals readily absorb odors from these products.

EGG FUNCTION

Processing facilities, retail foodservice operations, and the consumer depend on eggs for many uses in food preparation. A recipe formulation *without* eggs may not exhibit the same qualities as one that contains eggs, depending on the function of the egg in

TABLE 10.3 Some of the Functions of Eggs in Food Systems

- *Binder*

Eggs are viscous and they coagulate (to a solid or semisolid state); therefore they bind ingredients such as those in meatloaf or croquettes, and they bind breading.

- *Clarifying agent*

Raw egg whites coagulate around foreign particles in a hot liquid. For example, they seize loose coffee grounds from brewed coffee and clarify broth and soups.

- *Emulsifier*

Egg yolks contain phospholipid emulsifiers, including lecithin. Emulsifiers allow two ordinarily immiscible liquids, such as oil and water to mix in the preparation of mayonnaise.

- *Foaming, leavening agent, aeration*

Egg whites increase six to eight times in volume when beaten to a **foam.** As the egg white foam is heated, the protein coagulates around air cells, maintaining a stable foam structure. Egg white foams leaven angel food cake and are created for meringues and desserts.

- *Gel*

A two-phase system of liquids in solids forms as eggs coagulate, forming a gel in custards.

- *Thickening agent*

Eggs coagulate and thicken mixtures such as custards and hollandaise sauce.

- *Other:* color, flavor, nutritive value, etc. Eggs serve numerous other roles in foods. Egg yolk carotenoids add *color* to baked products and may be spread on doughs to impart a crusty *sheen*. Eggs provide *flavor;* the fat component *inhibits crystal formation* in sugars, and *inhibits staling*. Eggs *provide nutritional value.*

---

the food. Eggs are polyfunctional products. Some of the functions of eggs are listed in Table 10.3.

INSPECTIONS AND GRADING FOR EGG QUALITY

Unlike meat and poultry with two distinct inspection and grading processes, all shell eggs are *not* inspected and graded. Rather, there is one process of grading, which includes an evaluation of wholesomeness. Grading is voluntary, although most eggs on the retail market are graded under federal inspections (2), according to established standards. The 1970 Federal Egg Products Inspection Act provides the assurance that egg products are wholesome and unadulterated and that plants processing egg products are continuously inspected.

The United States Department of Agriculture (USDA) grades eggs on a fee-for-service basis in order to assign grades. Grading involves an evaluation of the *exterior* shell, its shape, texture, soundness (not broken), and cleanliness, as well as the *interior* white and yolk, and air cell size, and at least 80% of a dozen eggs must be the grade specified on the carton. Lesser grades and older eggs may be used successfully in cooked or baked food mixtures. A high quality egg that is fit for the consumer is one without blemishes and with a shell that is intact and clean

Candling

The USDA bases grades on candling quality, evaluated either by hand (Figure 10.2) or mass scanning (Figure 10.3). *Candling* is a technique that allows a view of the *shell* and *inside* of eggs without breaking the contents. The term came about because

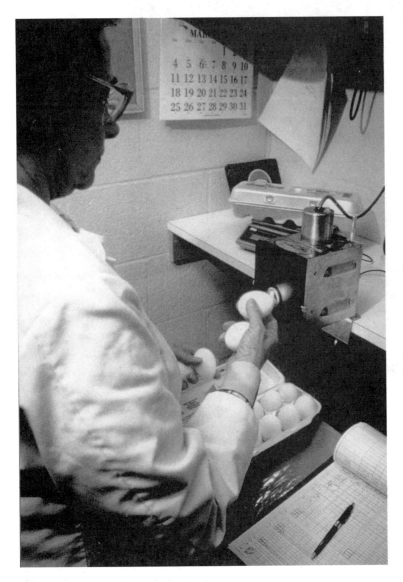

FIGURE 10.2   Candling eggs by hand
(*Source:* USDA).

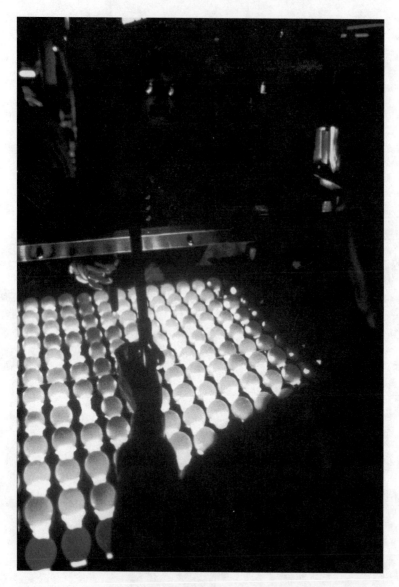

FIGURE 10.3   Candling by mass screening
(*Source:* USDA).

candlelight was once used for inspecting the interior of eggs, where egg contents could be seen when held up to a candle while being rapidly rotated.

Today, commercial eggs may be scanned in mass, with bright lights under trays of eggs. Candling may be completed either at the farm or at the egg distributor before eggs are sold to the consumer. Direct external observation of the shape and cleanliness of the shell may occur prior to or immediately following candling. A candler will also form occasional comparisons of broken-out appearance evaluation with candled appearance.

Blood spots are evidence of a ruptured blood vessel that formed during egg development, and do not always appear during candling. They may be undesirable to some consumers but pose no health hazard. The noticeable presence of blood spots decreases with age, as water movement from the white dilutes their appearance in the yolk.

Letter Grades

The *voluntary* USDA grading is based on candling quality. Grade shields on the carton indicate that the eggs were graded for quality and checked for size under the supervision of a technically trained packer. Packers who do not use the USDA grading service are monitored by *state* agencies, and may not use the *USDA* grade shield. The USDA grade shields are shown in Figure 10.4. The USDA assigns a grade of "AA" to the highest quality egg. Even this high quality may quickly diminish if eggs are exposed to improper storage conditions (2).

Occasional micrometer measurements of thick albumen egg height may also be carried out in a grading office where samples are tested (See Figures 10.5 and 10.6).

An "AA" egg has:

- A thick white, prominent, chalazae cord. The height of the broken-out white is measured in Haugh Units (with a micrometer) and compared to weight.
- A yolk must be round, high, and free from apparent defects. A flattened yolk indicates that the vitelline membrane has weakened with age or by poor storage conditions. The height is measured in relation to width.
- An air cell that may not exceed 1/18 inch in depth.
- A shell that must be clean and unbroken.

  "A" grade indicates that:

- An egg is clear, reasonably thick, and stands high.
- The yolk must be practically free from apparent defects.
- The air cell must not exceed 3/16 inch in depth.
- The shell must be unbroken.

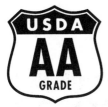 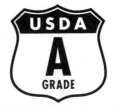

FIGURE 10.4 USDA emblem certifying quality (*Source*: USDA).

GRADES

Grade AA

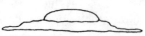

A Grade AA egg will stand up tall. The yolk is firm and the area covered by the white is small. There is a large proportion of thick white to thin white.

Grade A

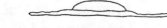

A Grade A egg covers a relatively small area. The yolk is round and upstanding. The thick white is large in proportion to the thin white and stands fairly well around the yolk.

Grade B

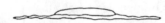

A Grade B egg spreads out more. The yolk is flattened and there is about as much (or more) thin white as thick white.

FIGURE 10.5 Grades of eggs (*Source:* California Egg Commission).

"B" grade eggs:

- Cover a wider area when broken open and are thinner and more flattened, possibly containing blood spots.
- Contain a yolk that may be slightly flattened and enlarged.

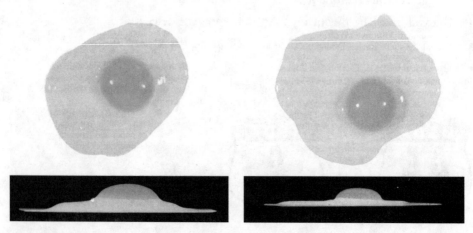

FIGURE 10.6 Quality standards for grades (*Source:* USDA).

- Are given to abnormally misshapen eggs.
- Have an air cell size that must not exceed 3/8 inch in depth.
- Have a shell that must be unbroken and show no adhering dirt.

    "C" grades are also given but are not made available to the consumer.

Air cell

The **air cell,** also known as the air sac or air pocket (Figure 10.1), is formed between the two shell membranes after the egg is laid, and it enlarges during storage. Initially, there is either no air cell or a small one, and it then becomes apparent to the eye via candling, at the large blunt end of the egg when the egg contents shrink and the *inner* membrane pulls away from the *outer* membrane. It increases with age, cooling, and moisture loss. An acceptable air-cell size for the different grades is contained in the letter grades: 1/18 inch for Grade AA, 3/16 inch for Grade A, and 3/8 inch for Grade B quality eggs.

   For control of air-cell size and the possible microbial spoilage that may follow, as oxygen migrates to the yolk, eggs should be packed with the large end of the egg up. If packed and stored in this manner, air movement from the cell to the yolk is minimized. As a consequence of a large air-cell size, eggs will float if placed in a bowl of water.

EGG SIZE

Egg-size comparisons are shown in Figure 10.7. The USDA does not include an evaluation of egg size as a part of egg quality. Eggs are classified by the USDA according to size and weight as follows:

- Jumbo 30 ounces minimum weight per dozen
- Extra large 27 ounces minimum weight per dozen
- Large 24 ounces minimum weight per dozen
- Medium 21 ounces minimum weight per dozen
- Small 18 ounces minimum weight per dozen
- Pee wee 15 ounces minimum weight per dozen

   There is a difference of 3 ounces per dozen between each class, with the best value per dozen computed by comparing selling price per ounce, although *large* eggs are the standard size egg used in published recipes. The *major* factor in determining egg size is the age of the hen; an older hen produces a larger egg. *Secondary* factors influencing size are the breed and weight of the hen. The quality of the feed as well as overcrowding and stress impact size, perhaps negatively. USDA services available to volume purchases of eggs appear in Figure 10.8.

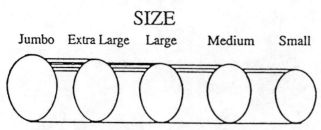

Several factors influence the size of an egg. The major factor is the age of the hen. As the hen ages, her eggs increase in size. Although any size egg may be used for frying, scrambling, cooking in the shell or poaching, most recipes for baked dishes such as custards and cakes are based on the use of Large eggs. To substitute another size, use this chart:

Large		Small	Medium	X-Large	Jumbo
1	=	1	1	1	1
2	=	3	2	2	2
3	=	4	3	3	2
4	=	5	5	4	3

FIGURE 10.7 Egg sizes
(*Source*: California Egg Commission).

PROCESSING/PRESERVATION OF EGGS

Eggs are laid at a hen's body temperature and require subsequent refrigeration, both for food safety purposes and in order to limit negative quality changes. It is possible to hold an egg for 6 months in cold [29–32°F(0°C)] storage if the shell pores are closed. Shell eggs or egg products may be preserved in the following manner.

Mineral Oil

Shell eggs may be sprayed or dipped in mineral oil on the same day they are laid. The mineral oil partially closes the shell pores and allows less microorganism (bacteria, mold) permeability. It also allows an egg to hold more moisture, retain CO_2, and be protected against a pH rise in storage. Mineral oil dips or sprays may cause a hard cooked egg to be more difficult to peel.

Pasteurization

The FDA requires **pasteurization** of all commercial liquid, dry, or frozen egg products out of the shell. This treatment destroys microorganisms such as *Salmonella* bacteria that can travel from the digestive tract and droppings of birds into the egg, causing foodborne illness infection.

The USDA requires a process of pasteurization that achieves a temperature of 140–143°F (60–62°C), for 30 minutes or longer. In addition to reaching

USDA Shell Egg Certification

The following USDA services are available to volume purchasers of shell eggs—food service operators, retailers, manufacturers, brokers, wholesalers, and exporters:

☑ Independent, third party certification of shell egg quality based on U.S. standards.

☑ Certification that purchases meet contract specifications for quality, grade, weight, quantity, temperature, packaging, transportation, or other desired product characteristics.

☑ Assurance of product quality on a continuous basis regardless of supplier.

☑ Continuous monitoring of plant facilities and processing equipment to ensure appropriate sanitary standards are met.

☑ Assurance that plants use only USDA approved chemicals, compounds, insecticides, and rodenticides.

☑ Identification of eggs with a USDA plant number and code date to facilitate an immediate traceback, if necessary.

☑ Establishment of a common language that enables buyers and sellers to communicate about egg quality and other characteristics without actually seeing the product.

☑ Establishment of a basis for fair, competitive bidding between suppliers.

Figure 10.8   USDA shell egg certification
(*Source:* USDA).

the required temperature for the destruction of pathogenic bacteria, pasteurization must maintain the functional properties of the egg. For example, following pasteurization, *whites* may still be whipped for use in a meringue (although they need a longer time period to beat to a foam) and *yolks* or *whole eggs* must retain their function as emulsifiers.

Ultrapasteurization combined with aseptic packaging of liquid whole eggs creates a commercial product with numerous advantages over frozen or shell eggs (3,4). According to a market leader in refrigerated ultrapasteurized liquid whole eggs and scrambled egg mixture (5), the eggs have a shelf life of 10 weeks when stored between 33 and 40°F (1–4°C). The eggs are *Salmonella, Listeria,* and *E. coli* negative. The eggs should not be frozen, so that they are not subjected to freezer-to-refrigerator storage, which can result in a loss of functional properties.

Ultrapasteurized liquid whole egg products (UPLWEP), developed by a university food science department and foods company (4,5), were awarded a previous Institute of Food Technologists' Food Technology Industrial Achievement Award. The award recognized UPLWEP as a significant advance in the application of food technology to commercial food production.

Freezing

Egg products are pasteurized prior to freezing. *Uncooked whites* retain their functional properties after freezing and thawing, whereas *cooked whites* exhibit **syneresis** (water leakage) upon thawing. *Whole eggs* and *yolks* may gel and become gummy upon thawing, possibly as a result of an aggregation of low-density lipoproteins in the yolk. Processors may control this by adding papain (an enzyme) to hydrolyze the protein. A 10% sugar solution (1 tablespoon of sugar per cup of eggs, household measure), a 5% syrup of corn syrup, or 1 teaspoon of salt per cup of eggs may be added to yolks before freezing as a control against aggregation. As water is bound to the enzyme, sugar, or salt, the defrosted product exhibits less gel formation.

Dehydration

Egg dehydration is a process of preservation that began in 1870s. Dehydration offers microbial control to egg products, as water levels are reduced commonly by spray drying or drying on trays (producing a flaked, granular form). The dehydrated whole egg, white, yolk, or blend is then packaged in various sized packages or drums. Subsequently, it may be reconstituted and cooked, or added as an ingredient to packaged foods such as cake mixes or pasta.

Whites require the removal of glucose prior to dehydration in order to improve storage stability because glucose in the whites leads to unacceptable browning and flavor changes. The browning is a result of the Maillard reaction (nonenzymatic) of proteins and sugars in long or hot storage. Glucose may be removed by lactobacillus microbial fermentation or by enzymatic fermentation with commercial enzymes such as glucose oxidase or catalase.

Yolks undergo irreversible changes in their lipoprotein structure when dehydrated. They should be kept at temperatures of less than 50°F (10°C) to maintain quality.

STORING EGGS

The USDA graded eggs are washed, sanitized, oiled, graded, and packaged soon after they are laid, and it is usually a matter of days between the egg leaving the hen house and reaching the supermarket. Cold temperatures, high humidity, and proper handling are required in storage, and when kept cold, eggs may be safely stored for 4–5 weeks past the pack date. The pack date is stamped on egg cartons as a number of 001 through 365, which corresponds to the day of the year that the eggs were packed. An expiration date of 30 days past the pack date may appear on eggs with the federal grade mark.

It is recommended that the consumer should store eggs on an inside shelf of the refrigerator, large end up, *not* on the door where the temperature is warmer. Whether it is 1 dozen eggs or flats of 30 dozen or more, eggs should be kept in the carton in which they were obtained, in order to prevent moisture loss and the absorption of odors and flavors from other refrigerated ingredients. Hard cooked eggs may be retained in a refrigerated unit for up to 1 week. Any break-out portions of egg may be safely stored under refrigeration: yolks in water, for 1–2 days, in a covered container; whites for up to 4 days in a covered container.

DENATURATION AND COAGULATION

When a protein molecule retains the peptide linkages between amino acids (its primary structure), yet unfolds, **denaturation** occurs producing *irreversible* changes in the specific folding and shape that a protein assumes in space. This may occur due to heat, mechanical action such as beating or whipping, or an acidic pH. The helical chains with *intramolecular* bonds uncoil and align in a parallel fashion, forming *intermolecular* bonds, and the protein chains shrink. Denaturation may be mild or extensive. In the process, the egg changes in appearance from translucent to opaque.

Coagulation represents the process that occurs when denatured protein molecules from either the white or yolk form a solid mass. The liquid/fluid egg (which is a sol) is converted into a solid or semisolid state (which is a gel). This coagulation occurs over a wide temperature range and is influenced by factors, such as heat, beating, pH, use of sugar and salt. Coagulation results in the precipitation of the protein, such as is evidenced by the formation of a curd in cheesemaking. Beyond denaturation and coagulation, undesirable curdling occurs. In **curdling,** the precipitate shrinks and becomes tough. Some factors involved in the mild denaturation, subsequent coagulation, and curdling are as follows:

- **Heat**. The egg *white* denatures, coagulates, and becomes solid at temperatures 144–149°F (62–65°C). Whites are more heat sensitive than *yolks,* which begin to coagulate at 149°F (65°C) and become solid at 158°F (70°C). Whole eggs coagulate at an intermediate temperature. In the preparation of an egg mixture such as an egg custard, the rate of heating and intensity of heat must be controlled. A *slow* rate of heating coagulates the egg mixture at a lower temperature than a rapid rate of heating. Additionally, it provides the margin of error between the coagulation temperature and undesirable curdling, because the coagulation temperature is close to the curdling point. A *rapid* rate of heating may quickly exceed the desired temperature and result in undesirable curdling.

  With *mild heating,* an egg protein denatures and molecular associations form in the protein structure coagulating the egg. Prolonged or *intense heating* causes curdling with negative changes such as water loss and shrinkage (Chapter 8).

Baking in a water bath controls both the rate of heating and the heat intensity. Water baths do not allow the product temperature to exceed the boiling temperature of water.

- **Surface changes by mechanical beating,** and so forth. The changes denature the helical protein structure.
- **Acid pH.** An acid pH coagulates eggs. For example, adding acid to the water used for poaching eggs coagulates the egg white, and acid in the water controls leakage from cracks in eggs that are hard cooked. Acidic cooking water may cause difficulty in peeling an older, more alkaline egg.

EFFECT OF ADDED INGREDIENTS ON COAGULATION

The addition of other ingredients to an egg, such as sugar and salt, affect the denaturation and coagulation process.

Sugar. The addition of sugar exerts a protective effect on the egg by controlling the rate of denaturation and ultimate formation of intermolecular bonds. For example, in the preparation of meringues, the foam in the meringue will not be as large if sugar is added early, *prior* to denaturation, rather than late, *after* the egg white has denatured. Sugar also raises the temperature required for coagulation. A custard, prepared with sugar has a higher coagulation temperature than a similar egg–milk mixture without sugar but produces no change in the finished gel (Chapter 14).

Salt. When salt is added, it promotes denaturation, coagulation, and gelation. Salt may be a constituent of food, such as the milk salts in milk, or it may be added to a product formulation. Milk salts contribute to custard gelation, whereas the addition of water to eggs does *not* promote gelation.

Acid level. As the pH decreases and becomes more acidic, coagulation of the white occurs more readily. An older, more alkaline egg will result in less coagulation than a fresh, neutral pH egg. Vinegar may be added to the water of poached and hard cooked egg to aid in denaturation and coagulation and to prevent spreading. Coagulation depends on which egg protein is involved, and its isoelectric point (pI)—the point at which a protein is least soluble and usually precipitates.

Dilution. Egg is often *diluted* by the addition of other substances in a food system. The coagulation temperature is elevated if an egg mixture is made dilute by water or milk. If a mix is diluted, a less firm finished product results.

COOKING CHANGES

Cooking methods that produce tender, high-quality products should be selected. Some examples are provided in the following:

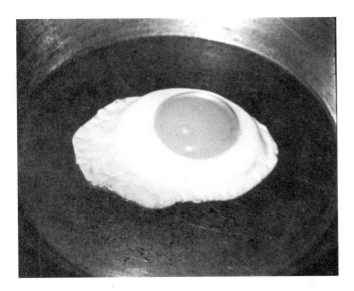

Figure 10.9   Pan fried egg.

Pan Frying: (Figure 10.9)

- Pan frying coagulates the egg proteins.

- A preheated pan allows coagulation before the egg has an opportunity to spread; an overheated pan may overcoagulate the egg and produce a tough product.

- Frying eggs in a measurable amount of fat and basting the top of the egg with fat produces a tender egg, but may not be desirable in terms of the calorie and fat contribution that is offered.

- Eggs may be pan "fried" in liquids other than fat or oil, and the pan lid may remain in use to create steam that cooks the egg's upper surface.

Hard Cooked Eggs:

- *Method:* "Boiled eggs" are tenderer when they reach a *simmering, not boiling* temperature. Too many eggs (more than one layer deep) or placing eggs in cold water at the start of cooking may retard the "doneness" of hard cooked eggs, therefore it is recommended that eggs be placed one layer deep in a covered saucepan of *boiling* water, and then *simmered*, not boiled, for 15–18 minutes for a hard cooked egg, or just 2 1/2–5 minutes for a soft "boiled" egg.

- *Peeling:* Eggs should be cooled rapidly to facilitate easier peeling. Fresh eggs, 1–1 1/2 weeks old, may be difficult to peel, in part because an alkaline pH has not yet been achieved.

- *Cracking:* In order to prevent cracking from an expansion of internal pressure, it may be recommended that the air cell at the large end of an egg be punctured. This is especially true for older eggs. Acid may be added to the cooking water in order to coagulate any egg that escapes through cracks, or the egg may be warmed slightly prior to cooking.

- *Color:* Green discoloration of hard cooked eggs occurs with long and high heat exposure. The green color is due to the formation of *ferrous sulfide* from sulfur in the egg white protein combining with iron from the yolk.

Custard:

- *Method:* Custards (served plain or incorporated into cream desserts, flan, or quiche) are cooked with a slow rate of heating. This provides a margin of error that protects against a rapid temperature elevation from the point of coagulation to undesirable curdling where the protein structure shrinks and releases water. Custards may be stirred or baked. Soft, *stirred* custard will cling to a stirring spoon, as it thickens. It remains pourable and does *not* form a gel. If overheated, or heated too quickly, the mixture curdles and separates into curds and whey. Therefore, the use of a double boiler or cooking over water is recommended in order to control temperature and the rate of cooking. A *baked* custard reaches a higher temperature than stirred custard and gels. Baking in a water bath is recommended in order to control heat and prevent the mixture from burning (Figure 10.10).

- *Texture:* The texture of an egg custard is dependent on a number of factors, including the extent of egg coagulation and added ingredients. A well-coagulated

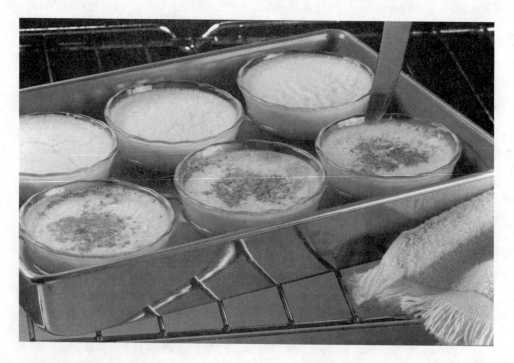

Figure 10.10 Custard baked in water bath
(*Source:* American Egg Board).

custard is fine textured; a curdled custard is extremely porous and watery. Milk assists in coagulating the egg; sugar raises the coagulation temperature, and custards prepared with starch (such as arrowroot, cornstarch, flour, tapioca) control curdling.

EGG WHITE FOAMS AND MERINGUES

An egg white *foam* is created as whites are beaten to incorporate air. A foam holds its shape as protein coagulates around air cells, and thus, beaten whites are used in numerous food applications, as meringues, or incorporated into a recipe to lighten the structure. The volume and stability of egg white foams is dependent on the temperature of the egg and other added substances, as shown in Table 10.4. If the

TABLE 10.4   Some Factors Affecting the Volume and Stability of Egg White Foams

Temperature—The temperature of eggs influences beating ability. At room temperature, eggs have less surface tension and are more easily beaten than if they were cold. Yet, at warm temperatures, *Salmonella* may grow and cause illness in susceptible individuals.

pH—If acid substances such as cream of tartar are added to raw egg whites at the beginning of the beating process, there is less volume but greater stability due to intramolecular bond coagulation. Acid should be added in the whipping process *after* eggs reach the *foamy stage* and have large air cells.

Salt—Salt adds flavor. Its presence delays foam formation, and if added early in the beating process, it produces a drier foam with less volume and stability. Salt should be added to egg white foams *at the foamy stage* or later.

Sugar—The protective effect of sugar on eggs has been discussed. The addition of sugar causes less intermolecular bonding of the egg proteins than would occur in the absence of sugar. Therefore, the addition of sugar results in an egg foam that is stable, but has less volume. A fine-textured, more stable foam develops if finely ground (NOT confectioners sugar as it contains cornstarch) sugar is added early in the beating process. Sugar (2–4 tablespoons per egg white) should be added to foams gradually, *at the soft peak* or stiff peak stage of development, *after* large air cells have formed and denaturation has begun.

Fat—Traces of fat may remain in the equipment used for beating egg white foams; fat may originate from the egg yolk or be introduced by another added ingredient in the product formulation. If fat enters the egg white, there will be substantially less foaming, thus less volume of the beaten white. Fat interferes with the foaming that would occur if protein aligned itself around the air cell and coagulated.

Liquid—The addition of liquid dilutes the egg white. Added liquid, such as water, will increase volume and tenderness of foams, yet it results in a less stable, softer foam and an increased likelihood of syneresis. Dried egg white that has been reconstituted requires a longer beating time than fresh egg whites, due to some protein breakdown in the drying process.

foam is not immediately incorporated into a formulation, it may lose some of its characteristic elasticity, and upon standing, become stiff and brittle.

When egg whites are over-beaten to the *dry foam* stage, they are not as effective a leavening agent as eggs beaten to a *stiff peak* because, with additional beating, the eggs become inelastic and are not able to expand. Also, leavening is diminished if *older* eggs are used for creation of foams. While they whip up more easily, protein does not coagulate around air cells as well in older eggs as fresh eggs, and there is a higher percentage of thin whites that create large, unstable foams. Additionally, eggs that are *cold* have a high surface tension and do not beat to as high a volume as room temperature eggs. To solve this dilemma, and prevent Salmonella risks, rather than setting eggs out to warm to room temperature, eggs may be slightly warmed by placing them in a bowl of warm water prior to use.

Egg *yolks* contain fat that physically interferes with the alignment of protein around air cells. Therefore, the yolks should be completely separated from the whites that are intended to create a foam. Although egg yolks cannot form foams, they may be beaten to become thicker. Commercial *egg substitutes,* aside from imparting their yellowish color, may be successfully used in the preparation of foams if they consist primarily of whites and contain no fat.

A variety of food products are created using egg white foams, including cakes, dessert shells, sweet or savory soufflés, and pies. A sweet, beaten, and baked egg white foam is known as a meringue and may be either soft or hard, the latter prepared with more sugar. Examples of sweet meringue confections include pies, cookies, and candies. The majority of these require that egg whites be beaten to either the soft or stiff peak stage, and added immediately to the recipe. Care should be taken to gently *fold*, not stir the beaten egg whites into the other recipe ingredients (see Figure 10.11). Processors use egg white foams to create special appearance and volume.

The special problems that may arise with meringues are *weeping* and *beading*. A hot oven and cold pie filling may be responsible for both of these problems in the same meringue. **Weeping** is the release of water from *undercoagulated* (perhaps

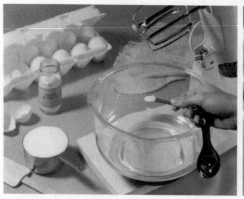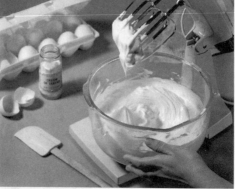

Figure 10.11 Unbeaten (left) and beaten egg whites (right) after addition of acid and sugar (*Source*: American Egg Board).

underbeaten) *or undercooked* egg whites. It may occur at the bottom of the meringue, at the interface of meringue and filling if the meringue is not placed on a hot filling.

Beading is apparent in *overcoagulated* or overcooked meringues. It may be the result of insufficient incorporation of sugar into the beaten egg whites, or baking too long, whereby proteins reach high temperatures and release water. Beading appears as drops of amber colored syrup on top of meringue. A brief look at the stages of denaturation appears in Table 10.5 when egg whites are beaten to foams.

EGG PRODUCTS AND EGG SUBSTITUTES

Egg products include pasteurized, processed, convenient, refrigerated liquid, frozen, and dried eggs that are available in the marketplace to commercial and retail users.

TABLE 10.5   Beaten Egg White Foam

Stage	Description
Unbeaten raw egg white	• small volume of thick and thin whites • no initial additives
Foamy	• unstable, large air-cell volume, transparent • bubbles coalesce if beating is halted • acid coagulates protein around air cell • add cream of tartar (acid) now
Soft rounded peaks	• air cells subdivide in size and are whiter • volume is increased • add sugar now • may be used for food applications • used for soft meringue
Stiff pointed peaks	• many small air cells, volume is increased • egg protein coagulates around fine air cells • ready for most food applications • used for hard meringue
Dry peak foam	• brittle, inelastic; less volume as air cells break • denatured, water escapes, **flocculated** • not as effective as a leavening agent • overcoagulated, curdled appearance

They are inspected by the USDA. If in liquid form, eggs may be ultrapasteurized (see Milk and Milk Products Chapter 11) or aseptically packaged (see Packaging of Food Products, Chapter 19) to extend shelf life. ***Egg substitutes*** have *no* yolks and may contain 80% egg white. The "yolk" is made of corn oil, nonfat milk solids (NFMS), calcium caseinate, soy protein isolate, soybean oil, and other substances, including vitamins and minerals. The egg substitute also contains no cholesterol, less fat, and more *unsaturated* fat than whole egg, and many U.S. egg patents have been issued relating to low-fat and low or decholesterized egg products (6,7).

The egg-white proteins of egg substitutes are heat-sensitive, and denaturation may be controlled with the addition of other ingredients. However, the use of egg substitutes in scrambled eggs and omelets (Figure 10.12) requires an equipment surface cooking temperature of 250–280°F (121–138°C), well below the typical restaurant griddle temperature of 350–375°F (177–191°C). Use of an omelet pan or aluminum pan on the griddle reduces the temperature of the pan interior to an appropriate level without turning down the griddle (5). Many egg substitutes (those containing no fat) although yellowish in color, may be beaten for use in foams.

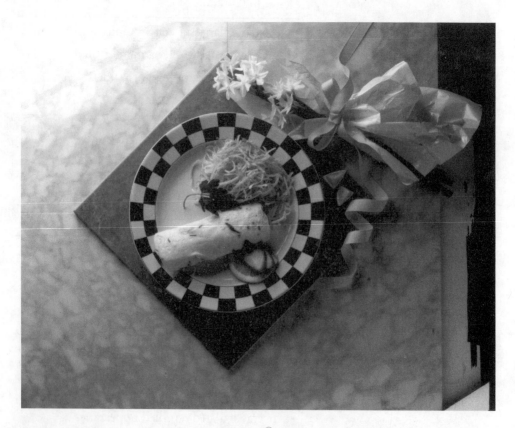

Figure 10.12 Egg product (Courtesy of SYSCO® Incorporated).

NUTRITIVE VALUE OF EGGS

Eggs contain *vitamins* A, D, E, the water-soluble B's, and *minerals* such as iron, phosphorus, and zinc as well as iodine, potassium, and sulfur. Eggs are low in calories—75 cal per large egg—and are used to fortify many foods low in protein.

Eggs are a complete *protein*, with a **biological value** of 100, which indicates that all the absorbed protein is retained by the body, and all other protein sources are evaluated against this standard. That is not to say that eggs are "the perfect *food.*" Egg *whites* are given the highest **protein-digestibility-corrected amino acid score** (PDCAAS) of 1.0, which corrects the amino acid composition with its digestibility. For FDA labeling purposes, the PDCAAS method of determining protein quality is used. The % Daily Value for protein that appears on labels reflects both the quantity (in grams) and quality of protein (Table 10.6).

Egg yolks contain cholesterol, which must be restricted by some individuals, and over the past years, the American Heart Association (AHA) has changed its recommendations from eating no more than *three* eggs per week to eating *four* eggs per week. Technology has made the determination of cholesterol content more accurate and reflective of the actual amount, and has produced eggs that are lower than the USDA analysis of 215 mg cholesterol that is calculated for the majority of eggs. These developments may be achieved by control of animal feed, without using drugs, hormones, or antibiotics. Additional data on dietary cholesterol and its effect on lipoprotein metabolism are reported in Refs. (6–8).

SAFETY OF EGGS

The contents of freshly laid eggs are generally sterile, although **Salmonella enteritidis** (SE) has been found inside some eggs. Eggs are usually protected from bacteria by the shell and the two shell membranes, however, the surface of *shell eggs* contains a high level of bacteria, especially when it is soiled, and these bacteria may enter the shell through the pores. If bacteria travel to the internal portion of the egg, it is typically the egg yolk membrane (i.e., the vitellin membrane), not the yolk or white that harbors the bacteria.

The Egg Safety Action Plan, a joint effort by the FDA and USDA, was announced in late, 1999. Its intent is to reduce the incidence of SE, and it contains *two* important requirements. 1) The *refrigeration* requirement in this Plan is that eggs

TABLE 10.6 PDCAAS of Selected Foods

Egg white	1	Chick peas	0.66
Casein (milk)	1	Pinto beans	0.63
Soybean isolate	0.99	Rolled oats	0.57
Beef	0.92	Lentils	0.52
Kidney beans	0.68	Whole wheat	0.40

delivered to a retail establishment (restaurants, hospitals, schools, nursing homes grocery stores, delis, and vending operations) be quickly stored at an ambient temperature of 45°F (7°C) or less upon receipt, and 2) There is a required *statement* on shell-egg cartons that reads as follows:

"**SAFE HANDLING INSTRUCTIONS**: To prevent illness from bacteria: keep eggs refrigerated, cook eggs until yolks are firm, and cook foods containing eggs thoroughly."

The FDA Commissioner added to this November, 2000 press and broadcast media release saying: "... no sunny side up, no over easy." (Dr. Jane E. Henney, FDA Commissioner.)

The FDA prohibits the use of raw or lightly cooked eggs in food production or manufacturing facilities. Eggs must reach an internal temperature of 145°F (63°C) or higher to be considered safe for consumption (check local jurisdiction).

As well, The President's Council on Food Safety has encouraged developments in science and technology by companies and universities to reduce the incidence of SE. For example, methods are being investigated/employed to bring an egg temperature down form 109°F (43°C) (the internal temperature of hens) to a cold temperature of 45°F (7°C) to control SE. One such method utilizes cryogenic carbon dioxide, another uses a clean warm-water bath to kill bacteria without cooking (10,11).

International contamination of eggs with SE is very low, even from a known positive flock (9). Yet, the safety of eggs must be ensured. For example, only clean, uncracked eggs should be purchased from a reputable supplier. Exterior surface bacteria can enter shells of dirty eggs, or even clean ones, especially through cracks causing the egg to be unsafe. Also, since washing is a routine step in commercial egg processing, *rewashing* eggs prior to use is not necessary or recommended. When eggs are washed in warm water and then refrigerated, pressure changes in a cooling egg draw harmful exterior microbes in through the pores. One more safety consideration involves the common restaurant practice of "pooling" (commingling), which is not recommended. (Pooled eggs are many eggs cracked together and stored ahead, ready to use.) Eggs should be stored cold at temperatures of approximately 40°F (4.4°C).

Prior to incorporation into recipes, either egg yolks, or the egg white to be used for meringue, may be *partially cooked* over direct heat or water bath to control SE. If the egg is *refrigerated*, bacterial growth is extremely slow, and disease is not likely to result. Egg *products* are pasteurized and free of *Salmonella*.

Hard cooked eggs reach a final cooking temperature that is sufficient to kill the natural bacteria of an egg, yet *recontamination* may occur. For example, if the egg is hidden, the oil coating of the egg may be lost, and the pores of the egg may open. Subsequently, the egg may be contaminated with substances such as lawn chemicals, fertilizers, or droppings from household pets, birds, reptiles, and rodents (7). Thus, for consumers who follow the traditional practices of decorating and hiding Easter eggs, the USDA caution remains: Keep perishables at room temperature for no longer than 2 hours. Decorated eggs may be very inexpensive and are, thus, included in many celebrations, but the recommendation is that separate eggs be used for eating and decorating or "hiding."

Egg White Resistance to Bacterial Growth

Egg *whites* have natural protection against microorganisms by several chemical substances, but cannot be considered 100% safe once the shell has been broken. Avidin, lysozyme, and conalbumin of egg white provide protection against microbial growth. *Avidin,* in the raw egg, binds the vitamin biotin required for some microorganism growth. *Lysozyme* hydrolyzes cell walls of some bacteria and thus demonstrates antibacterial action, especially at lower pH levels (reminder: prevention of CO_2 loss is a good control as CO_2 loss leads to higher pH). *Conalbumin* binds with the iron of the yolk preventing growth of the microorganisms that require iron for growth.

Pasteurized raw eggs in uncooked foods such as mayonnaise do not support the growth of bacteria as do *unpasteurized* shell eggs. Thus, only pasteurized egg products may be used in manufacturing or retail operations, where a food containing eggs is not subject to adequate heat treatment. Uncooked meringues prepared by shell egg whites that are *not* pasteurized are considered a *"low*-risk" food though, because they contain a large amount of sugar that ties up the water needed for bacterial growth. The water activity needs of the bacteria are not met, and the bacteria do not grow. Yet, some risk of bacterial presence remains and, again, it is recommended that all eggs including egg whites be cooked prior to use (Chapter 16). It is not recommended that raw eggs or egg parts remain raw in a recipe.

USDA Sampling

The USDA-administered Egg Products Inspection Act of 1970 requires routine sampling and analysis, and routine inspection for wholesome, unadulterated eggs and egg products. Plants are inspected regardless of whether the shipment is intrastate, interstate, or out of the country. State standards, regulated by the state's Department of Agriculture must be equivalent to federal standards.

CONCLUSION

Whole eggs, and their component parts, are important for their nutritive value and array of functional properties such as binding, emulsification, foaming, gelling, and thickening. These properties change with cooking as the egg protein denatures. The processes of grading and evaluation of quality, although not mandatory, are officially carried out by the USDA and their state counterparts. Evaluation of quality and freshness is also an industry and consumer concern. Eggs are candled in order to evaluate and assign grades. In candling, the yolk, white, and air-cell size as well as the integrity of the shell are viewed prior to sale. Egg size is not a part of egg quality evaluation. The color of an egg shell is dependent on the breed of hen, and the yolk color is dependent on the feed.

Processing and preservation of eggs occurs with the use of mineral oil and the techniques of pasteurization, freezing, and dehydration, after which proper storage is important in maintaining safety and other aspects of food quality. The addition of other ingredients to an egg, such as salt and acid, promote denaturation. Sugar exerts a protective effect, controlling the denaturation and coagulation processes. Some factors affecting the volume and stability of egg white foams include temperature, pH, salt, sugar, fat, and addition of liquid. The recommendation is that eggs not be old or cold.

Various forms of eggs, including pasteurized shelled eggs, are available, and egg substitutes may be purchased in the marketplace. Eggs have a biological value of 100, and are given the highest PDCAAS score. Vigilance is necessary in the handling and use of eggs, as the growth of *Salmonella* may occur in this potentially hazardous food.

GLOSSARY

Air cell or air pocket: A space between shell membranes where air is found within the shell, typically at the large end of an egg.

Biological value: Eggs contain a score of 100 based on its efficiency in supporting the body's needs; reflects the amount of nitrogen retained in the body, due to the completeness of the protein. (An incomplete protein is deaminated and nitrogen is not retained.)

Beading: Amber colored syrup beads on top of baked meringue as a result of overcoagulation.

Binder: Holds the ingredients of a mixture or its breading together.

Candling: Viewing the inside and shell of an egg by holding it up to a bright light.

Clarify: To remove foreign particles from a hot liquid.

Coagulation: Extensive denaturation of protein molecules yielding a solid mass or gel.

Curdling: The protein precipitates, shrinks, releases water, and becomes tough.

Denaturation: Changes in the conformation of a protein caused by changes in temperature, an acidic pH, or by surface changes such as mechanical beating.

Egg substitute: Liquid or frozen egg white product with a "yolk" typically consisting of corn oil, nonfat milk solids, calcium caseinate, soy protein isolate, soybean oil, and other substances.

Emulsifier: Material that allows two ordinarily immiscible substances to mix.

Flocculated: Separation of overbeaten egg white foam into small masses.

Foam: Increased volume of beaten egg white that holds shape as protein coagulates around air cells.

Gel: A two-phase system where egg coagulates with liquid in a solid.

Pasteurization: Heating for a specific time at a temperature that eliminates pathogens.

Protein-digestibility-corrected amino acid score (PDCAAS): A measure of protein quality that compares the amino acid balance with requirements of preschoolers and corrects for digestibility. Used by the FDA for labeling and by the WHO.

Salmonella enteritidus (SE): Pathogenic, infection-causing bacteria especially prevalent in poultry and eggs.

Syneresis: "Weeping" or water leakage from coagulated egg.

Thickening agent: Increases viscosity.

Ultrapasteurization: High temperature, short time heat to kill pathogenic microorganisms.

Weeping: Syneresis or release of water from undercoagulated or underbeaten egg whites.

REFERENCES

1. Jordan R, Barr AT, Wilson MC. *Shell eggs: Quality and Properties As Affected by Temperature and Length of Storage.* Purdue University Agricultural Experiment Station: West Lafayette, IN. Bulletin #612.
2. *Egg Grading Manual.* Handbook No. 75. Washington, DC: USDA. 1983.
3. Giese J. Ultrapasteurized Liquid Whole Eggs Earn 1994 IFT Food Technology Industrial Achievement Award. *Food Technology.* 1994; 48(9): 94–96.
4. Department of Food Science, North Carolina State University, Raleigh, North Carolina.
5. Michael Foods Inc, Minneapolis, MN.
6. Binge NA, Cheng J. Low-fat, low-cholesterol egg yolk in food applications. *Food Technology.* 1995; 49(5): 94–101.
7. American Egg Board. Park Ridge, IL.
8. Whitney EN, Rolfes SR. *Understanding Nutrition,* 9th ed. St. Paul, MN: West Publishing Co., 2001.
9. California Egg Commission. Upland, CA.
10. Praxair Inc. Technologies target Salmonella in eggs. *Food Engineering.* 2000; July/August: 14.
11. Mermelstein NH. Cryogenic system rapidly cools eggs. *Food Technology.* 2000; 54 (6): 100–102.

BIBLIOGRAPHY

Agri-Dairy Products. Purchase, NY.
How to Buy Eggs. Home and Garden Bulletin No. 144. Washington, DC: USDA.
Stadleman WH, Cotterill OJ. *Egg Science and Technology,* 3rd ed. Binghampton, NY: Food Products Press, 1990.
USDA. Washington, DC.

CHAPTER 11

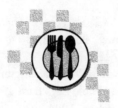

Milk and Milk Products

INTRODUCTION

Milk is the first food of young mammals produced by the mammary glands of female mammals. It is a mixture of fat and high quality protein in water, and contains some carbohydrate (lactose), vitamins, and minerals. Milk and milk products may be obtained from different species, such as goats and sheep, but the focus of this chapter is on cow milk and milk products. While fluid milk contains a very large percentage of water, it may be concentrated to form evaporated milk and cheeses. Throughout the world, it is used in a variety of ways, such as a beverage, cheese, yogurt, or in soups and sauces. By law, milk and milk products must contain a designated percent of milk solids, not fat (MSNF), but the butterfat component is the most expensive component of milk and its level determines if milk is offered for retail sale as *whole* milk or at some lesser percentage of fat, such as 2% milk, 1%, 1/2%, or fat-free

Milk may be cultured, dried, fortified, homogenized, or pasteurized, and used to create products with different taste, texture, nutritive value, and shelf life. It may be processed into products such as buttermilk, cheese, cream, ice milk, ice cream, sour cream, and yogurt with different levels of fat content. Dried milk is added to a multitude of industrially manufactured or home-prepared foods. It may be added to foods to increase the protein or calcium value.

Milk is not well tolerated by a large portion of the population that does not have the enzyme to digest the milk sugar. High temperatures may curdle milk; therefore, care must be taken in the preparation of foods with milk. Milk requires safe handling and cold storage.

COMPOSITION OF MILK

Milk varies in physical and chemical composition depending on such factors as age, and breed of the cow, activity-level, stage of lactation, use of medication, and interval between milkings. On the average, the **total milk solids**, which are carbohydrates, fat, protein, and minerals in the milk, comprise 12–13% of milk. The bulk of that total is **milk solids** nonfat **(MSNF)**, including the serum solids lactose, caseins, whey proteins, and minerals, which comprises approximately 8.5% of milk. Fat content varies.

Water

Milk is composed primarily of water, which is present at a level of approximately 87–88%. (The remaining 12–13% of milk is termed *total milk solids,* described above). Since approximately 20% of milk protein is found in the aqueous phase of milk, if that water is removed, the shelf life of milk products is extended.

Carbohydrate

Carbohydrate is *water-soluble* and present in the aqueous phase of milk, at levels of approximately 5%. The disaccharide *lactose* is the main carbohydrate that exhibits low solubility and may precipitate out of solution as a grainy textured substance. It is converted to lactic acid 1) upon *souring* due to bacterial fermentation, and 2) in the process of *aging* cheese, therefore, aged cheese may be digested even in the absence of the enzyme lactase. (The lactose content of milk and some milk products appears in Table 11.2.)

Fat

The completeness of milking determines richness of the fat content. Fat has a low density, and may easily be centrifuged or skimmed off of the milk yielding low-fat or skim milk. The fat, or butterfat, exists at levels of 3–4% in *whole* milk (varying by state law), at lesser levels in reduced-fat milks, and at significantly higher percentages in cream. It is the expensive component of milk, and the basis on which farmers are paid for milk.

Fat globules are less dense than the water in the aqueous phase of milk and, therefore, rise to the top of the container in the **creaming** process. When emulsified during homogenization there is an *increase in the number* of fat cells and *greater viscosity* because the fat is distributed throughout the fluid, and creaming does not occur. Membranes of lipids and protein, including lecithin, from each fat globule remain in the milk as it is processed.

Fat content in milk may vary greatly in calories. However, it either carries, or may be fortified to contain the fat-soluble vitamins, and it contains the pigments carotene and xanthophyll. Fat contains lipids such as cholesterol and the phospholipids, but it is primarily triglyceride (95%) with saturated, polyunsaturated, and monounsaturated fatty acid components that have varying melting points and susceptibility to oxidation. The fatty acid chains vary from 4 to 22 carbons in length and contain many short-chain fatty acids such as the saturated butyric acid (4 C) and caproic, caprylic, and capric acids.

Protein

Protein represents 3–4% of the composition of milk and components may be fractioned out of milk by ultracentrifugation. ***Casein*** is the *primary* protein of milk, comprising approximately 80% of the milk protein. The caseins are actually a group of similar proteins, which can be separated from the other milk proteins by acidification to a pH of 4.6 (the isoelectric point). At this pH, the caseins aggregate, since they are hydrophobic, are poorly hydrated and carry no net charge. The other milk proteins, being more hydrophilic, remain dispersed in the aqueous phase.

There are three main casein fractions, known as alpha$_s$-, beta- and kappa-casein (α_s-, β- and κ-casein). Alpha$_s$-casein actually comprises two fractions: α_{s1}-casein and α_{s2}-casein. However, these two fractions are difficult to separate from each other. The four fractions α_{s1}-, β-, κ- and α_{s2}-casein occur in the weight ratio 3:3:1:0.8. All four fractions are phosphoproteins containing phosphate groups esterified to the amino acid serine. The α_s- and β-casein fractions contain several phosphate groups, and as a result are "calcium-sensitive," and may be coagulated by addition of calcium. Kappa-casein contains only one phosphate group and is not calcium sensitive. The α_s- and β-casein fractions are very hydrophobic. However, kappa-casein is a glycoprotein containing an acidic (charged) carbohydrate section, and so it is much more hydrophilic.

In milk, the casein fractions associate with each other and with colloidal calcium phosphate to from stable spherical structures known as ***casein micelles***. The more hydrophobic α_s- and β-casein fractions exist mainly in the interior of the micelles, whereas the more hydrophilic κ-casein exists mainly on the micelle surface. It is the κ-casein that gives the micelles their stability in milk under normal handling conditions. This is due to the negative charge and hydration of the kappa-casein, coupled with the fact that the charged hydrophilic carbohydrate section of the molecule tends to protrude from the micelle surface in hair-like structures, which confer *steric* (or spatial) stability on the micelles.

The casein micelles are coagulated by addition of acid at a pH of 4.6–5.2. As the micelles approach their isoelectric point, the charge and extent of hydration is reduced, and the κ-casein hair-like structures flatten, reducing steric hindrance. Hence, the micelles are no longer stable, and so they aggregate. This is the basis for the formation of cottage cheese, which is an acid cheese containing casein curds. Acid also causes some calcium to be removed from the micelles, and so cottage cheese is relatively low in calcium compared with some other dairy products.

The casein micelles may also be coagulated by addition of the enzyme rennin, which may be added to milk to prepare rennet custard or cheese. Rennin cleaves a specific bond in κ-casein, and causes the charged, hydrophilic hair-like structures to be removed from the micelles. As a result, the micelle surface is uncharged, hydrophobic, and unstable, and so the micelles aggregate to form curds. The curds may be separated from the whey and processed to form cheese (see section on Cheese). Coagulation by rennin does not cause calcium to be removed from the micelles.

Casein micelles are relatively heat stable, and are not denatured by heat (at neutral pH) unless temperatures are very high and heating is prolonged. This is not a problem under most cooking conditions. However, it is a potential problem in heated concentrated milk products such as evaporated milk. The problem is avoided by addition of carrageenan to protect the protein.

Caseins contain both hydrophobic and hydrophilic sections; in addition, they contain a high proportion of the amino acid proline, and so they are flexible proteins containing little regular, ordered secondary structure (see Chapter 8). As a result, they readily *adsorb* at an oil–water interface, forming a stable film that prevents coalescence of emulsion droplets (see Chapter 13), and so they make excellent emulsifiers.

A *second* protein fraction of milk is the **whey** or serum. It makes up approximately 20% of milk protein and includes the lactalbumins and lactoglobulins. Whey proteins are more hydrated than casein and are denatured and precipitated by *heat*, rather than by *acid*. (More information is contained in this chapter in the section entitled Whey.)

Other protein components of milk include enzymes such as lipase, protease, and alkaline phosphatase, which hydrolyze triglycerides, proteins, and phosphate esters, respectively. The average measures of protein quality, including biological value, digestibility, net protein utilization, protein efficiency, and chemical score, for milk and milk products appears in Table 11.1.

Vitamins and Minerals

Milk contains both water-soluble and fat-soluble *vitamins*. The nonfat portion of milk is especially plentiful in the B vitamin riboflavin, a greenish fluorescent colored

TABLE 11.1 Average Measures of Protein Quality for Milk and Milk Products

	BV	Digestibility	NPU	PER[a]	Chemical Score
Milk	84.5	96.9	81.6	3.09	60
Casein	79.7	96.3	72.1	2.86	58
Lactalbumin	82	97	79.5[b]	3.43	c
Nonfat dry milk	–	–	–	3.11	–

Note: Biological value (BV) is the proportion of absorbed protein that is retained. *Digestibility* (D) is the proportion of food protein that is absorbed. *Net protein utilization* (NPU) is the proportion of food protein intake that is retained (calculated as BV × D). *Protein efficiency ratio* (PER) is the gain in body weight divided by weight of protein consumed. *Chemical score* is the content of the most limiting amino acid expressed as a percentage of the content of the same amino acid in egg protein.

[a]Often PER values are adjusted relative to casein which may be given a value of 2.5.

[b]Calculated.

[c]Denotes no value compiled in Food and Agriculture Organization of the United Nations (FAO) report. *Source*: Adapted from the National Dairy Council.

vitamin. It acts as a photosynthesizer and is readily destroyed upon exposure to sunlight.

Vitamin A is naturally in the fat component of *whole* milk, but whole milk is fortified with vitamin D because it is naturally present only in small amounts. *Low-fat* and *nonfat milk* are fortified with both of these vitamins because fat is reduced or absent.

Minerals (ash) such as calcium and phosphorus are present at levels of approximately 1% of milk, with a third of calcium in solution, and two-thirds of calcium colloidally dispersed. Calcium is combined with the protein casein as calcium caseinate, and with phosphorus as calcium phosphate and as calcium citrate. Other minerals present in milk are chloride, magnesium, potassium, sodium, and sulfur.

Classification of Milk

Whole milk is considered to be the following:

- *Solution* that contains the sugar lactose, the water-soluble vitamins thiamin and riboflavin, and many mineral salts such calcium phosphate, citrates, and the minerals chloride, magnesium, potassium, and sodium

- *Colloidal dispersion* (sol) with casein and whey proteins, calcium phosphate, magnesium phosphate, and citrates

- *Emulsion* with fat globules suspended in the aqueous phase (serum) of milk. The fat globules are surrounded by a complex membrane, the milk fat globule membrane (MFGM), which contains mainly protein and phospholipids (and a few carbohydrate sidechains at the outer surface). This membrane prevents coalescence of the fat droplets.

SANITATION AND GRADING OF MILK

Milk is a potentially hazardous food that must be kept out of the temperature danger zone. With its high water content and plentiful protein, vitamins, and minerals, milk is an ideal medium for supporting bacterial growth. Production, processing, and distribution of milk must ensure that products are free from pathogenic bacteria and low in nonpathogens. Healthy cows and sanitary conditions of handling lead to low bacterial counts. Proper handling also contributes to satisfactory shelf life, as well as appearance, flavor, and nutritive value.

The temperature of raw milk should reach 40°F (4°C) or less within 2 hours of being drawn from the cow. It should be kept well chilled, as it is highly perishable and susceptible to bacterial growth. The shelf life for properly refrigerated milk is 14 days or perhaps 45 days for milk products (cream, lactose reduced milk) that are ultrapasteurized (see Pasteurization).

A contaminated cow, cross-contamination at the farm or from workers hands, or unsanitary equipment or utensils may lead to the spread of certain diseases by milk or milk products. Traditionally, the diseases of diphtheria, salmonellosis, typhoid fever, tuberculosis, and undulant fever were spread by consumption of unsafe milk. Today, the incidence of these diseases is rarely attributed to milk transmission, as milk is pasteurized to destroy pathogens. The control of insects and rodents, as well as separation of animal waste products from the milking area is also necessary for safe milk production.

The United States Department of Agriculture (USDA) and state Departments of Agriculture regulate milk and milk products in interstate and intrastate commerce. Grade "A" milk is available to the consumer for sale as fluid milk, although Grades "B" and "C," with higher bacterial counts, are also safe and wholesome. The grades of US Extra and US Standard are given to dried milk. USDA official grades are given to all inspected milk on a voluntary fee-for-service basis.

FLAVOR OF MILK

The mild, slightly sweet, pleasant flavor, and mouthfeel of milk is due to the presence of emulsified fat, colloidally dispersed proteins, the carbohydrate lactose, and milk salts. Fresh milk contains acetone, acetaldehyde, methyl ketones, and short-chain fatty acids that provide aroma. Less desirable, "barny" or rancid flavors, or other "off-flavors," may be due to the following:

- Slightly "cooked" flavor from excessive pasteurization temperatures.

- Animal feed, including ragweed and other weeds, or wild onion from the field.

- Formation of off-flavor, or off-odor, short-chain fatty acids in raw milk due to lipase activity, causes rancidity of the fat, and this is destroyed by the heat of pasteurization. (The short chain butyric acid may produce an off-odor or off-flavor due to bacteria in the emulsified water of milk, not lipase.)

- Oxidation of fat or phospholipids in the fat globule membrane, especially in emulsified, homogenized milk. Adequate pasteurization temperatures are necessary to destroy the enzyme which oxidizes fat.

- Light-induced flavor changes in the proteins and riboflavin because riboflavin acts as a photosynthesizer.

- Stage of lactation of the cow.

Following pasteurization, milk is typically subjected to "flavor treatment" to standardize the odor and flavor. Milk is instantly heated to 195°F (91°C) with live steam (injected directly into the product), and subsequently subject to a vacuum that removes volatile off-flavors and evaporates excess water produced from the steam.

MILK PROCESSING

Pasteurization

Fluid milk is not routinely *sterilized*, but rather, it is *pasteurized* to assure destruction of the *pathogenic* bacteria, yeasts, and molds, as well as 95–99% of *nonpathogenic* bacteria. **Pasteurization** minimizes the likelihood of disease and extends the storage life of milk. The US Public Health Service of the FDA has developed model ordinances (not the law) that may be adopted by state and local jurisdictions.

Pasteurization temperatures do not change milk components to any great extent (see Nutritive Value). Vitamin destruction and protein denaturation are minimal, and the result is that milk is made safe for consumption. Several acceptable methods of *pasteurization* include thermal processing according to the following.

Pasteurization

- 145°F (63°C) for 30 or more minutes—the batch or holding method and is considered Low-Temperature Longer Time **(LTLT)** pasteurization.
- 161°F (72°C) for 15 seconds—the flash method and is the High-Temperature Short-Time **(HTST)** method of pasteurization.
- 191°F (88°C) for 1 second.
- 194°F (90°C) for 0.5 second.
- 201°F (94°C) for 0.1 second.
- 204°F (96°C) for 0.05 second.
- 212°F (100°C) for 0.01 second.

Pasteurization (or sterilization) is required of all Grade A fluid milk or milk products subject to interstate commerce for retail sale.Traditionally, prevention of tuberculosis (TB) was the primary concern in pasteurization; thus, temperatures of 143°F (62°C) were used to destroy *Mycobacterium tuberculosis,* the bacteria causing TB in humans. Actually, *Coxiella burnetii* that causes Q fever requires an even higher temperature for destruction; thus the required 145°F (63°C) for pasteurization. Rapid cooling controls nonpathogenic growth.

A large U.S. foodborne illness outbreak in recent years, where many thousands of people became ill, was attributed to raw milk that entered the wrong pipeline and contaminated already pasteurized milk. *Inadequate* pasteurization, or the presence of trace amounts (less than 0.1%) of *raw* milk, may be detected by a simple test revealing the presence of a *high* alkaline phosphatase activity. Inversely, *adequate* pasteurization is demonstrated by the absence of the alkaline phosphatase enzyme, which is naturally present in milk, but destroyed at temperatures similar to those required for pasteurization.

Sterilization of milk occurs at the following time and temperature:

- 280–302°F (138–150°C) for 2–6 seconds—**ultrapasteurization** or ultrahigh-temperature **(UHT)** processing (sterile, aseptic). With this treatment, milk is *sterilized* by reaching temperatures beyond the normal pasteurization temperature, and packaging too, is sterilized. Thus, it is *aseptically* packaged, and the milk does not require refrigeration until it is opened.

Sterilization *temperatures* in combination with the use of presterilized *containers*, under sterile *conditions* do not allow spoilage or pathogenic bacteria to enter the milk.

Thus, milk treated in this manner may be safely stored up to 3 months or longer. An example of this is milk in packaging similar to "juice boxes."

Homogenization

The primary function of **homogenization** is to prevent creaming, or the rising of fat to the top of the container of milk (whole or some low-fat milk, *not* fat-free milk). The result is that milk maintains a more uniform composition with improved body and texture, a whiter appearance, richer flavor, and more digestible curd. Homogenization mechanically increases the *number*, and reduces the *size* of the fat globules. The size is reduced from 18 μ to less than 2 μ, or 1/10 of their original size. The process of homogenization permanently emulsifies the fine fat globules by a method that pumps milk under high pressure [2000–2500 lbs/in.^{2} (psi)] through small mesh orifices of a homogenizer.

As the surfaces of many new fat globules are formed, each fat globule becomes coated with a lipoprotein membrane and additional proteins from casein and whey. These proteins adsorb onto the freshly created oil surface preventing globules from reuniting and the fat remains homogeneously distributed throughout milk.

Milk may be homogenized prior to or subsequent to pasteurization. The homogenization process is completed at a fast rate to ensure the control of bacteria and loss of quality.

Some characteristics of homogenized milk include the following:

- No creaming or separation of cream to the top of the container.
- Whiter milk due to a finer dispersions of fat. There is an increase in the absorption and reflection of light due to the smaller fat particles.
- More viscous and creamy milk due to a greater number of fat particles.
- More bland due to smaller fat particles.
- Decreased fat stability as fat globule membranes are broken.
- Less stable to light and may exhibit light-induced flavor deterioration by sunlight or fluorescent light. Thus, paperboard cartons and clouded plastic bottles are used for milk.

Fortification

The addition of fat-soluble vitamins A and D to *whole* milk is optional. Low-fat milk, nonfat milk, and low-fat chocolate milk must be **fortified** (usually before pasteurization) to carry 2000 International Units (IU) or 140 Retinol Equivalents (RE) vitamin A per quart. It is required for milk subjected to interstate commerce.

The addition of vitamin D to reach levels of 400 IUs of vitamin D per quart is optional but routinely practiced. Vitamin D is naturally present in milk to some extent due to the synthesis of vitamin D by the cow as it is exposed to sunlight, and because vitamin D may be present in animal feed.

To increase the viscosity and appearance, as well as the nutritive value of low-fat milk, nonfat milk solids may be added to milk. This addition allows milk to reach a 10% MSNF (versus 8.25% usually present), and it will state "protein fortified" or "fortified with protein" on the label.

Bleaching

The FDA allows benzoyl peroxide, or a mixture of benzoyl peroxide with potassium alum, calcium sulfate, and magnesium carbonate to be used as a bleaching agent in milk to remove pigments such as carotenoids and chlorophylls. The weight of *benzoyl peroxide* must not exceed 0.002% of the weight of the milk, and the *potassium alum, calcium sulfate*, and *magnesium carbonate*, individually or combined must not be more than six times the weight of the benzoyl peroxide. Vitamin A or its precursors may be destroyed in the bleaching process; therefore, sufficient vitamin A is added into the milk, or in the case of cheesemaking to the curd.

TYPES OF MILK

Fluid Milk

Milk may come from goats (Mediterranian countries), sheep (southern Europe), reindeer (northern Europe), and other animal sources throughout the world. It is Holstein cows that typically produce the greatest quantity of milk, and are therefore, the primary milk cow in the U.S. The Guernsey and Jersey breeds produce milk with the highest percentage of fat—approximately 5% fat.

Milk appears *white* due to the reflection of light from colloidally dispersed casein protein and calcium phosphate particles in the milk dispersion; however, an *off-white* color may be due to carotenoid pigment in the animal feed. A *bluish* color may be observed in milk skimmed of fat.

Both the fat content and percent of MSNF of fluid milk are subject to FDA regulations and new technological developments. The butterfat and caloric content of milk are as follows:

Type of Milk	Fat Percent	Calories
Whole	3.25%	150 cal/8 oz.
Reduced fat	2%	120 cal/8 oz.
Low-fat or light	0.5, 1.0%	100 cal/8 oz. (1%)
Nonfat, fat-free/skim	< 0.5%	90 cal/8 oz.

Flavored milk contains fat, protein, vitamin, and mineral contents similar to the milk to which the flavoring was added. It will vary in caloric and carbohydrate values according to added ingredients, yet there is *no* appreciable effect on the availability of calcium or protein to humans when normal quantities of chocolate are added to milk (National Dairy Council).

Evaporated and Concentrated Milks

Evaporation and condensation, coupled with packaging in cans, extends the shelf life of milk. Cans of evaporated milk may be adequately stored for extended time periods, although undesirable color or flavor changes may occur after one year. Once the can has been opened, it should be refrigerated and can be held for up to 1 week.

Evaporated milk is concentrated through the process of evaporation [at 122–131°F (50–55°C)] in a vacuum chamber. Either whole or nonfat milk with 60% of the water removed is then homogenized, fortified with vitamins A and D, canned, and *sterilized* in the can [240–245°F (115–118°C)] in a pressure canner.

Whole evaporated milk must contain not less than 25% total milk solids and not less than 7.5%, milkfat. Evaporated *nonfat* milk must contain not less than 20% milk solids and no more than 0.5% milkfat. It must be fortified with 125 and 25 IU of vitamins A and D, respectively.

Milk is increasingly less stable with the progression of concentration and heat and it may coagulate, so the stabilization of milk proteins is better assured by preheating (forewarming) milk prior to sterilization at temperatures of 203°F (95°C) for 10–20 minutes. This forewarming is designed to denature colloidally dispersed serum proteins and to shift salt balance of calcium chloride and phosphates that are in solution. Disodium phosphate or carrageenan may be added to stabilize casein against precipitation (Chapter 5).

The high temperature used in processing evaporated milk or long storage of the product may produce a light tan color due to the early stages of the **Maillard reaction** between the milk protein and the milk sugar, lactose.

Evaporated milk is reconstituted (rehydrated) at a 1:1 ratio of evaporated milk and water, adding slightly less water than was removed in the 60% evaporation.

Sweetened condensed milk is concentrated whole or nonfat milk with approximately 60% of the water removed, and sugar levels of 40–45% in the finished product. There is a calorie difference in this milk processing, as *whole* sweetened condensed milk contain no less than 8% milkfat and 28% total milk solids, and *nonfat* contains no more than 0.5% milkfat and 24% total milk solids.

Sweetened condensed milk is pasteurized, but *not sterilized*, because the high sugar content (usually at least 60% in the water phase) plays a role in preventing bacterial growth. This is due to the osmotic effect of the sugar that competes with the bacteria for water and, thus, controls bacterial growth.

Dried Milk

Dried milk powder may be processed from either pasteurized whole or, more commonly, from nonfat milk. It is first condensed by removing two-thirds of the water and is typically sprayed into a heated vacuum chamber (spray drying) to dry to less than 5% moisture levels. Milk may also be dried by spraying a jet of hot air into concentrated nonfat milk (foam spray drying). The drying process has no appreciable effect on the nutritive value of milk (National Dairy Council). Most nonfat dry milk is fortified with vitamins A and D.

"Instant" nonfat dry milk, or "agglomerated" milk has some moisture added back to the spray-dried milk powder. It is easily pourable and dispersible in cold water. Three and a half ounces (1–1/3 cups) of dried milk powder is needed to yield 1 quart of fluid milk. Nonfat dried milk (NDM) may be added to foods to increase the protein or calcium content.

Buttermilk and whey may also be dried. *Whey* is of high biological value containing lactalbumins and lactoglobulins, with one-half of the protein and slightly more lactose than NDM. Dried milk is an economical form of milk for shipping, has an extended shelf life, and is useful for addition to numerous other foods. A more acceptable flavor is developed when the milk is reconstituted and chilled several hours before consumption.

Cultured Milk/Fermentation

Cultured products are *fermented* by the addition of bacterial cultures, such as *Lactobacilli* and *Streptococci*, to fluid dairy products. Earlier, warm milk from various animals (cows, sheep, goats, camels) was preserved for several days or weeks, with no need for refrigeration, by the addition of a small milk culture from a preceding batch. The introduction of the harmless lactic acid bacteria (or *bacterial enzymes*) induced a chemical change in the organic substrates of milk solids. Lactose was fermented to lactic acid creating a low pH in the process, which controlled both spoilage and pathogenic bacterial growth, and caused the casein to coagulate.

Acidified products are produced by souring milk with an acid such as lactic, citric, phosphoric, or tartaric acid with or without microorganisms. The addition of lactic-acid-producing bacteria is optional, and because *cultured* and *acidified* products contain different amounts of lactic acid, they differ in flavor.

The following are examples of some commonly cultured milk products:

- **Buttermilk** was traditionally the liquid that *remained* when cream was churned to form butter. Today, this is not the case commercially, because low-fat or skim milk begins the process. Although its name may mistakenly signify a high-fat content, yet because of the type of milk used, it is more correctly named "cultured low-fat milk" or "cultured nonfat milk." Buttermilk differs from nonfat milk in that it contains phospholipids and protein from the fat globule *membrane*, whereas nonfat milk does not.

- **Cultured buttermilk** is pasteurized low-fat or nonfat milk to which a starter culture of *Lactobacilli* and *Streptococci* (*S. lactis*) is added. These bacteria ferment lactose, producing lactic acid, which clots the milk. Butter flakes or liquid butter, or low levels (0.01–0.15%) of salt, may be added. *Leuconostoc citrovorum* and *L. destranicum* bacteria, 0.2% citric acid, or sodium citrate may be added for flavor.

- **Sour cream** was made traditionally from heavy (whipping) cream that was *soured*. Today, it is made from pasteurized, homogenized, fresh, light cream (approximately 18% fat, depending on law) that is coagulated by a method similar to buttermilk (recall that while buttermilk starts with low-fat or skim milk, sour cream production begins with 18% fat, cream). *S. lactis* and *Leuconostoc* bacteria may be added for flavor, and stabilizers such as gelatin or gums may be present. Nonfat milk solids may be added to thicken the cream. A bitter taste in sour cream that is stored more than 3–4 weeks may form due to proteolytic bacterial enzyme activity.

- **Yogurt** is the food produced by culturing one or more of the pasteurized *optional dairy* ingredients such as cream, milk, partially skimmed milk, or skim milk (used alone or in combination) with a bacteria culture. The production process used to make yogurt is similar to buttermilk and sour cream, but the incubation temperature and types of bacteria are different. The culture used for yogurt production contains the lactic-acid producing bacteria, *L. bulgaricus* and *S. thermophilus*.

  Yogurt may be made using whole, low-fat or skim milk. The formulation may include nonfat dry milk or condensed skim milk so that it contains not less than 8.5% MSNF and not less than 3.25% milkfat. Or it may be prepared to be a *reduced* or *low-fat* yogurt, and have levels of 0.5–2.0% milkfat, or less. Other optional ingredients include buttermilk, whey, lactose, lactalbumins, lactoglobulins, or whey modified by partial or complete removal of lactose and/or minerals to increase the nonfat solid contents of the food. New research and development continues to explore additional optional ingredients.

  Nutritive or non-nutritive sweeteners may be added, as well as flavoring agents, color additives, and stabilizers such as gelatin, gums, and pectin (Chapter 17). Vitamin addition is optional—2000 IU vitamin A per quart. *Frozen* yogurt may contain stabilizers for freezer stability, sugar, and added milk solids. The different types of yogurt, sundae-style, or blended, swiss yogurt are cultured and stored in different manners.

  Microorganisms in yogurt exist in a "friendly" form, known as *probiotic flora*. Such probiotic yogurt is able to survive destruction during gastrointestinal (GI) passage and offer health benefits such as immune stimulation, and positive balance to the GI microflora (4). In combination with *L. acidophilis*, it is thought that lactase is enabled to pass successfully through the stomach acids and reach the small intestine where it functions in lactose digestion, preventing the discomfort experienced by those individuals who are lactose intolerant (National Dairy Council).

  The National Yogurt Association's "LIVE and active cultures" seal indicates that the yogurt contains at least 100 million *L. acidophilis* bacteria per gram at the time it is manufactured, although this number diminishes with time (1), and the microbial enzyme lactase.

- **Acidophilus milk** is made from pasteurized low-fat or nonfat milk to which *L. acidophilus* is added and incubated. Although not proven yet, a possible benefit of consumption is that ingestion of this bacteria can produce a number of B vitamins, thereby replacing what may have been destroyed during antibiotic treatment.

Specialty milks include lactose-reduced milk, calcium-fortified, as well as flavored milks, and shakes.

OTHER MILK PRODUCTS

Butter

Butter is a concentrated form of fluid milk, produced through churning of pasteurized cream. **Churning** involves agitation that breaks fat globule membranes so the emulsion breaks, fat coalesces, and water (buttermilk) escapes. The original 20/80 *oil-in-water* emulsion of milk becomes a 20/80 *water-in-oil* emulsion. It may have a yellow color due to the fat-soluble animal pigment, carotene.

Sweet cream butter is made by the addition of *S. diacetyllactis*, which ferments the citrate in milk to acetaldehyde, acetic acid, and diacetyl, the last being the major flavor compound of butter. Commercially, it may contain salt, yet, is known as "sweet cream" butter, because today, the butter is prepared from *sweet*, not the traditional *soured* cream. The USDA Grade AA is of superior quality, USDA Grade A is very good, and Grade B is standard.

Today, there are various blends of butter and margarine in the market. The fat composition and taste differ from the original. *Margarine*, or oleomargarine, is the food in plastic form or liquid emulsion containing not less than 80% fat. It may be produced from water and/or milk and/or milk product, be unsalted, or lactose-free. It contains vitamin A and may contain vitamin D.

Spreads contain a higher percentage of water and may not be suitable for some baking and cooking applications.

Cream

Cream is the high-fat component separated from whole milk as a result of the creaming process. It has a higher proportion of fat droplets to milk than regular fluid milk, and according to federal standards of identity, cream must contain 18% milkfat or more. Due to this high fat content of cream compared to milk, some yellow, fat-soluble pigments may be apparent. Some animal milk does not require homogenization as fats are naturally small and do not coalesce.

Various liquid creams available for use in foods include the following:

- Light (coffee) cream—18–30% butterfat.
- Light whipping cream—30–36% butterfat.
- Heavy cream—36% butterfat, minimum.
- "Half-and-Half" cream diluted with nonfat milk—10.5% butterfat.
- Whipping cream packaged under pressure in aerosol cans may contain sugar, flavoring, emulsifiers, and a stabilizer.

Cheese

The FDA's definition of cheese is "a product made from curd obtained from the whole, partly skimmed, or skimmed milk of cows, or from milk of other animals, with or without added cream, by coagulating with rennet, lactic acid, or other suitable enzyme or acid, and with or without further treatment of the separated curd by heat or pressure, or by means of ripening ferments, special molds, or seasoning." According to USDA 2000 statistics, the commercial volume jumped 6%, with the average personal consumption rising to 30.3 pounds. In descending order, American, cheddar, and mozzarella cheese are by far the leaders in sales, followed by a distant sales of Monterey Jack, swiss, and colby cheese.

Cheese (Fig. 11.1) is a concentrated form of milk that contains casein, various percentages of fat, primarily saturated fat, mineral salts, and a small portion of milk serum (whey proteins, lactose, and water-soluble vitamins). It is the curd that forms as a result of casein coagulation by the enzyme rennin (also known as chymosin) or lactic acid.

Several animal or plant *enzymes* that may be used in cheesemaking include the following:

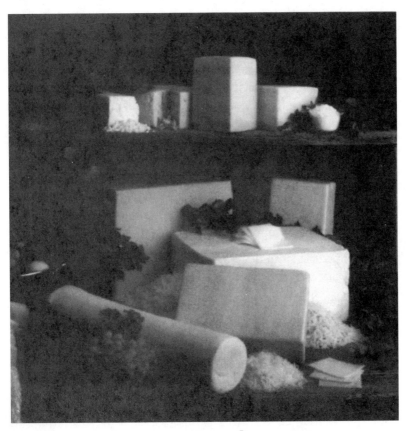

FIGURE. 11.1   Cheeses. (Courtesy of SYSCO® Incorporated)

- Rennet, from the stomach of milk-fed calves, contains mainly *rennin*. (Pepsin is also present, but in small quantities.) Although **rennin** is active at neutral pH, the enzyme clots milk much faster in acidic conditions, and so lactic acid is often added. Starter cultures that produce lactic acid may also be added. (The action of rennin was described in the earlier section on proteins.) Although calf rennet may be preferred, it is not available in sufficient quantities, and so other sources of milk-clotting enzymes are also used.
- Industry may use *pepsin* from the stomach of pigs, *proteases* from fungi, as well as plant enzymes such as *papain* (from papaya) and *ficin* (from figs) to clot milk casein and form some cheeses.

An example of a cheese made with lactic acid is cottage cheese.

Cottage cheese is a low-fat, soft, acid cheese formed by coagulation of casein with lactic acid. It is made from pasteurized skim milk, to which is added either lactic acid, or a bacterial culture that produces lactic acid to reduce the pH to 4.6. The caseins aggregate to form curds, which are separated from the whey by cutting, stirring, and draining. The curds may also be heated, to cause shrinkage and facilitate removal of the whey. They are then washed to reduce acidity. They may be mildly salted to give flavor. Sweet or soured cream may also be blended with the curds to give products containing 2 or 4% fat. Cottage cheese is packaged as loose curd particles (which may be designated large or small) and it is not aged or ripened. It is highly perishable and must be kept refrigerated.

As mentioned, a starter culture may be added to milk in order to begin curd development. Once a curd has formed, it is cut, cooked to shrink the curd, and drained of any remaining whey (syneresis), salted to provide flavor, draw whey from the curd, and retard microbial growth, pressed, and fermented with various microorganisms at 40–55°F (4–13°C).

Cheese is classified according to 1) the *moisture* content, producing either very hard, hard, semisoft, or soft cheeses, and 2) the kind and extent of *ripening*:

- *Hard cheese* contains 30–40% water. It has very tiny fat globules and is a near-perfect emulsion. *Soft cheese* contains 40–75% water and has large fat globules. It is only slightly emulsified.
- **Ripening** may require 2–12 months and may be the result of bacterial, mold, or yeast activity. In that time, *lactose* is fermented by lactase to lactic acid, *fat* is hydrolyzed by lipase, and *protein* undergoes some proteolysis to amino acids by rennin. It refers to the chemical and physical changes that occur in the cheese in the time between curd precipitation and satisfactory completion of texture, flavor, and color development.

Some cheeses, such as cottage cheese or cream cheese, are not ripened, whereas other cheese may be ripened to develop its own characteristic flavor, color, aroma, or appearance. Cheeses may be ripened with *bacteria*. For example, the holes or eye formation in Swiss cheese is evidence of gas- producing bacteria that exist throughout the interior of the cheese. Some cheeses, such as brick and Limburger, are ripened by inoculation of the milk with *bacteria* and *yeast*. These microorganisms ripen from the surface to the interior of the cheese.

Other cheeses such as Camembert and Brie, for example, are ripened by *mold* that is sprayed onto the surface of the cheese, or mold may be introduced internally as in the ripening of blue cheese that is inoculated with *Penicillium roqueforti*. (Blue cheese is made from cow milk; Roquefort cheese is made from sheep milk).

Despite the abundance of names given to various cheeses throughout the world, there are only approximately 18 types that differ in flavor and texture. These types are listed as follows:

- Brick (USA)—semisoft, ripened primarily by bacteria
- Camembert (France)—soft, mold externally applied (*Oidum lactis* and then *P. camemberti*); thin edible crust
- Cheddar (England)—hard, bacteria-ripened (*S. lactis* and *S. cremoris*); most common cheese used for cooking in the United States, colored by annatto (a seed pod extract)
- Cottage cheese—soft, unripened; creamed, low-fat, nonfat, or dry curd
- Cream cheese (USA)—soft, unripened; may be flavored
- Edam (The Netherlands)—hard, ripened; ball shaped with a red- paraffin coating
- Gouda (The Netherlands)—semisoft to hard, ripened; similar to Edam
- Hand—soft
- Limburger (Belgium)—soft, surface bacteria ripened (*Bacterium linens*)
- Neufchatel (France)—soft, unripened in the United States; ripened in France
- Parmesan (Italy)—hard, bacteria ripened
- Provolone (Italy)—hard, ripened
- Romano (Italy)—very hard, ripened
- Roquefort (France)—semisoft, internally mold ripened (*P. roqueforti*)
- Sap Sago (Switzerland)—very hard, ripened by bacteria
- Swiss, Emmentaler (Switzerland)—hard, ripened by gas-forming bacteria (*S. lactis* or *S. cremoris*, and *S. thermophilus*, *S. bulgaricus*, and *P. shermani*).
- Trapist—semisoft, ripened by bacteria and surface microorganisms
- Whey cheeses, such as Ricotta (Italy), which may be a combination of whole and low-fat milk, or whey; coagulated by heating, not rennin.

In the United States, the FDA has requirements for specific standardized cheese that must be followed by manufacturers, packers, and distributors. In addition to the list above, some other standardized cheese types include Asiago, Caciocavello siciliano, Colby, Gammelost, Gorgonzola, Gruyere, Monterey Jack, Mozzarella, Muenster, Nuworld, and Samsoe.

To differentiate between some types of cheese, the following explanations are given:

- *Natural cheese* is the curd of precipitated casein. It may be overcoagulated and allows water to be squeezed out when exposed to high heat, in which case it shows a separated appearance and stringy texture. Therefore, low heat should be used when cooking with natural cheese.

- *Pasteurized process(ed) cheese* is the most common cheese produced in the United States. By FDA ruling, it is "prepared by comminuting and mixing, with the aid of heat, one or more cheeses of the same, or two or more varieties, except cream cheese, neufchatel cheese, cottage cheese, low-fat cottage cheese, cottage cheese dry curd, cook cheese, hard grating cheese, semisoft, part-skim cheese, part-skim spiced cheese, and skim milk cheese for manufacturing with an emulsifying agent ... into a homogeneous plastic mass" (CFR 21).

The mixture is pasteurized (which halts ripening and it flavor development) for 3 minutes at 150°F (66°C), and salt is added. An emulsifier such as disodium phosphate or sodium citrate is incorporated to bind the calcium and produce a more soluble, homogeneous, and smooth cheese that can withstand higher heat than natural cheese, without coagulating. The melted cheese is placed in jars or molds such as foil-lined cardboard boxes or single-slice plastic wrap.

This cheese may also contain an optional mold-inhibiting ingredient consisting of not more than 0.2% by weight of sorbic acid, potassium sorbate, sodium sorbate, or any combination of two or more of these, or consisting of not more than 0.3% by weight of sodium propionate, calcium propionate, or a combination of sodium and calcium propionate.

The moisture content of a process cheese made from a *single* variety of cheese is not more than 1% greater than the maximum moisture content prescribed by the definition and standard of identity, for the variety of cheese used, if there is one. In no case is the moisture to be more than 43% (except 40% for process washed curd and process Colby cheese, and 44% process Swiss and Gruyere).

The moisture content of a process cheese made from *two* or *more* varieties of cheese is not more than 1% greater than the arithmetical average of the maximum moisture contents prescribed by the definitions and standards of identity, if there is one, for the cheeses used. In no case is the moisture content more than 43% (40% cheddar, Colby, 44% Swiss and Gruyere).

The fat content of process cheese made from a *single* variety of cheese is not less than the minimum prescribed by the definition and standard of identity for the variety of cheese used, and in no case is less than 47% (except process Swiss 43% and process Gruyere 45%). The fat content of process cheese made from *two* or *more* varieties of cheese is not less than the arithmetical average of the two cheeses, as described above, and in no case is less than 47% (except the mixture of Swiss and Gruyere 45%).

Low-fat processed cheese demonstrates an improvement in texture and meltability when Oatrim, a glucan-amylodextrin, is added at low levels.

- *Pasteurized process(ed) cheese food* is comminuted and mixed and contains not less than 51% cheese by weight. The moisture is not more than 44%, and the fat content is not less than 23%. Thus, it contains *less cheese* and *more moisture* than process cheese. It may contain cream, milk, nonfat milk, NDM, whey, and other color or flavoring agents. It has a soft texture and melts easily.

An emulsifying agent may be added in such quantity that the weight of the solids of such an emulsifying agent is not more than 3% of the weight of the pasteurized process cheese food (FDA).

- *Pasteurized process cheese spread* is comminuted and mixed. It has a moisture content of 44–60%, and a milkfat level of not less than 20%. Therefore, it has *more moisture* and *less fat* than processed cheese food and can be spread. Gelatin and gums such as carob bean, cellulose gum (carboxymethylcellulose), guar, tragacanth, and xanthan, as well as carrageenan may be added if such substances are not more than 0.8% of the weight of the finished product (FDA). Sodium may be added to retain moisture, and sugar or corn syrup may be added for sweetness.

- *Cold-pack cheese* preparation involves grinding and mixing natural cheese without heat. The moisture content of a cold-pack cheese made from a *single* variety of cheese is not more than the maximum prescribed for the variety of cheese used (if there is a standard of identity), and the fat content is not less than the minimum prescribed for that cheese, but is not less than 47% (except 43% cold-pack Swiss, and 45% Gruyere).

While it is typically cold-pack cheeses that may contain various flavor combinations, manufacturers have the technology to create custom-colored and custom-flavored specialty cheeses as needed (5). When made from *two* or *more* varieties of cheese, the moisture content should be the arithmetical average of the maximum of the two cheeses, as prescribed by the definition or standard of identity, but in no case more than 42%. The fat content is not less than the arithmetical average of the minimum percent of fat prescribed for the cheeses, if there is a standard of identity or definition, but in no case less than 47% (cold-pack Swiss and Gruyere 45%).

The lactose content of ripened cheese decreases during ripening and is virtually absent for several weeks. It is the whey that contains lactose, which some individuals cannot consume (lactose intolerance). The majority of vitamins and minerals remain after ripening, some protein is hydrolyzed by rennin or proteases, and some fat is digested. Grades of US Grade AA and A are assigned to some commonly consumed cheeses such as cheddar and Swiss cheese.

Ice Cream

Ice cream is a food produced by freezing, while stirring a pasteurized mix containing dairy product. While ice mixes were enjoyed for centuries prior to this, the first commercial, wholesale ice cream was manufactured in 1851, in Baltimore, Maryland. The mix consists of one or more of the optional dairy ingredients such as cream, milk, skim milk, sweet cream buttermilk or sweetened condensed milk, and optional caseinates.

In addition to the dairy ingredient, sherbet, low-fat ice cream, and ice creams contain other ingredients. Typically, sugar (sucrose, dextrose, which flavors and depresses the freezing point), cookies, eggs, fruit, nuts, and other ingredients such as coloring or flavoring agents, emulsifiers [such as egg yolks, Polysorbate 80 (a sorbitol ester consisting of a glucose molecule bound to the fatty acid; oleic acid), or mono- and di-glycerides], stabilizers (gelatin, vegetable gum), and water are added.

The ice cream mix is subject to pasteurization, homogenization, holding (for aging), and *quick* freezing. *Slow* freezing creates larger ice crystals. Air is naturally incorporated into an ice cream mixture by agitation, but excessive air may not be whipped into a mix as specified by federal and state standards. The increase in volume due to air is **overrun**, and is calculated as

$$\%\text{Overrun} = (\text{Volume of ice cream} - \text{Volume of mix}) \times 100/\text{Volume of mix}$$

For example, if a 1-gallon container of ice cream contains an equal measure of ice cream mix and air, it has 100% overrun. Overrun in ice creams may range from 60% to greater than 100%.

Ice cream contains not less than 10% milkfat, nor less than 10% MSNF, except when it contains milkfat at 1% increments above the 10% minimum:

Low-fat ice cream (formerly ice milk) contains *less* fat and *more* MSNF, and deluxe ice cream contains *more* milkfat and *less* MSNF. Other frozen desserts may include milk and varying percentages of milkfat or perhaps a fat substitute.

Blended milk products are fruit juices and milk, that may contain added lactic acid, or caffeine, plus other ingredients, and may be prepared using herb teas and additional sugars.

Sherbet contains 1–2% milk fat and 2–5% total milk solids. A greater amount of sugar and less air (hence 30–40% overrun) than ice cream are standard.

Percent milkfat	Minimum percent MSNF
10	10
11	9
12	8
13	7
14	6

WHEY

Whey has previously been discussed as the aqueous (serum) protein in milk, but it warrants further discussion due its increasing use in consumer products. Research is ongoing to target separating milk serum proteins from liquid milk prior to cheesemaking (6). It comprises approximately 20% of the protein in milk, contains the albumins and globulins, the majority of lactose (which is the primary ingredient of it solids component), and the water-soluble nutrients, such as riboflavin. Whey is the by-product of cheesemaking, the liquid that remains after curds are formed and drained (recall the nursery rhyme Little Miss Muffet). A tremendous quantity of cheese is manufactured, and, currently, more satisfactory ways of using whey are being explored.

Some cheese such as ricotta cheese may be made partially of whey. Whey may also be used in beverages, frozen dairy desserts, and baked goods. In a dried form, it may have useful applications as an emulsifier and in providing extra protein to foods. Yet, because it contains lactose, which the majority of the world cannot digest (see Lactose Intolerance), it cannot be used in worldwide feeding.

Whey begins to precipitate at temperatures *below* the coagulation temperature of casein, yet, is not precipitated at a pH of 4.6 or by rennin, as is casein. Evidence of whey precipitation is seen when the lactalbumin coagulum (as well as calcium phosphate) sticks to the bottom of the pan and scorches.

Whey is concentrated by ultrafiltration to yield *whey protein concentrates* (WPCs). WPCs are frequently added to yogurt, and dried for use in such items as coffee whitener, whipped toppings, meringue, fruit beverages, chocolate drinks, and processed meats. Other purification steps may be added to yield *whey protein isolates* (WPIs). WPIs are used in infant formulas, and whey refinery may yield proteins used to fortify clear bottled drinks, including sodas. Fractionation in the whey refining process could lead to products without phenylalanine, and thus to products useful ingredients to people with phenylketonuria (PKU) (7).

COOKING APPLICATIONS

Subsequent to the mild *denaturation* or change in molecular structure of proteins, cross-links are formed. **Coagulation** and precipitation of clumps or aggregates may occur with heat or when acid, enzymes, or salts are in a formulation. Some of these effects are as follows:

- **Heat**: Heat may denature, coagulate, or curdle whey proteins. Slow, low, or moderate heat such as indirect heating over a water bath should be used for milk-based products, because increasing temperatures and length of heating (especially of concentrated milks) form greater amounts of coagulum at the bottom of the pan. The same calcium phosphate compound that forms at the *bottom* of the pan by scorching also forms a skin (scum or film) at the *surface* of the food. Therefore, calcium phosphate levels are reduced in the heating of milk. Cooking with a cover is recommended in order to prevent this skin formation. Another effect of heat is that it may break the fat emulsion when the protein film around the fat globules breaks, causing the fat to coalesce.

- **Acid**: Acid may be added to food or be a part of a food, or it may be produced by bacteria. It coagulates milk mixtures by forming an unstable casein protein. Casein precipitates at a pH of approximately 4.6, but whey proteins are not precipitated by acid.

- **Enzyme coagulation**: The primary enzyme use to coagulate milk is rennin. Rennin requires a slightly acidic environment and functions best at temperatures of 104–108°F (40–42°C). Calcium is retained if the coagulation of milk is achieved by rennin, as calcium is not released to whey but is held by casein. Rennin is used in cooking custard-like desserts.

- **Salt coagulation**: Calcium and phosphorus salts present in milk are less soluble with heat and may coagulate milk protein. Salty foods such as ham that are cooked in milk frequently may curdle the milk. As with acid, a gelatinized starch buffer is used to prevent undesirable precipitation.

- **Polyphenolic compound coagulation**: Phenolic compounds (formerly called tannins) in some plant materials, including fruits and vegetables like potatoes, coagulate milk. Although baking soda (alkali) may be added to vegetable–milk combinations to shift the pH and control curdling, it is not recommended, as it destroys vitamin C. A gelatinized starch buffer may be used for controlling this undesirable coagulation.

MILK SUBSTITUTES AND IMITATION MILK PRODUCTS

In 1973, the FDA differentiated between *imitation* and *substitute* products by establishing regulations regarding the use of the two names. An ***imitation milk*** product may look and taste like the traditional product but is *nutritionally inferior*. Specifying the term "imitation" on labels is no longer a legal requirement. A milk ***substitute*** product is one that resembles the traditional product and is *nutritionally equal*. A substitute is pasteurized, homogenized, and packaged like milk. It is more economical than real dairy products because it does not contain the costly butterfat.

Milk and milk products with the "REAL" symbol on the package indicate that the product is made from real dairy products, not substitutes or imitations.

Filled Milk

Filled milk is a *milk substitute* that consists of a vegetable *fat* or *oil* (*no milk*), and nonfat *milk* solids. Therefore, it *cannot* be consumed by persons who have milk allergies. The vegetable fat has traditionally been coconut oil, but it may be partially hydrogenated corn, cottonseed, palm, or soy oil. In addition to the milk and oil, water, an emulsifier such as monoglycerides or diglycerides, color such as carotene, and flavoring may be added. Filled milk contains no cholesterol.

Imitation Milk

Imitation milk usually contains *no milk* products at all—*no milk fat or milk solids*. It is composed of water, vegetable oil, corn syrup, sugar, sodium caseinate, or soy, and stabilizers and emulsifiers. Vitamins and minerals may be added to the product to improve the nutritional value.

Flavored "milk," "butter," "cream cheese," whipped "cream," and other imitation products are available in marketplace. Nondairy "creamers," or whiteners are prevalent in fluid and dehydrated form. They may require refrigeration or freezing comparable to the dairy product that they resemble depending on the ingredients.

SAFETY/QUALITY OF MILK

Milk is a highly perishable substance, high in water, with significant amount of protein, and a near-neutral pH (6.6)—the qualities that support bacteria growth. Details of sanitation are previously mentioned, but it is important to know about the care and safety of milk.

Packaging contains a date on the carton that should be followed for a retail sale. Milk may remain fresh and usable for several days past this ''sell-by-date'' if the following directions, suggested by the Dairy Council, are observed:

- Use proper containers to protect milk from exposure to sunlight, bright daylight, and strong fluorescent light to prevent the development of off-flavor and a reduction in riboflavin, ascorbic acid, and vitamin B_6 content.
- Store milk at refrigerated temperatures [45°F (7°C)] or below as soon as possible after purchase.
- Keep milk containers closed to prevent absorption of other food flavors in the refrigerator. An absorbed flavor alters the taste but the milk is still safe.
- Use milk in the order purchased.
- Serve milk cold.
- Return milk container to the refrigerator immediately to prevent bacterial growth. Temperatures above 45°F (7°C) for fluid and cultured milk products for even a few minutes reduce shelf life. Never return unused milk to the original container.
- Keep canned milk in a cool, dry place. Once opened, it should be transferred to a clean opaque container and refrigerated.
- Store dry milk in a cool, dry place and reseal the container after opening. Humidity causes dry milk to lump and may affect flavor and color changes. If such changes occur, the milk should not be consumed. Once reconstituted, dry milk should be treated like any other fluid milk: covered and stored in the refrigerator.
- Serve UHT milk cold and store in the refrigerator after opening.

Carbohydrate Browning Reactions

Color and flavor changes are observed in canned or dry milk that has been subject to either long or high-temperature storage. The browning does *not* indicate contamination or spoilage, rather it is the nonenzymatic Maillard browning or ''carbonyl-amine browning'' reaction between the free carbonyl group of a reducing sugar and the free amino group of protein.

NUTRITIVE VALUE OF MILK AND MILK PRODUCTS

The FDA ruling for dairy products, in 1996 revoked the "Standard of Identity" (prescribed formulation or recipe that the manufacturer needed to follow). Thus nutrient claims such as "fat-free," and others, similar to those carried by other products became the rule for dairy labels.

Proteins

Milk contains high-quality proteins—casein and whey. According to the American Diabetes Association (ADA) Exchange List, an 8-ounce serving of fluid milk contains 8 g of protein regardless of fat content.

Fats and Cholesterol

Dairy products may be made into fat-free, low-fat, reduced fat, or cholesterol-free formulations (2, 3). For example, cholesterol-free milk is made by adding hydrolyzed oat flour (oatrim) to nonfat milk. Dairy products may also be used as a *fat replacer in other foods* (fat-free does not mean calorie- free). yogurtesse® is the dairy-based fat replacer, introduced in 1996, that is used in products such as baked goods, sauces, and dressings. It contains no fat and is cholesterol-free. Yogurtesse® contains nonfat milk solids, whey protein, pectin, locust bean gum, carrageenan, and other components.

Labeling changes have served both to benefit processors' creativity, such as in developing "light" milk, and to better assist consumers in lowering their fat and saturated fat intake. As shown above in section Types of Milk, a label may state whole milk, reduced fat, or fat-free. The calorie levels differ according to the fat content. For example, whole milk contains 150 cal per 8 ounces and skim milk contains 90 cal per 8 ounces. According to the USDA, milk sales have indicated an increase in the sales of reduced-fat and skim milk, while there has been a decrease in full-fat, whole milk, as shown below.

Milk sales (in billion pounds)		
	1976	1996
Full-fat	26.4	18.8
Reduced Fat	21.2	24.2
Fat-free	3.2	8.9

Carbohydrates

The carbohydrate content of 8 ounces of milk is 12 g regardless of the level of fat. A discussion of lactose intolerance follows.

Vitamins and Minerals

The fat-soluble vitamins A, D, E, and K are present in whole and some reduced-fat milk. Fortification beyond vitamin A and D is not allowed in current Standards of Identity. Milk is a major source of riboflavin (B_2) in the diet of many populations. Losses of B_2 may occur due to exposure to sunlight as riboflavin is a photosynthesizer. Milk also contains the amino acid tryptophan, a precursor to niacin.

No apparent undesirable effect on protein, fat, carbohydrates, minerals, and vitamins B_6, A, D, and E are observed with pasteurization. Vitamin K is slightly diminished, and there is less than 10% loss of thiamin and vitamin B_{12}.

TABLE 11.2 Composition of Milks from Different Species (100-g Portions)

Nutrient	Cow	Human	Buffalo	Goat	Sheep
Water (g)	87.99	87.50	83.39	87.03	80.70
Calories	61	70	97	69	108
Protein (N × 6.38) (g)	3.29	1.03	3.75	3.56	5.98
Fat (g)	3.34	4.38	6.89	4.14	7.00
Carbohydrate (g)	4.66	6.89	5.18	4.45	5.36
Fiber (g)	0	0	0	0	0
Cholesterol (mg)	14	14	19	11	–
Minerals					
Calcium (mg)	119	32	169	134	193
Iron (mg)	0.05	0.03	0.12	0.05	0.10
Magnesium (mg)	13	3	31	14	18
Phosphorus (mg)	93	14	117	111	158
Potassium (mg)	152	51	178	204	136
Sodium (mg)	49	17	52	50	44
Zinc (mg)	0.38	0.17	0.22	0.30	–
Vitamins					
Ascorbic acid (mg)	0.94	5.00	2.25	1.29	4.16
Thiamin (mg)	0.038	0.014	0.052	0.048	0.065
Riboflavin (mg)	0.162	0.036	0.135	0.138	0.355
Niacin (mg)	0.084	0.177	0.091	0.277	0.417
Pantothenic acid (mg)	0.314	0.223	0.192	0.310	0.407
B_6 (mg)	0.042	0.011	0.023	0.046	–
Folate (mcg)	5	5	6	1	–
B_{12} (mcg)	0.357	0.045	0.363	0.065	0.711
Vitamin A (RE)	31	64	53	56	42
Vitamin A (IU)	126	241	178	185	147

Source: National Dairy Council.

One 8-ounce cup (240 ml) of whole fluid cow's milk contains the following minerals: potassium, calcium, chlorine, phosphorus, sodium, sulfur, and magnesium. Milk does not contain iron. The composition of milks from different species appears in Table 11.2.

Low-sodium milk may be included in diets with sodium restrictions. Sodium may be reduced from a normal amount of 49 mg to about 2.5 mg per 100 g of milk by replacing the sodium with potassium in an ion exchange.

Trends in beverage intake from the late 1970s through the mid 1990s show a 31% decrease in young women (12–19 years old) drinking milk. A decrease in this period of years indicates a need for intervention, perhaps including the recommendation of consumption of calcium from other sources (8).

Recent trends have shown a *decrease* in consumption of milk, and consumption of *more* sugar-sweetened beverages. Flavored milks are an alternative to such beverages, and may assist in reversing recent trends (9).

LACTOSE INTOLERANCE

Many individuals demonstrate a permanent loss of the enzyme used to digest the principal milk sugar lactose; they are *lactose intolerant*. Lactose intolerance may be due to the absence of or insufficient amount of lactase, a birth deficit, or physical impairment. Caucasians are among the few population groups who can digest lactose.

If lactose remains undigested by lactase in the intestine, it is fermented by microflora to short-chain fatty acids and gasses such as carbon dioxide, hydrogen, and in some individuals to methane. Symptoms of lactose intolerance include flatulence, abdominal pain, and diarrhea due to the high solute concentration of undigested lactose. A correct understanding of tolerable dose is needed by the lactose-intolerant individual, and the food industry that develops lactose-free food.

Lactose assists in the absorption of calcium, phosphorus, magnesium, zinc, and other minerals from the small intestine brush border. Nondairy "milk" such as soy or imitation milk contains no lactose; therefore, it may be consumed by individuals with milk allergies and by those who would otherwise not drink milk.

The loss of lactase activity in the intestine affects, to some extent, approximately 75% of the world's population (10). Individuals with lactose intolerance may compensate by consuming lactase-treated milk (which reduces lactose by 70%) or purchase the lactase enzyme and administer it directly to milk prior to consumption. It has been shown that small servings (120 ml = 6 g of lactose) of milk, and hard cheeses (less than 2 g of lactose) may be consumed without an increase in intolerance symptoms. Up to 12 g of lactose are tolerated, especially if the individual consumes other foods with the source of lactose (11). Some fermented products, such as cheese, are tolerated if lactose has sufficiently been converted to lactic acid. Aged cheese is an example of such food. The lactose content of some milk and milk products is given in Table 11.3.

TABLE 11.3 Lactose Content of Milk and Milk Products

Type of Milk	Weight 1 Cup (g)	Average Percentage	Grams/Cup
Whole milk	244	4.7	11.5
Reduced fat milk (2%)	245	4.7	11.5
Low-fat milk (1%)	245	5	12.3
Nonfat milk	245	5	12.5
Chocolate milk	250	4.5	11.3
Evaporated milk	252	10.3	26.0
Sweetened condensed milk	306	12.9	39.5
Nonfat dry milk (unreconstituted)	120	51.3	61.6
Whole dry milk (unreconstituted)	128	37.5	47.9
Acidophilus milk (nonfat)	245	4.4	10.8
Buttermilk	244	4.3	10.5
Sour cream	230	3.9	8.9
Yogurt (plain)	277	4.4	10.0
Half-and-Half	242	4.2	10.0
Light cream	240	3.9	9.3
Whipping cream	239	2.9	6.9

Source: National Dairy Council.

CONCLUSION

Milk is the first food of mammals. It contains major nutrients, carbohydrate, fat, and protein, with water being predominant (88%). The two major proteins in milk are casein and whey, with additional protein found in enzymes. The fat content of milk varies and is designated by law according to the specific product and jurisdiction.

Milk is *pasteurized* to destroy pathogens, and is *homogenized* to emulsify fat and prevent creaming. Grade A milk must be treated in this manner if subjected to interstate commerce. Milk may be fluid, evaporated, condensed, dried, or cultured, and made into butter, cheese, cream, ice cream, or a variety of other products. It is a potentially hazardous food due to its high protein, water activity, and neutral pH and must be kept cold.

GLOSSARY

Buttermilk, cultured: Pasteurized low-fat or nonfat milk to which bacteria are added to ferment lactose to the more acidic lactic acid that clots the casein in milk.
Casein: Primary protein of milk, colloidally dispersed.
Casein micelles: Stable spherical particles in milk containing α_s-,β- and κ-casein, and also colloidal calcium phosphate. The micelles are stabilized by κ-casein, which exists mainly at the surface; the α_s- and β-casein fractions are located mainly in the interior of the micelles.
Cheese: Coagulated product formed from the coagulation of casein by lactic acid or rennin; may be unripened or bacteria ripened; made from concentrated milk.

Churning: Agitation breaks fat globule membranes so the emulsion breaks, fat coalesces, and water escapes.

Coagulate: The formation of new cross-links subsequent to the denaturation of a protein. This forms a clot, gel, or semisolid material as macromolecules of protein aggregate.

Creaming: Fat globules coalesce (less dense than the aqueous phase of milk) and rise to the surface of unhomogenized, whole, and some low-fat milk.

Cultured: See fermented.

Evaporated milk: Concentrated to remove 60% of the water of ordinary fluid milk; canned.

Fermented: (Cultured) enzymes from microorganisms, or acid that reduce the pH and clot milk by breaking down the organic substrates to smaller molecules.

Fortified: Increasing the vitamin content of fresh milk to contain vitamins A and D to levels not ordinarily found in milk.

Homogenization: Dispersion of an increased number and smaller fat globules to prevent creaming.

Imitation milk: Resembles (looks, tastes like) the traditional product but is nutritionally inferior; contains no butterfat or milk products.

Lactose intolerance: Inability to digest lactose due to the absence or insufficient level of intestinal lactase enzyme.

Maillard reaction: The first step of browning that occurs due to a reaction between the free amino group of an amino acid and a reducing sugar; nonenzymatic browning.

Milk solids nonfat (MSNF): All of the components of milk solids except fat.

Milk substitute: Resembles (looks, tastes like) traditional product and is nutritionally equal; contains no butterfat (e.g., filled milk).

Overrun: The increase in volume of ice cream over the volume of ice cream mix due to the incorporation of air.

Pasteurization: Heat treatment to destroy both pathogenic bacteria, fungi (mold and yeast), and most nonpathogenic bacteria.

Rennin: Enzyme from the stomach of milk-fed calves used to clot milk and form many cheeses.

Ripening: The time between curd precipitation and completion of texture, flavor, and color development in cheese. Lactose is fermented, fat is hydrolyzed, and protein goes through some hydrolysis to amino acids.

Sterilization: Temperature higher than that required for pasteurization, which leaves the product free from all bacteria.

Sweetened, condensed milk: Concentrated to remove 60% of the water, contains 40–45% sugar.

Total milk solids: All of the components of milk except for water.

Whey: Secondary protein of milk, contained in serum or aqueous solution; contains lactalbumins and lactoglobulins.

References

1. Yogurt, the health food it's cracked up to be? *Tufts University Diet and Nutrition Letter* 1996; 14(9) November: 3–5.
2. Pszczola DE. Low-fat dairy products: Getting a new lease on life. *Food Technology*. 1996; 50(9): 32.

3. Pszczola DE. Oatrim finds application in fat-free, cholesterol-free milk. *Food Technology*. 1996; 50(9): 80–81.

4. Hollingsworth P. Food Technology Special Report. Yogurt reinvents itself. *Food Technology*. 2001; 55(3): 43–49.

5. Research yields new reasons to say cheese. *Food Engineering*. 2000; November: 16.

6. Manufacturing news. New processing technique yields new protein concentrate. *Food Engineering*. 2001; February: 14.

7. A new way to separate whey proteins. *Food Engineering*. 2000; December: 13.

8. Bowman S. Beverage choices of young females: Change and nutrient impact on nutrient intakes. *J Am Diet Assoc*. 2002; 102: 1234–1239.

9. Johnson RK, Frary C, Wang MQ. The nutritional consequences of flavored-milk consumption by school-aged children and adolescents in the United States. *J Am Diet Assoc*. 2002; 102: 853–855.

10. Savaiano DA, Levitt MD. Milk intolerance and microbe-containing dairy foods. *Journal of Dairy Science*. 1987; 70: 397–406.

11. Hertzler SR, Huynh, BL, Savaiano DA. How much lactose is low lactase? *Journal of the American Dietetic Association*. 1996; 96: 243–246.

BIBLIOGRAPHY

Agri-Dairy Products. Purchase, NY.

American Dairy Products. Chicago, IL.

American Whey. Paramus, NJ.

Associated Milk Producers. New Ulm, NM.

Cheese Varieties and Descriptions. Handbook 54. Washington, DC: USDA, 1974.

Dairy and Food Industries Supply Association, Inc. McLean, VA.

How to Buy Cheese. Home and Garden Bulletin No. 193. Washington, DC: USDA, 1977.

How to Buy Dairy Products. Home and Garden Bulletin No. 201. Washington, DC: USDA, 1979.

Market Place. BST declared safe. *Food Engineering*. 1994; 66(1): 15.

National Dairy Council. Rosemont, IL.

National Yogurt Association. McLean, VA.

Potter NN, Hotchkiss JH. Food Science, 5th ed. New York: Chapman & Hall, 1996.

Robinson RK. *Modern Dairy Technology*, 2nd ed. New York: Chapman & Hall, 1994.

Swartz M, Wong C. Milk proteins: Nutritional and functional uses. *Cereal Foods World*. 1985; 30: 173.

Viera ER. *Elementary Food Science*, 4th ed. New York: Chapman & Hall, 1996.

PART IV

Fats in the Food Guide Pyramid

CHAPTER 12

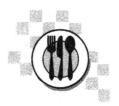

Fat and Oil Products

INTRODUCTION

Fats and oils are triglycerides, the major component of lipids. Lipids also include the phospholipids and sterols. Fats and oils are *insoluble* in water and have a greasy feel that the consumer may feel or see evidence of on a napkin or dinner plate. Fats may be processed into monoglycerides and diglycerides—glycerol units that have one or two fatty acid chains, respectively, and they may be added to many food products functioning as emulsifiers.

Some of the functions of fat in food preparation are as follows:

- Add or modify flavor, texture
- Aerate (leaven) batters and doughs
- Contribute flakiness
- Contribute tenderness
- Emulsify (See Chapter 13)
- Transfer heat, such as in frying
- Provide satiety
- Prevent sticking

Fat is enjoyed in the diet due to its flavor, texture, aroma, and palatability. Fats also carry the fat-soluble vitamins A, D, E, and K.

Sources of fats and oils may be animal, vegetable, or marine that may be manufactured in some combination in industrial processing. *Fats* appear solid at room temperature, whereas *oils* are liquid at room temperature.

Oils used in margarines, spreads, dressings, retail bottled oils, as well as frying oils are the largest market segments of edible oils (1). Soybean oil is the highest volume vegetable oil used in the United States. It is incorporated into a variety of products.

Various fat replacements attempt to mimic fat in mouthfeel and perception, and their caloric and cholesterol level are significantly less than fat. Fats and oils are contained in foods that appear throughout the Food Guide Pyramid, although they are not part of the composition of fruits. As a group, fats and oils appear with sweets at the top of the pyramid, with the recommendation that they should be used sparingly in the diet.

STRUCTURE AND COMPOSITION OF FATS

Glycerides

Glycerides include *monoglycerides*, *diglycerides*, and *triglycerides*. The first two act as emulsifiers, and more than 95% of fats and oils are *triglycerides*—the most abundant fatty substances in food. Triglycerides are insoluble in water and may be either liquid or solid at room temperature, with liquid forms generally referred to as *oils*, and solid forms as *fats*. Structurally, glycerides contain a glycerol molecule backbone joined to one or more fatty acid molecules. A *monoglyceride* contains glycerol esterified to *one* fatty acid molecule, and the equation for that reaction is given in Figure 12.1. (The general formula for a fatty acid is used where R represents the hydrocarbon chain.)

If *two* fatty acids are esterified to glycerol, a *diglyceride* is formed, and *three* fatty acids undergoing the same reaction make a *triglycerides*. If a triglyceride contains three identical fatty acids, it is called a *simple triglyceride,* if it contains two or three different fatty acids it is called a *mixed triglyceride*. Spatially, there is no room for all three fatty acids to exist on the same side of the glycerol molecule; thus, triglycerides are thought to exist in either a stair-step (chair) or a tuning-fork arrangement (Figure 12.2). The arrangement and specific type of fatty acids on the glycerol determine the chemical and physical properties of a fat.

Minor Components of Fats and Oils

In addition to glycerides and free fatty acids, lipids may contain small amounts of phospholipids, sterols, tocopherols, fat-soluble pigments, and vitamins, as discussed in this section of the text.

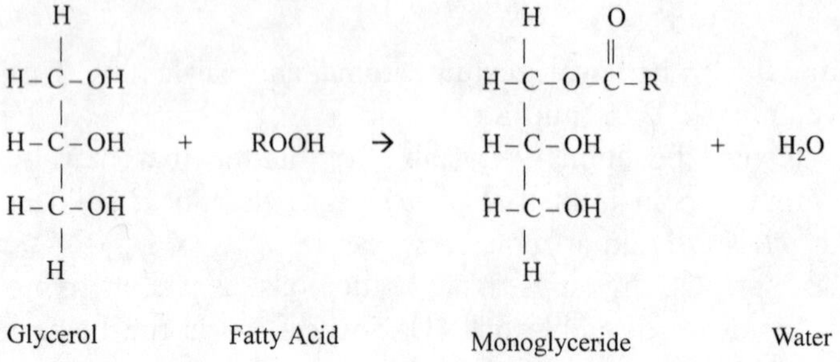

FIGURE 12.1   Formation of a monoglyceride.

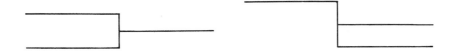

FIGURE 12.2   Fatty acid tuning-fork (left) and stair-step or chair arrangements (right).

Phospholipids are similar to triglycerides but contain only *two* fatty acids esterified to glycerol. In place of the third fatty acid, there is a polar group containing phosphoric acid and a nitrogen-containing group, the most common is known as **lecithin** (Figure 12.3). Lecithin is found in nearly every living cell. The word is derived from the Greek *lekithos* that means "yolk of an egg," and lecithin is in egg yolk. However, the primary *commercial* source of lecithin is the soybean (2). The two fatty acids of a phospholipid are attracted to fat, whereas the phosphorus and nitrogen are attracted to water. Therefore, a phospholipid forms a bridge between fat and water, two ordinarily immiscible substances, and emulsification is observed (see Emulsification and Chapter 13). "Refined" lecithins are modified to provide important surface active properties to a variety of foods such as instant drink mixes, infant formulas, meat sauces and gravies, dispersible oleoresins, pan releases, chewing gum, and fat-replacer systems (2).

Sterols contain a common steroid nucleus, an 8–10 carbon side chain and an alcohol group. The chemists view of sterols is *unlike* triglycerides or phospholipids—they are round in shape. Cholesterol is the primary *animal sterol* (Figure 12.4) although *plant sterols,* or stanols also exist; the most common ones are sitosterol and stigmasterol. Other plant sterols are found in "margarine" type products, including those marketed under the trade name Benecol[R].

Tocopherols are important minor constituents of most *vegetable oils; animal fats* contain little or no tocopherols. Tocopherols are antioxidants, helping to prevent oxidative rancidity, and are also sources of vitamin E. They are partially removed by the heat of processing and may be added after processing to improve oxidative stability of oils. If vitamin E is added to oil, for example, the oil is frequently marketed as a source of vitamin E, or as an antioxidant-containing oil.

Fats are not good sources of vitamins, apart from vitamin E, but fat-soluble vitamins A and D may be added to foods such as margarine and milk in order to

$$
\begin{array}{l}
H-\underset{|}{C}-O-\underset{\parallel}{C}-(CH_2)_n-CH_3 \\
\\
H-\underset{|}{C}-O-\underset{\parallel}{C}-(CH_2)_7 CH=CH(CH_2)_7-CH_3 \\
\\
H-\underset{|}{C}-O-\underset{\parallel}{P}-O-CH_2-CH_2-N^+(CH_3)_3 \\
\quad\; H \qquad O^-
\end{array}
$$

FIGURE 12.3   Lecithin (phosphatidyl choline).

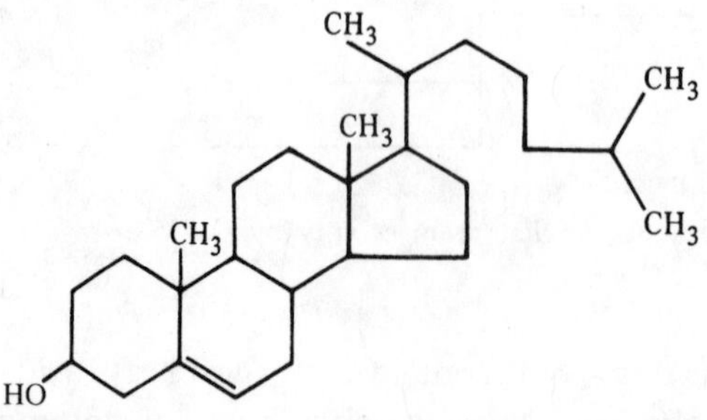

FIGURE 12.4 Cholesterol, phytosterols.

increase nutritive value. Fat must be present in the diet for, among other reasons, the absorption of fat-soluble vitamins.

Pigments such as carotenoids and chlorophylls may be present in fats, and these may impart a distinct color to a fat. Such colors are normally removed during processing.

STRUCTURE OF FATTY ACIDS

Fatty acids are long hydrocarbon chains, with a methyl group (CH_3) at one end of the chain and a carboxylic acid group (COOH) at the other. Most natural fatty acids contain from 4 to 24 carbon atoms, and most contain an even number of carbon atoms in the chain. For example, butyric acid is the smallest fatty acid, having four carbon atoms, and it is found in butter; lard and tallow contain longer fatty acids. Fatty acids may be *saturated*, in which case they contain only single carbon-to-carbon bonds and have the general formula $CH_3(CH_2)_nCOOH$. They have a linear shape, as shown in Figure 12.5.

Fatty acids may also be *unsaturated*, containing one or more carbon-to-carbon double bonds. *Monounsaturated* fatty acids such as oleic acid, contain only one double bond, *polyunsaturated* fatty acids, such as linoleic and linolenic acids, contain two or more double bonds. Generally, *unsaturated* fats are *liquid* at room temperature and have low melting points.

The double bonds in fatty acids occur in either *cis* or the *trans* configuration (Figure 12.6), representing different isomeric structures. In the **cis** form, the hydrogen atoms attached to the carbon atoms of the double bond are located on the

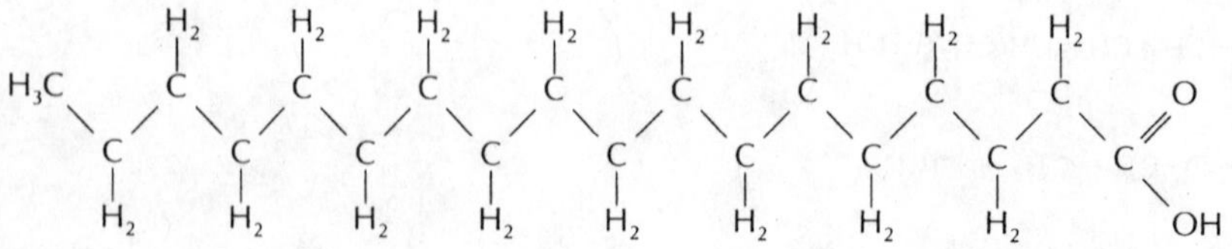

FIGURE 12.5 Example of a fatty acid.

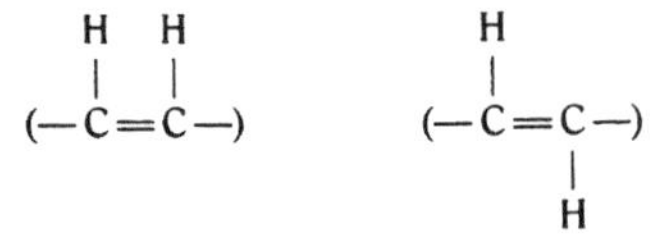

FIGURE 12.6   *Cis* (left) and *trans* (right) configurations representing isomeric structures of fatty acids.

same side of the double bond. In the **trans** configuration of the isomer, the hydrogen atoms are located on opposite sides of the double bond.

The configuration of the double bonds affects both melting point, and shape of a fatty acid molecule. The *trans* double bonds have a higher melting point than the *cis* configurations, and *trans* configurations do not significantly change the linear shape of the molecule. However, a *cis* double bond causes a kink in the chain. (A *cis* double bond introduces a bend of about 42° into the linear hydrocarbon chain.) Such kinks affect some of the properties of fatty acids, including their melting points.

All naturally occurring fats and oils that are used in food exist in the *cis* configuration. However, hydrogenation of oils causes conversion of some double bonds to the *trans* configuration.

While current labels and advertisements do not include trans fatty acids, the National Cholesterol Education Program (NCEP) has stated that "trans fatty acids are another LDL-raising fat that should be kept to a low intake". More specific labeling, which includes trans fatty acids content, is desired by some nutrition activists (3).

Isomerism

Fatty acids may have geometric or positional **isomers**, which are similar in number of C, H, and O, but form different arrangements, thus offering different chemical and physical properties. Oleic and elaidic acids are examples of *geometric* isomers, existing in the *cis* and *trans* forms, respectively. *Positional* isomers have the same chemical formula, but the position of the double bonds varies. Examples include alpha-linolenic acid, which has double bonds at carbons 9, 12, and 15, counting from the acid end of the chain, and the rare isomer gamma-linolenic acid, which has double bonds at positions 6, 9, and 12.

Commercial modification of fats may produce either geometric or positional fatty acid isomers. Geometric isomers tend to be produced during hydrogenation of fats, and positional isomers may be formed during interesterification or rearrangement of fats.

NOMENCLATURE OF FATTY ACIDS

Fatty acids are named in three ways; 1) each has a *common* or *trivial* name, which has been used for many years, and they also have 2) a *systematic* or *Geneva* name, which is more recent, and has the advantage of describing the structure of the fatty acid to which it belongs. In addition, there is 3) the *omega* system, which classifies fatty acids according to the position of the first double bond, counting from the methyl

TABLE 12.1   Nomenclature of Some Common Fatty Acids

Systematic Name	Common Name	No. of Carbons	Melting Point °F (°C)
Ethanoic	Acetic	2	
Butanoic	Butyric	4	18 (−7.9)
Hexanoic	Caproic	6	26 (−3.4)
Octanoic	Caprylic	8	62 (16.7)
Decanoic	Capric	10	89 (31.6)
Dodecanoic	Lauric	12	112 (44.2)
Tetradecanoic	Myristic	14	130 (54.4)
Hexadecanoic	Palmitic	16	145 (62.9)
Octadecanoic	Stearic	18	157 (69.6)
Eicosanoic	Arachidic	20	168 (75.4)
Docosanoic	Behenic	22	176 (80.0)
9-Octadecenoic	Oleic	18-1	61 (16.3)
9,12-Octadecadienoic	Linoleic omega-6	18-2	20 (−6.5)
9,12,15-Octadecatrienoic	Linolenic omega-3	18-3	9 (−12.8)

Source: Adapted from Institute of Shortening and Edible Oils.

end of the molecule. This system was developed to classify families of fatty acids that can be synthesized from each other in the body. Examples of all three names for some of the most common fatty acids are given in Table 12.1.

Fatty acids are also be denoted by two numbers, the first signifying the number of carbon atoms in the chain and the second indicating the number of double bonds present. For example, oleic acid, which contains eighteen carbon atoms and one double bond, could be written as 18:1 (Table 12.1).

Geneva or Systematic Nomenclature

The Geneva naming system is a systematic method of naming the fatty acids, and each name completely describes the structure of the fatty acid to which it belongs. Each unsaturated fatty acid is named according to the number of carbon atoms in the chain, as shown in Table 12.1. For example, stearic acid, which has 18 carbon atoms in its chain, has the name octadecanoic acid; **Octadec** means 18. The *oic* ending signifies that there is an acid group (COOH) present, and **anoic** signifies that there are no double bonds in the chain. Palmitic acid, which contains 16 carbon atoms, is named hexadecanoic acid. **Hexadec** means 16, and the **anoic** ending again shows that there are no double bonds in this fatty acid chain (the **oic** equals presence of an acid group).

Fatty acids that contain double bonds are also named according to the number of carbon atoms they contain. Therefore, oleic acid (18:1), linoleic acid (18:2) and linolenic acid (18:3) all have **octadec** as part of their name, signifying that they each contain 18 carbon atoms. The rest of the name differs, however, because they contain one, two, or three double bonds, respectively. The number of double bonds and their position in the fatty acid chain are both specified in the name.

It is important to note that the position of each double bond is specified counting from the functional group or **acid end** of the molecule, not from the methyl end. Thus, oleic acid has the name 9-octadecenoic acid. The number 9 refers to the position of the double bond between carbon-9 and carbon-10, counting from the acid end. Note that the name ends with **enoic** acid, the **en** signifying that there is a double bond present.

Linoleic acid is named 9,12-*octadecadienoic* acid. Again, the position of double bonds is specified, counting from the acid end. **Octadeca** means that there are 18 carbon atoms in the chain, and **dien** signifies that there are two double bonds in the chain. Similarly, linolenic acid, which contains three double bonds, is named 9,12,15-*octadecatrienoic* acid. The letters **trien** indicate that there are three double bonds in the chain, and again their positions are specified counting from the acid end of the molecule.

The configuration of the double bonds may also be specified in the name. For example, oleic acid and elaidic acid are geometric isomers, because the double bond in oleic acid exists in the *cis* configuration, whereas elaidic acid contains a double bond in the *trans* configuration. The complete name for oleic acid is ***cis*, 9-octadecenoic acid**, and elaidic acid is named ***trans*, 9-octadecenoic acid**.

By looking at a systematic name for a fatty acid, it is possible to tell how many carbon atoms it contains, and how many double bonds and where they are located. Each name gives important information about the fatty acid that is not available just by looking at the trivial or omega name of the acid.

The Omega Naming System

The omega naming system is used for unsaturated fatty acids and denotes the position of the first double bond in the molecule, counting from the **methyl** (CH_3) end, not the acid (as in the Geneva system). This is because the body lengthens fatty acid chains by adding carbons at the acid end of the chain. Using the omega system, a family of fatty acids can be developed which can be made from each other in the body. For example, an omega-6 fatty acid contains its first double bond between carbon-6 and carbon-7, counting from the methyl end. Linoleic acid is an example of an omega-6 fatty acid, and it is the primary member of the omega-6 family. Given linoleic acid, the body can add two carbon atoms to make arachidonic acid (20:4), which is also an omega-6 fatty acid.

The primary omega-3 fatty acid is linolenic acid, which contains three double bonds. The first double bond is located on carbon-3, counting from the methyl end. The body can synthesize both eicosapentaenoic acid (EPA: 20:5) and docosahexaenoic acid (DHA: 22: 6) from linolenic acid. Both EPA and DHA are omega-3 fatty acids, because their first double bond is located at carbon-3 (again, counting from the methyl end of the molecule).

PROPERTIES OF FATS AND OILS

Crystal Formation

When liquid fat is cooled, the molecular movement slows down as energy is removed, and the molecules are attracted to each other by Van der Waals forces. These forces are weak and of minor significance in small molecules. However, their effect is cumulative, and in large or long-chain molecules, the total attractive force is appreciable. Consequently, fat molecules can align and bond to form crystals.

Symmetrical molecules and molecules with fatty acids that are similar in chain length align most easily to form crystals. Fats containing *asymmetrical* molecules and molecules containing kinks due to double bonds align less easily, because they cannot pack together closely in space. Molecules that align easily need less energy to be removed before they will crystallize, and so they have high melting points. They also tend to form *large* crystals. Molecules that do not align easily have low melting points, because more energy must be removed before they crystallize and they tend to form *small* crystals.

Polymorphism

Fats can exist in different crystalline forms, and this phenomenon is known as *polymorphism*. A fat may crystallize in one of four different crystal forms, depending on the conditions during crystallization, and on the composition of the fat. The smallest, and least stable crystals are called **alpha (α) crystals**. These are formed if fats are chilled rapidly. The alpha crystals of most fats are unstable, and change readily to **beta prime (β') crystals**. These are small needlelike crystals, approximately 1 μm long. Fats that can form stable β-crystals are good for use as shortenings, as they can be creamed easily, and give a smooth texture. Unstable β' crystals change to the **intermediate crystal** form, about 3–5 μm in size, and finally convert to **coarse beta (β) crystals**, which can range from 25 to 100 μm in length. Beta crystals have the highest melting point.

Formation of small crystals is favored by rapid cooling with agitation. This allows formation of many small crystals, instead of slow growth of fewer large crystals. (Smaller crystals are desirable if a fat contributes aeration to a food.) Growth of large crystals occurs if cooling is slow.

The more heterogeneous the fat, the more likely that the molecules form small stable crystals. Homogeneous fats readily form large crystals. Lard is an example of a homogeneous fat; more than 25% of the molecules contain stearic acid, palmitic acid, and one unsaturated fatty acid molecule (usually oleic acid). Therefore, lard exists in the coarse *beta* crystalline form. However, lard can be modified by interesterification, which causes the fatty acids to migrate and recombine with glycerol in a more random manner. Rearranged lard forms stable β'-crystals, because it is more heterogeneous. Acetoglycerides are able to form stable α-crystals, because they contain acetic acid esterified to glycerol, in place of one or two fatty acids. This increases the heterogeneity of the fatty acid composition of each individual triglyceride, which hinders the formation of large crystals.

All other things being equal, a fat with small crystals contains many more crystals and a much greater total crystal surface area than does a fat containing large crystals. Fats with small crystals are harder fats, have a smooth, fine texture, and appear to be less oily because the oil is present as a fine film surrounding the crystals, whereas the reverse is true of fats with large crystals.

The food industry uses controlled polymorphism to obtain fats with crystal sizes that improve their functional properties in foods. For example, fats used for creaming must contain small, stable crystals in the β' form; thus, crystallization is controlled during the manufacturing process.

Melting Points

The melting point is an index of the force of attraction between molecules. The greater the attractive forces between molecules, the more easily they will associate to form a solid, and the harder it is to separate them when they are in the crystalline form and convert them to a liquid. A lot of energy in the form of heat must be put in to convert a solid to a liquid; thus, the melting point will be high. In other words, a high melting point indicates a strong attractive force between molecules. A strong attractive force indicates a good degree of fit between the molecules. Molecules that do not fit together well do not have strong attractive forces holding them together, and so they have lower melting points.

A fat or oil, which is a mixture of several triglycerides, has a lower melting point and a broader melting range than would be expected based on the melting points of the individual components. However, the melting range is dependent on the fatty acids of the component triglycerides. Fats may also be plastic at room temperature, containing some triglycerides that are liquid and some that are solid.

Generally speaking, oils, liquid at room temperature tend to be more unsaturated, have shorter chains, and have lower melting points than fats, which are plastic or solid, with long chains and high melting points at room temperature. However, this is not the case always, as illustrated by coconut oil (see Tropical Oils), which has a high level of saturates (90%), but a low melting range [75–80°F (24–27°C)]. It is liquid at room temperature because it contains an appreciable number of relatively short-chain (12 carbons) fatty acids, as is the case with palm and palm kernel oils. Lard, on the other hand, contains only about 37% saturates, but mostly long-chain fatty acids, and so it is semisolid at 80°F (27°C).

The melting point of a fat or oil is actually a range, not a sharply defined temperature. The melting range depends on the composition of the fat. Each fat or oil contains triglycerides that melt at different temperatures, depending on their component fatty acids. Some fats have a wide melting range, whereas others, such as butter or chocolate, have a narrow melting range. Chocolate has a narrow melting range that is close to body temperature, and this accounts for its characteristic melt-in-your-mouth property.

The melting points of individual fatty acids depend on such factors as *chain length, number of double bonds* (degree of saturation), and *isomeric configuration,* because all these factors affect the degree of fit and the force of attraction between fatty acid molecules.

Chain length: *Long-chain* fatty acids have a higher melting point than *short-chain* fatty acids, because there is more potential for attraction between long chains than there is between short chains. The attractive forces are cumulative and can be appreciable if the chain is long enough. (In other words, you can think of them as having a zipper effect. A long zipper is much stronger than a short one, because more teeth are intersecting with each other.) For example, butyric acid (4:0) has a melting point of 18°F (-7.9°C), whereas stearic acid (18:0) has a higher melting point of 157°F (69.6°C). Stearic acid is a crystalline solid at room temperature, whereas butyric acid is a liquid unless the temperature drops below the freezing point of water.

Number of double bonds: A second factor that determines melting point is the *number of double bonds*. As the number of double bonds *increases,* the melting point *decreases.* Double bonds introduce kinks into the chain, and it is harder for molecules to fit together to form crystals; thus, the attractive forces between the molecules are weaker. This is demonstrated by comparing the melting points of stearic, oleic, linoleic, and linolenic acids, as shown in Table 12.1.

Isomeric configuration: A third influence on melting point is *isomeric configuration.* Geometric isomers have different melting points, because the cis double bond configuration introduces a much bigger kink into the molecule than does the *trans* configuration. Consequently, the *cis* isomer has a lower melting point than the *trans* isomer, because molecules in the *cis* configuration do not fit together as well as molecules in the *trans* configuration. This can be seen by comparing the melting points of oleic and elaidic acids. Oleic acid (*cis*) has a lower melting point than elaidic acid (*trans*). Low-*trans* liquid shortening such as the high oleic, monounsaturated sunflower oil require no *trans* or "hydrogenated" reporting on labels, because it has a level of less than 2% *trans* fatty acids. A standard shortening may contain more than 30% *trans* fat levels.

The melting point of a triglyceride depends on the melting point of the component *fatty acids* as discussed above. *Simple* triglycerides can fit together easily, because the three fatty acid chains are identical and therefore allow for close packing of the molecules and high melting points. In general, the more *heterogeneous* triglycerides will not fit together as well, and so will have lower melting points. The melting point of a fat increases with each shift in polymorphic form, from alpha to coarse beta crystals.

Plastic Fats

Fats may either be liquid, plastic, or solid at room temperature. A ***plastic fat*** is moldable because it contains both liquid oil and solid crystals of triglycerides. Its consistency depends on the ratio of solid to liquid triglycerides: the more liquid triglycerides, the softer the fat will be, and the more solid triglycerides, the harder it will be. A plastic fat is a two-phase system, containing solid fat crystals surrounded by liquid oil. The liquid phase acts as a lubricant, enabling the solid crystals to slide past one another, and thus conferring moldability to the fat. A fat that contains only solid triglycerides is hard and brittle and cannot be molded, because the crystals cannot move past each other.

Fats that are creamed, for example in shortened cakes, must be plastic, so that they are easily workable (Chapter 14) and incorporate air into a mixture without breaking. Ideally, they should be plastic over a wide temperature range, so that creaming can be carried out at different temperatures. Fats with a wide plastic range contain some triglycerides that are solid at high temperatures and some triglycerides that are liquid at low temperatures. Therefore, the melting range is wide, and so the fat is semisolid or plastic over a wide temperature range. Butter has a narrow plastic range and is, therefore, not a good choice for a fat that needs to be creamed. It cannot be creamed if taken straight out of the refrigerator, because it is too hard; neither can it be creamed if it sits on the counter on a warm day, because it will be too liquid.

Fats with a wide plastic range are obtained by commercial modification, including hydrogenation and interesterification. Examples of such fats include partially hydrogenated soybean oil (found in margarine) and interesterified lard. Shortenings that are to be creamed must also contain small crystals, preferably in the β' form. Rearranged lard forms stable β'-crystals, and so has a fine-grained texture that is suitable for creamed fats.

COMPOSITION OF DIETARY FATS AND OILS

A table showing fatty acid composition of various fats and oils frequently used by the consumer in food preparation is shown in Figure 12.7.

Polyunsaturated fats are liquid at room temperature and found primarily in *plants*. Safflower oil is 76% polyunsaturated, sunflower oil is 71%, soybean oil 54%, and corn oil 57% ("partially hydrogenated" oils are hydrogenated to have a greater degree of saturation).

Monounsaturated fats are liquid at room temperature and found chiefly in *plants*. Olive oil is 75% monounsaturated, high-oleic safflower oil is 80% (versus 76% polyunsaturated safflower oil), and canola (rapeseed oil) is 61% monounsaturated. These fats are associated with a decrease in serum cholesterol and a decreased risk of coronary heart disease (CHD).

Saturated fats are solid at room temperature and found primarily in *animals*, although it is found in some tropical oils. These fats are implicated in a greater rise in serum cholesterol than in dietary cholesterol.

Overall, it is not a simple categorization of the type of fatty acids that raise, lower, or show no effect on serum cholesterol.

Animal Fats

Animal fats typically have 18 carbons in the fatty acid chain. These long chains are made of various fatty acids and are chiefly saturated. Such fats may be *rendered* for

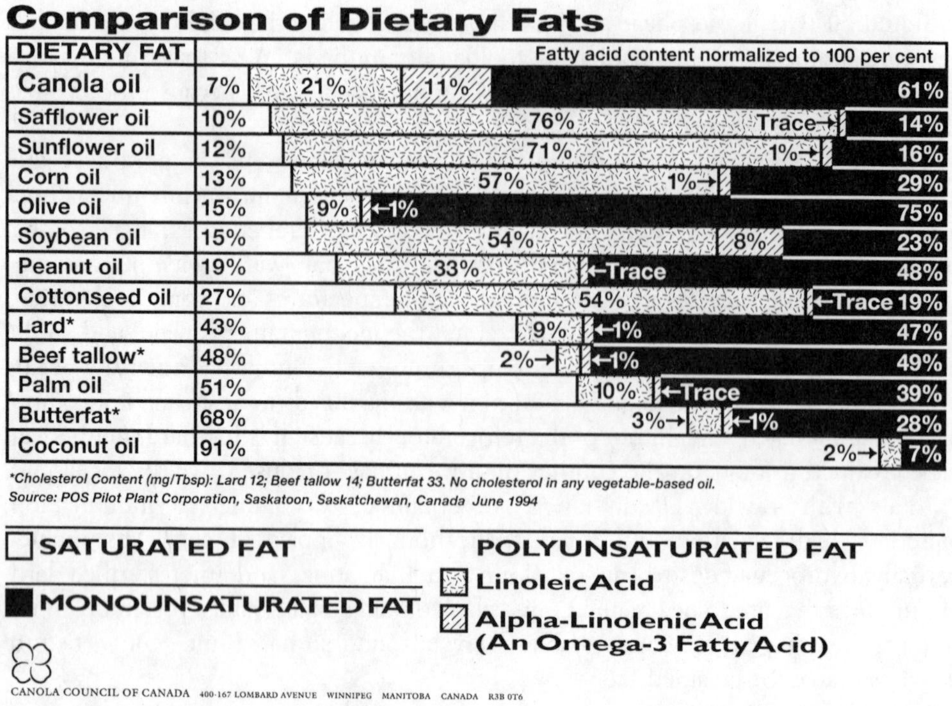

Comparison of Dietary Fats

DIETARY FAT	Fatty acid content normalized to 100 per cent
Canola oil	7% · 21% · 11% · · · · · · · 61%
Safflower oil	10% · · · · 76% · · · Trace→ · 14%
Sunflower oil	12% · · · 71% · · · 1%→ · 16%
Corn oil	13% · · · 57% · · · 1%→ · 29%
Olive oil	15% · 9% · ←1% · · · · · 75%
Soybean oil	15% · · · 54% · · · 8% · 23%
Peanut oil	19% · · 33% · ←Trace · · 48%
Cottonseed oil	27% · · 54% · · ←Trace 19%
Lard*	43% · · 9% · ←1% · · 47%
Beef tallow*	48% · 2%→ · ←1% · · 49%
Palm oil	51% · 10% · ←Trace · 39%
Butterfat*	68% · 3%→ · ←1% · 28%
Coconut oil	91% · · 2%→ · 7%

*Cholesterol Content (mg/Tbsp): Lard 12; Beef tallow 14; Butterfat 33. No cholesterol in any vegetable-based oil.
Source: POS Pilot Plant Corporation, Saskatoon, Saskatchewan, Canada June 1994

☐ SATURATED FAT

■ MONOUNSATURATED FAT

POLYUNSATURATED FAT

▨ Linoleic Acid

▨ Alpha-Linolenic Acid
(An Omega-3 Fatty Acid)

CANOLA COUNCIL OF CANADA 400-167 LOMBARD AVENUE WINNIPEG MANITOBA CANADA R3B 0T6

FIGURE 12.7 Comparison of composition of dietary fat
(*Source:* Canola Council of Canada).

use in baking and cooking applications (see Rendered Fat). Animal fats derived from hogs and cattle include the following:

- **Lard**. Rendered from hogs, 43% saturated fatty acids. It lacks natural antioxidants and is therefore less stable than equally saturated vegetable oils that have been partially hydrogenated (4).

- **Tallow (Suet)**. Rendered from cattle, 48% saturated fatty acids.

In part due to the fact that animal fats contain cholesterol and saturated fat and a pronounced flavor, the use of lard and tallow in foods has declined in favor of vegetable oils.

Tropical Oils

Oils derived from plants grown in tropical areas of the world are referred to as *tropical oil*. Unlike most plants, these in particular are high in saturated fat content and contain an appreciable amount of short-chain fatty acids. Examples of tropical oils include the following:

- **Cocoa butter**. Extracted from cocoa beans, typically used in candies and chocolate confections.

- **Coconut oil**. Highest saturated fat vegetable oil—over 90% saturated; very stable against oxidation, and, to a lesser degree, stable against hydrolysis.

- **Palm oil**. 50% saturated fatty acids; stable against oxidation.

- **Palm kernel oil**. 84% saturated fatty acids; derived from the kernel of the palm tree; stable against oxidation.

PRODUCTION AND PROCESSING METHODS

Crops are bred to increase the grower's yield while offering health benefits because growers want high yield, and *consumers* want desirable health features in fats and oils. Both groups desire shelf stability. A brief discussion of the conventional as well as nonconventional approaches to breeding appears in the following text. Techniques are provided by the molecular geneticist and are available to growers and oilseed processors so that suppliers of edible oils can make both shelf stability and consumer health their priorities.

For example, ordinary soybean oil is not shelf stable because it contains 7.6% linolenic acid, an unstable, 18-3, polyunsaturated fatty acid. To improve on this, *conventional* cross-breeding and selection has developed a low-linolenic soybean oil (LLSO), containing 2.5–3% linolenic content (5). This lower-linolenic soybean oil, derived from selected soybeans, is more stable than ordinary soybean oil, and does not require hydrogenation for protection against rancidity. Consumers who want less saturated oil may make this oil their choice.

Unconventional approaches to breeding include gene modification, which produces a more stable oil that does not require hydrogenation. Then, stability as well as lower saturated fat may be achieved in a product. Cross-breeding or genetic modification that offers increased shelf stability without loss of health benefits may be desirable. [To make oils more shelf-stable and solid during storage, oil is treated by hydrogenation (see hydrogenation). This adds hydrogen and produces a more saturated fat. Some consumers may find this to be an undesirable treatment from a health point of view because, in fact, saturated fat intake contributes more toward the elevation of serum cholesterol than does dietary cholesterol intake.]

Some production methods are discussed below.

Deodorized Oils

Deodorized oils are those that have undergone the process of removing odors by heat and vacuum or by adsorption onto charcoal. For example, olive oil may be deodorized to provide broader use in baking applications, without imparting its characteristic odor and flavor to food.

Rendered Fat

Rendered fat is the fat derived from animal fat and then freed from connective tissue by heat. Food manufacturers render *hog* fat and process it to become *lard*, or *cattle* fat to become *tallow*. On a small scale, the consumer may render fat by cutting it into small pieces and gently boiling the pieces to extract liquid fat, and then cooling, until it becomes solid. The leftover rind, devoid of usable fat, has uses outside the scope of a discussion of fats.

As previously mentioned, lard and tallow are not as commonly used in cooking as they were in the past, partially because of the pronounced flavor, saturated fat, and cholesterol content. As well, animals are now bred to be leaner, so lard is less available. Today, there are many convenient, commercially prepared shortenings on the market that replace lard in cooking.

The large crystalline structure of lard is composed of many similar triglycerides that are used to produce a highly desirable, flaky pie crust. Lard may be processed to contain smaller crystals, and then it functions more like a hydrogenated shortening. The addition of antioxidants such as BHA and BHT protect it against rancidity.

MODIFICATION OF FATS

Hydrogenation

Hydrogenation is the process of adding hydrogen to unsaturated fatty acids to reduce the number of double bonds. The purpose of hydrogenation is twofold:

- To convert liquid oils to semisolid or plastic fats
- To increase the thermal and oxidative stability of the fat, and thus the shelf life

Hydrogenation of unsaturated fatty acid occurs when hydrogen gas is reacted with *oil* under controlled conditions of temperature and pressure, and in the presence of a nickel catalyst. The reaction is carefully controlled and stopped when the desired extent of hydrogenation has been reached. As the reaction progresses, there is a gradual production of *trans* fatty acids (discussed herein), which increases the melting point of the fat or oil and creates a more solid product.

The extent of the hydrogenation process is controlled to achieve stability and/or the physical properties required in the finished food. If the reaction is taken to completion, a saturated fat is obtained, and the product is hard and brittle at room temperature. However, this is not usually the aim of hydrogenation, as *partial* hydrogenation is normally desired, providing an intermediate degree of solidification, reducing, but not eliminating the number of double bonds. In fact, approximately 50% of the total fatty acids present in partially hydrogenated vegetable shortening products are monounsaturated and about 25% are polyunsaturated.

The process of hydrogenation causes conversion of some *cis* double bonds to the *trans* configuration. Most of the *trans* fatty acids formed are monounsaturated, and tub margarines, for examples, typically contain *trans* fatty acid levels of 13–20%. There is debate about the safety of *trans* fatty acids in the diet, and it is possible that they may raise cholesterol levels in the body. However, more research is needed before any firm conclusions can be drawn. Positional isomers are also formed to some extent during hydrogenation (food labels may chose to include information on *trans* content).

[A Federation of American Societies for Experimental Biology (FASEB) report published in 1985 (6) concluded that there was little cause for concern with the safety of dietary *trans* fatty acids, both at present and expected levels of consumption. However, this was challenged by later research, which indicated that a high *trans* fatty acid diet raised total and LDL cholesterol (low-density lipids or "bad" cholesterol) levels, and lowered HDL-cholesterol (high density lipids or "good" cholesterol) levels in humans.]

In foods, plastic fats have useful functional properties for use in margarines or shortenings that are to be creamed. Polyunsaturated fats are subject to oxidative rancidity; thus, reducing the number of double bonds by hydrogenation increases their stability. Hydrogenated fats are frequently specified in batter and dough recipes that depend of the creaming ability of solid fats for eration (Chapter 14). Creaming increases volume by incorporating air and results in numerous air cells. As a result, the grain of the crumb in baked products is small and even.

Interesterification

Interesterification, or *rearrangement*, causes the fatty acids to migrate and recombine with glycerol in a more random manner. This causes new glycerides to form and increases the heterogeneity of the fat. However, it does not change the degree of unsaturation or the isomeric state of the fatty acids.

Lard is an example of a fat that is modified in this way to improve its functional properties. In its natural state, lard is a relatively homogeneous fat, as has already been mentioned. Therefore, it has a narrow plastic range and is too firm to be used straight from refrigerator but too soft at temperatures above normal room temperature. Lard also contains coarse β-crystals. Rearrangement increases the heterogeneity of lard, enabling it to form stable β′-crystals and increasing the temperature range over which it is plastic or workable. This significantly enhances its use as a shortening product.

Hydrogenation may be used in conjunction with interesterification and may either precede or follow it. This gives a shortening manufacturer the ability to produce fats with a wide range of properties.

Acetylation

Acetoglycerides or *acetin fats* are formed when one or two fatty acids in a triglyceride are replaced by acetic acid (CH_3COOH). Acetin fats may be liquid or plastic at room temperature depending on the component fatty acids. However, the presence of acetic acid lowers the melting point of the fat, because the molecules do not pack together as readily. It also enables the fat to form stable α-crystals.

Acetin fats are used as edible lubricants; they also form flexible films and are used as coating agents for selected foods such as dried raisins and produce to prevent moisture loss (Chapter 17).

Winterization

Winterized oil is oil that has been pretreated to control undesirable cloudiness from the large, high-melting-point triglyceride crystals in oil that crystallize (forming solids) at refrigeration temperatures. In the process of winterization, oil is refrigerated and subsequently filtered to remove the undesirable crystals, which could readily disrupt a salad dressing emulsion. The treated oil is called *salad oil*, which is specially used in salad dressing. *Salad oils* are clear and are bleached, deodorized, and refined, in addition to undergoing winterization. Salad oils differ from *cooking oils*, which do not undergo winterization.

DETERIORATION OF FATS

Fats deteriorate either by absorbing odors or by becoming rancid. For example, deterioration by *absorbing odors* becomes evident when chocolate fat absorbs the odor of smoke in a candy store environment, or the odor of soap packaged in the same grocery bag. Butter may deteriorate by readily absorbing refrigerator odors. When *rancidity* causes deterioration, it produces a disagreeable odor and flavor in fatty substances. Processing does not remove *all* chance of fat and oil deterioration and rancidity, but it prolongs the life of a fat or oil.

Rancidity can occur in two ways (below) that make fats undesirable for use in foods. **Hydrolytic rancidity** involves reaction of fats with water and liberation of free fatty acids. **Oxidative rancidity** is a more complex and potentially more damaging reaction. In this case, the fat is oxidized and decomposes into compounds with shorter carbon chains such as fatty acids, aldehydes, and ketones all of which are volatile and contribute to the unpleasant odor of rancid fats.

Hydrolytic Rancidity

Fats may become rancid when the triglycerides react with water and free their fatty acids from glycerol. The reaction is shown in Figure 12.8. If one molecule of water reacts with a triglyceride, one fatty acid is liberated and a diglyceride remains. To liberate glycerol, all three fatty acids must be removed from the molecule. The reaction is catalyzed by heat and by enzymes known as lipases. Butter contains lipase, and if left on the kitchen counter on a warm day, a characteristic rancid smell

$$
\begin{array}{l}
CH_2-OOC-R \\
| \\
CH-OOC-R + 3H_2O \longrightarrow \\
| \\
CH_2-OOC-R
\end{array}
\qquad
\begin{array}{l}
CH_2-OH \\
| \\
CH-OH + 3RCOOH \\
| \\
CH_2-OH
\end{array}
$$

FIGURE 12.8 Hydrolytic rancidity.

frequently develops due to liberation of the short-chain butyric acid. (Unlike long-chain fatty acids, these short-chain fatty acids may form an unpleasant odor and flavor.) Hydrolytic rancidity is also a problem with deep-fat frying, where the temperature is high and wet foods are often introduced into the hot fat. The continued use of rancid oil results in additional breakdown of the oil.

To avoid this type of rancidity, fats should be stored in a cool place and, if possible, lipases should be inactivated. Fats should be kept away from water, and foods to be fried should be as dry as possible before they are added to hot fat. The kind of fat used for frying should be selected based on stability.

Oxidative Rancidity or Autoxidation

The predominant type of rancidity is oxidative rancidity. In this process, the unsaturated fatty acids are subjected to oxidative rancidity or autoxidation, and the more double bonds there are, the greater the opportunity for addition of oxygen to double bonds, increasing risk that the fat or oil will become rancid. **Autoxidation** is complex and is promoted by heat, light, certain metals (iron and copper), and enzymes known as lipoxygenases. The reaction can be separated into three stages: initiation, propagation, and termination.

The **initiation stage** of the reaction involves formation of a free radical. A hydrogen on a carbon atom adjacent to one carrying a double bond is displaced to give a free radical, as shown in Figure 12.9. There is chemical activity around and in the double bonds. (The bold type indicates the atoms or groups of atoms involved in the reactions.) As previously mentioned, this reaction is catalyzed by heat, light, certain metals such as copper and iron, and lipoxygenases. The free radicals that form are unstable and very reactive.

The **propagation stage** follows the initiation stage and involves oxidation of the free radical to yield activated peroxide. This, in turn, displaces hydrogen from another unsaturated fatty acid, forming another free radical. The liberated hydrogen unites with the peroxide to form a hydroperoxide, and the free radical can be oxidized as just described. Thus, the reaction repeats, or propagates, itself. Formation of one free radical, therefore, leads to the oxidation of many unsaturated fatty acids.

Hydroperoxides are very unstable and decompose into compounds with shorter carbon chains, such as volatile fatty acids, aldehydes, and ketones. These are

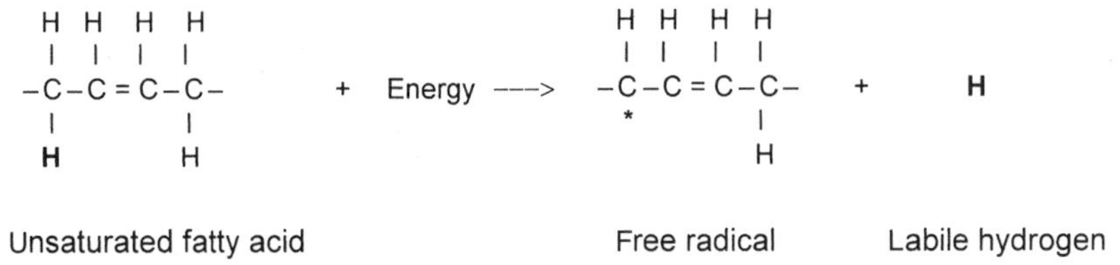

FIGURE 12.9 The initiation stage of autoxidation.

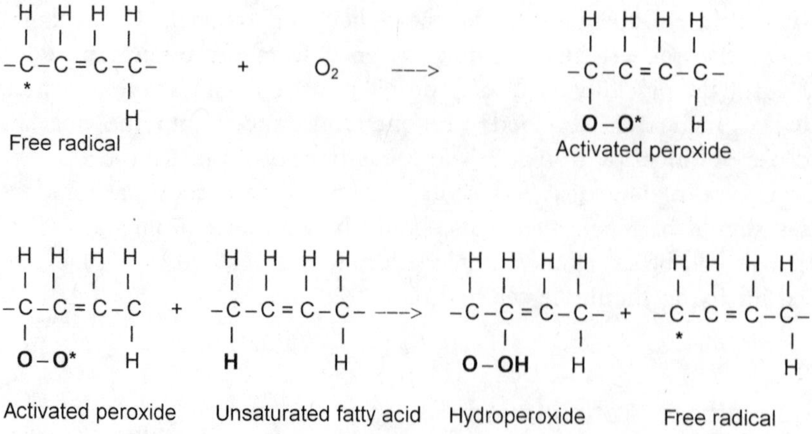

```
 H  H  H  H                                    H  H  H  H
 |  |  |  |                                    |  |  |  |
-C –C = C –C –        +      O₂     --->      –C –C = C –C –
 *           |                                      |
             H                                      O – O*    H
 Free radical                                 Activated peroxide
```

```
 H  H  H  H          H  H  H  H                H  H  H  H          H  H  H  H
 |  |  |  |          |  |  |  |                |  |  |  |          |  |  |  |
-C –C = C –C    +   –C –C = C –C –   --->    –C –C = C –C –   +   –C –C = C –C –
 |           |       |           |            |           |       *           |
 O – O*      H       H           H            O – OH      H                   H

 Activated peroxide  Unsaturated fatty acid   Hydroperoxide       Free radical
```

FIGURE 12.10   The two reactions of the propagation stage of autoxidation.

responsible for the characteristic odor of rancid fats and oils. The two reactions of the propagation stage of autoxidation are shown in Figure 12.10.

The **termination stage** of the reaction involves the reaction of free radicals to form nonradical products. Elimination of all free radicals is the only way to halt the oxidation reaction.

Prevention of Autoxidation

Oxidation can be prevented or delayed by avoiding situations that would serve as catalysts for the reaction. For example, fats and oils must be stored in a cool dark environment (offering temperature and light change controls) and in a closed container (to minimize oxygen availability). Vacuum packaging of fat-containing products controls oxygen exposure, and colored glass or wraps control fluctuations in light intensity. Fats must also be stored away from metals that could catalyze the reaction, and any cooking utensils used must be free of copper or iron. Lipoxygenases should be inactivated.

In addition, *sequestering agents* and *antioxidants* can be added to fats to prevent autoxidation (Chapter 17).

Sequestering agents bind metals, thus preventing them from catalyzing autoxidation. Examples of sequestering agents include EDTA (ethylenediaminetetraacetic acid) and citric acid.

Antioxidants help prevent autoxidation with its formation of fatty acid free radicals. Antioxidants prevent rancidity by donating a hydrogen atom to the double bond in a fatty acid and preventing the oxidation of any unsaturated bond. They halt the chain reaction along the fatty acid, which leads to rancidity.

Most antioxidants are phenolic compounds. Those approved for use in foods include **BHA** (butylated hydroxyanisole), **BHT** (butylated hydroxytoluene), **TBHQ** (tertiary-butyl hydroquinone), and propyl gallate. These are all synthetic antioxidants. The effectiveness of antioxidants may be increased if they are used together. For example, propyl gallate and BHA are more effective when combined than if used separately.

BHA is a waxy white solid that survives processing to create a stable product. It is effective in preventing oxidation of animal fats but not vegetable oils. BHT is a white crystalline solid that may be combined with BHA. It is effective in preventing oxidation of animal fats. TBHQ is a white-to-tan-colored powder that functions best in frying processes rather than baking applications (7).

Tocopherols are naturally occurring antioxidants that are present in vegetable oils. They can be added to both animal and vegetable oils to prevent oxidation. The tocopherols are also sources of essential nutrient vitamin E.

Use of antioxidants in foods containing fat increases their keeping quality and shelf life. Examination of food labels reveals that antioxidants are widely used in many food products, from potato chips to cereals. Without them, the quality of fat-containing foods would not be as good, and off-flavors and odors due to oxidative rancidity would be commonplace.

SHORTENING AND SHORTENING POWER OF VARIOUS FATS AND OILS

Plant, animal, or numerous plant–animal blends of fats and oils may be used for shortening, and, typically, the blend is creamy. The shortening potential of a fat or oil is influenced by its fatty acid composition (see Figure 12.5), and various fats and oils may function as shortenings. "Shortenings" may include many types, from pourable liquids to stiff solids, with the latter being most commonly considered shortening. A shortening functions to physically shorten platelets of protein–starch structure developed in manipulated wheat flour mixtures.

Lard has a large fatty acid crystal structure, unless it is interesterified, and forms a desirable flaky product. This solid fat when cut into pea-sized chunks or smaller melts within the gluten structure of flour, creating many layers, or *flakes* in pie crusts or biscuits.

Butter and margarine contain water and milk (20%) in addition to a variety of fat or oils (80%). Therefore, butter and margarine have less shortening potential than lard, hydrogenated shortening, or oil that contains 100% fat. When butter or margarine is incorporated into flour-based formulations, they toughen the mixture, as its water component hydrates the starch, causing it to swell. A recipe substituting butter or margarine for lard or hydrogenated shortening requires less additional water, and yields a *less flaky* pie crust.

The work on a replacement for butter originated in 1869 when margarine was formulated. Margarine contains part skim milk or whey and optional fat ingredient(s) and may include added salt and vitamin A. Today, margarine *substitutes* may be milk-free, sodium-free, or even fat-free. The margarine is likely to be high in polyunsaturated fatty acids (PUFA), if oil is listed as the first ingredient on a margarine label. If partially hydrogenated oil is listed first, there is less PUFA.

A product must be labeled "spread" if it does not meet the Standard of Identity for margarine.

Hydrogenated fats are saturated and easily workable. When creamed, they incorporate air into a mixture. They are processed to be without a pronounced flavor and have a wide plastic range. Hydrogenated fats contain 100% fat and have greater shortening power than butter or margarine. Finished food products may be *flaky*.

Oils contain a high liquid to fat crystal ratio and are unsaturated. They shorten strands of protein mechanically by coating the platelets. Oil controls gluten development and subsequent toughness because less water contacts the gluten proteins. Oil helps produce a *tender* product, but in pastries, flakiness may be sacrificed. Flakes are not readily obtained because there are no large chunks of fat to melt between layers of dough.

Tenderization Versus Flakiness Provided by Fats and Oils

Lipids provide either **tenderization** or **flakiness**, as discussed, and impart distinct characteristics of a food product. The differences are especially evident in finished pie crusts and can also be observed in biscuits. *Tender* products are easily crushed or chewed; they are soft and fragile—i.e., oil pie crusts. *Flaky* products contain many thin pieces or layers of cooked dough, i.e., puff pastry, lard pie crusts.

Some factors that affect these two distinct attributes are presented in Table 12.2. The *type of fat or oil* chosen to be incorporated into food, its *concentration, degree of manipulation,* and *temperature* each affect the flakiness and tenderness of a product. Fats and oils should be selected, and used with knowledge of these factors. Yet, health attributes of a fat or oil may supersede other quality attributes creating products that do not meet traditional product standards. For example, for health reasons, a pie crust may not incorporate solid fat but may be prepared using oil. If that is the case, the finished pie crust will sacrifice flakiness but will be tender and crumbly.

In order to control formation of an undesirable crumbly food product, some gluten formation may be needed prior to the addition of the fat or oil. This may be achieved by adding fat to a recipe, *after* some hydration and manipulation has formed gluten.

EMULSIFICATION (SEE CHAPTER 13)

Fats and oils are not emulsifiers; however, in addition to providing flavor, aerating batters and doughs, and shortening, fats and oils are important constituents of emulsions. An emulsion consists of a three-phase system composed of 1) a **continuous phase**—the phase or medium in which the dispersed phase is suspended, 2) a **dispersed phase**—the phase which is disrupted or finely divided within the emulsion, and 3) an **emulsifier**—the emulsifier is present at the interface between the dispersed phase and the continuous phase, and keeps them apart. An emulsifier acts in the following ways:

TABLE 12.2   Factors Affecting the Tenderness and Flakiness of a Product

---

The type of fat or oil—Chunks of *solid fat* create layers or flakes in the gluten starch mixture as they melt, whereas *oil* coats flour particles more thoroughly, *creating less layers* and a mealy product. Substituting one fat or oil for another may not produce acceptable or expected results.

Fat concentration—Fat may be reduced or omitted in a formulation, or the fat that *is* used may not be 100% fat, it may be a butter, margarine or "spread." Adequate levels of fat or oil must be present in foods if they are to meet acceptable standards. For example, sufficient fat in flour-based mixtures is needed to control gluten development and generate a tender crumb. Imitation "butters" or "spreads" have a high water content and may not have the high percentage of fat needed to perform satisfactorily in all baking, sautéing, or "buttering" processes.

Degree of manipulation—An insufficient degree of manipulation may result in poor distribution of fat throughout the food mixture. Inversely, excess manipulation may cause the fat to spread or be softened, thus minimizing the possibility of flakes. For example, a flaky pie crust is produced when solid fat is incorporated in the formulation as pea-sized chunks.

Temperature—Depending on the type of fat, *cold* shortenings (solid or liquid) provide less covering potential than *room temperature* shortenings and produce more flaky biscuits and pie crusts. Food items prepared with cold shortenings also remain slightly more solid in the hot oven while the item bakes. When a shortening is *melted,* it displays a greater shortening potential than an *unmelted* solid shortening; it coats better than the same amount of unmelted solid fat. Melted shortening produces a more tender, less flaky product.

- It adsorbs at the interface between two immiscible liquids such as oil and water.
- It reduces the interfacial tension between two liquids, enabling one liquid to spread more easily around the other.
- It forms a stable, coherent, viscoelastic interfacial film, which prevents or delays coalescence of the dispersed emulsion droplets.

Molecules that can act as emulsifiers contain both a polar, **hydrophilic** (water-loving) section, which is attracted to water, and a **hydrophobic** (or water-hating) section, which is attracted to hydrophobic solvents such as oil. In order for the hydrophilic section to be dispersed in the water phase and for the hydrophobic section to be dispersed in the oil phase, the molecule must adsorb at the interface between the two phases, instead of being dispersed in either bulk phase.

Good emulsifiers are able to interact at the interface to form a coherent film that does not break easily. Therefore, when two droplets collide, the emulsifier film remains intact, and the droplets do not coalesce to form one big droplet. Instead, they drift away from each other.

The best emulsifiers are proteins, such as egg yolk (lipoproteins) or milk proteins, because they are able to interact at the interface to form stable films, and hence to form stable emulsions. However, many other types of molecules are used as emulsifiers.

Mono- and diglycerides are examples of emulsifiers that are added to products in order to provide ease of mixing. They adsorb at the interface, reducing **interfacial tension**, and increasing the spreadability of the continuous phase, or the wettability of the dispersed phase.

In some cases, finely divided powders such as dry mustard or spices are used to emulsify an oil-in-water mixture. The mustard and spices adsorb at the interface and reduce interfacial tension. However, they cannot form a stable film around oil droplets, and so they are unable to form a stable emulsion. Therefore they should not really be considered as emulsifiers.

Emulsions may be temporary or permanent. A *temporary emulsion* separates upon standing. The emulsion is not permanent because the hydrophobic oil and hydrophilic water components separate upon standing. This is because the emulsifiers used are unable to form a stable interfacial film to prevent coalescence and of the droplets of the dispersed phase. As coalescence occurs, the droplets combine to form bigger ones, and eventually the two phases separate out completely. An example of a temporary emulsion would be French Dressing, which separates out a few seconds after it has been shaken.

A *permanent emulsion* is formed when two ordinarily non-miscible phases, such as water and oil, are combined with an emulsifier. One phase (usually the oil phase) is dispersed within the other as small droplets. These remain dispersed in the continuous phase (usually water), because they are surrounded by a stable film of emulsifier that resists coalescence, and so prevents separation of the two phases.

Thus, the time of separation of oil and water is dependent upon the effectiveness of an emulsifier, and the degree of agitation. As mentioned, more detail on emulsification is provided in Chapter 13, but some examples of emulsified mixes are cake mixes, mayonnaise, and salad dressings.

Cake mixes contain an emulsifier that aids in incorporation of air upon stirring or beating. The emulsifiers are usually monoglycerides and diglycerides, which act by dispersing shortening in smaller particles. This creates a maximum number of air cells that increase cake volume and creates a more even grain in the baked product (Chapter 14).

Mayonnaise is an emulsified product. The 1952 Standard of Identity describes mayonnaise as an emulsified semi-solid, with not less than 65% by weight, edible vegetable oil.

Salad dressings are typically emulsified, containing oil, vinegar, water, salts, and so on. Some dressings are available in no-fat formulations. Except for bacon dressing, which uses bacon fat, solid fats are generally not acceptable for use in a dressing. Oil coats the salad contents and it disperses herbs, spices, and other substances contained in the liquid.

Hydrocolloids (see Fat replacements, and Chapter 5) such as gelatin, gums, pectin, and starch pastes may be added in the preparation of salad dressings, but they contain only a hydrophilic section and are not considered emulsifiers. Rather, they act as stabilizers in emulsions, and help to prevent or lessen coalescence, because they increase the viscosity of the continuous phase.

FRYING

Frying with melted fat or oil is a common cooking technique because frying is a rapid heat transfer method that achieves a higher temperature than boiling or dry heat temperature. The characteristics of fats for frying include that the fat must be colorless, odorless, and bland and have a high smoke point.

Smoke Point

The smoke point is the temperature at which fat may be heated before continuous puffs of blue smoke come from the surface of the fat under controlled conditions. The presence of smoke indicates that free glycerol has been further hydrolyzed to yield *acrolein*, a mucous membrane irritant. Monoglycerides, in hydrogenated shortenings, and diglycerides are hydrolyzed more easily than triglycerides and they tend to have a low smoke point. Therefore, they are not recommended in frying oils. When fat exceeds the smoke point, it may reach *flash point*, when fire begins in the oil. Subsequently, it reaches the *fire point* where a fire is sustained in the oil. Oils such as cottonseed or peanut oil have a high smoke point of 444 or 446°F (229 or 230°C), respectively. Other oils with a lower smoking point may not perform satisfactorily when exposed, for example, to the high heat of a wok. Lard, butter, margarine, and animal fats have a low smoke point and less tolerance of heat compared to hydrogenated fat and oils.

Changes During Frying

Frying exposes the food product to high temperatures, removes water, and allows oil absorption. The duration of frying, composition of the food, surface treatment, and other factors have been studied to determine their effect on oil uptake. Additionally, increased gel strength, primarily in restructured snack products, and porosity require more study in order to determine their effect on oil uptake.

Thermal decomposition of oil occurs in fat as air, water, and prolonged high temperature leads to fat oxidation and hydrolysis. Oil may become an unwanted orange or brown color or it may become more viscous and foam. The smoke point decreases as oil is repeatedly used for frying.

Many factors are reported to affect oil uptake during frying (8), and a better understanding of how oil is absorbed during frying can lead to improved food quality of fried foods. Some of these factors are addressed in Table 12.3.

LOW-FAT AND NO-FAT FOODS

Consumer interest in eating reduced-fat or fat-free foods has increased, as is evidenced by the trend for more healthy foods. Yet, the per capita consumption of fats and oils has not decreased to meet the Surgeon General's recommendation (< 30% of a day's calories from fat) in the Report on Nutrition and Health. This may be in part

TABLE 12.3 Selected Factors That Affect Oil Uptake During Deep-Fat Frying

Frying temperature, Duration, and Product shape—Increases in temperature decreases oil uptake due to short frying duration.

Pressure frying decreases duration and oil uptake.

A high surface-to-mass ratio or surface roughness increases oil absorption.

Composition—The addition of soy protein, egg protein, or powdered cellulose decreases oil uptake. High sugar, soft flour, or developed gluten increase oil uptake.

Prefrying treatments—Blanching, prewashing with oil containing emulsifiers, freezing, and steam pretreatment have been shown to decrease oil uptake.

Surface treatment—Hydrocolloids (see Fat Replacements) and amylose coatings may function as barriers to fat uptake.

---

due to the fact that the function, flavor, and mouthfeel of fat has not been duplicated by a nonfat component in the diet.

Product developers of reduced-fat food "need to consider the sensory experience of full-fat products" (9). A report on overcoming flavor challenges in low-fat frozen desserts states that the removal of fat in ice cream products affects flavor and aroma, texture, and mouthfeel. In overcoming flavor challenges, the following points must be considered:

> "Removing any significant amount of fat (above 25%) from a product changes the flavor profile. As the concentration is further reduced, the flavor challenges are increased significantly. As more fat is removed, the differences become much more apparent and the challenges to the product developer increase." (9).

The USDA Agricultural Research Station had developed an encapsulated technology that allows the reduction of fat in foods, while releasing flavors and oils. The commercial ingredient is *Fanstek*®. Utilizing a starch lipid ratio varying from 10:1 to 2:1, oil droplets are suspended in cooked starch dispersions and then added as an ingredient to embellish flavor, texture and mouthfeel (USDA).

> "When fat is removed from a formulation, the only ingredients available to replace it are water, protein, carbohydrates, minerals, or air. Even if nothing new is added to the formula, these items increase automatically and proportionally. Each of these components interacts differently with flavor than fat does. A combination of these ingredients may mimic part of fat's function, but they cannot totally replace fat's functionality." (10).

FAT REPLACEMENTS

Fat replacements in a formulation may be protein, carbohydrates or fat-based. Emulsifiers (same calorie level as fat) and synthetic fat replacements (zero calories) are true fat replacers for fat in a formulation. Glicksman (8) reports that there are currently eight other categories of fat replacers that are basically hydrocolloid materials or contain hydrocolloids as an important part of their ingredient composition.

Hydrocolloids are long-chain polymers, principally carbohydrate, that thicken or gel in aqueous systems, creating the creamy viscosity that mimics fat. They include the starch derivatives, hemicelluloses, β-glucans, soluble bulking agents, microparticulates, composite materials [i.e., carboxymethyl cellulose (CMC) and microcrystalline cellulose or xanthan gum and whey], and functional blends (gums, modified starches, nonfat milk solids, and vegetable protein).

The use of a particular fat replacement may be determined by answering the question: What properties of fat are fat replacers attempting to simulate?

"Organoleptically, fatty or oily mouthfeel can be described as a combination of several basic parameters that together form the recognizable edible sensation of fattiness or oiliness. These parameters are viscosity (thickness, body, fullness), lubricity (creaminess, smoothness), absorption/adsorption (physiological effect on tastebuds), and others (not yet defined but may include such factors as cohesiveness, adhesiveness, waxiness, mouthcoating, etc.)" (10).

"Ingredients which provide these organoleptic stimuli can and do mimic fatty mouthfeel and perception and can be used to replace fat in many food products" (10). Today, there are many materials designed to replace fat; they are derived from several different categories of substances. Some replacers that attempt to simulate fat include protein-, carbohydrate-, and fat-derived fat replacements.

Protein-Derived Fat Replacements

Simplesse®is an all natural fat substitute developed by the NutraSweet Company and approved by the Food and Drug Administration (FDA) in 1990. It is a microparticulated protein (MPP). Simplesse® uses a patented process that heats and intensely blends naturally occurring food proteins such as egg white and milk proteins, along with water, pectin, and citric acid. The protein remains chemically unchanged, but aggregates under controlled conditions that allow formation of small aggregates or microparticles.

The blending process produces small, round uniformly shaped protein particles—about 50 billion per teaspoon—that create the creamy mouthfeel of full fat. The microparticulated particle size is near the lower range of MPPs that *naturally* occur in milk, egg white, grains, and legumes. For example, casein (milk protein) micelles range in size from 0.1 to 3.0 μm in diameter and are perceived as creamy to the tongue. In comparison a larger particle size, 10–30 μm in diameter, is found in powdered (confectionery) sugar, which is perceived as more powdery and gritty.

Initially, Simplesse® was an ingredient approved by the FDA for use in *dairy*-based frozen desserts. Today, it has many more food applications in products such as butter spreads, cheese (creamed, natural, processed, baked cheesecakes), creamers, dips, ice cream, and sour cream. It is also successfully incorporated into *oil*-based products such as margarine spreads, mayonnaise, and salad dressings.

Simplesse® has applications in some aspects of cooking and baking. It may be used in heat processes such as canning or pasteurization, but due to its protein composition, it is subject to denaturation and cannot be used in frying applications. NutraSweet has also created a series of three bakery blends using Simplesse® for specific fat-free, low-fat, or reduced-fat bakery applications. The blends create a fat reduction of 83–93% in muffins, pound cakes, and brownies and are used at levels of 1.0–3.0%. Powdered bakery blends are used for muffins, sweet dough products, and frostings. They are Kosher approved, and with proper storage, they have a shelf life of 9 months (11).

Due to its milk and egg protein composition, individuals allergic to milk or eggs cannot eat this fat substitute. It contains 1.2 cal/g (not a zero-calorie food), approximately one-third the calories of protein, and significantly lowers fat intake. Simplesse® is a Generally Recognized as Safe (GRAS) substance.

Whey protein concentrates (WPCs), and *isolates (WPIs)*, and *isolated soy protein* (legumes) are proteins that can be used to provide some of the functional properties of fat without the same number of fat calories. Soy may be used for emulsification or gelling and is approved for addition of up to 2% in cooked sausage and cured pork. It may be used at higher levels in ground meat and poultry.

Fat-Derived Fat Replacements

Fat-derived fat replacements, such as Olestra, offer 0 cal/g. Other replacements offer less than 9 cal/g of fat. *Olestra*, marketed under the brand name *Olean*®, differs from fats and oils in its chemical composition and properties. Olestra is a sucrose polyester (SPE), predominantly sucrose octaester, which is synthesized by reacting six to eight fatty acids with the eight free hydroxyl groups of *sucrose*. (Recall that fats are a *glycerol* backbone with three fatty acids attached). Each fatty acids may be 12–20 or more carbons in length and may be either saturated or unsaturated. Fatty acids may be derived from corn, coconut, palm, or soybean sources. Olestra became the latest of several food ingredients approved without GRAS status [others are TBHQ (1972), aspartame (1981), polydextrose (1981), and acesulfame K (1988) (Chapter 17)]. Its chemical makeup and configuration make olestra indigestible and it is not absorbed. Its numerous fatty acids are attached to the sucrose in a manner that cannot be easily penetrated by digestive enzymes in the length of time it is in the digestive tract. As a result, Olestra provides no calories.

Unlike Simplesse®, it may be used for frying applications. It was first patented in 1971 and sought FDA approval as a cholesterol-lowering drug. Approval was denied, because such a use was not shown. A subsequent petition in 1987 requested use of olestra as a direct food additive. It was to be used as a fat replacement for 1) up to 35% of the fat in home-use cooking oils and shortenings, and 2) up to 75% of the fat in commercial deep-fat frying of snack foods. The petition was amended in 1990 and approved in 1996 to allow the Proctor and Gamble Olean® to be used as a 100% replacement for fats in savory snacks (salty, piquant, but not sweet, such as potato chips, cheese puffs, and crackers), including the frying oil and any fat sources in the dough (conditioners, flavors, etc.). All other uses of olestra require separate petitions.

The FDA conclusions regarding the major chemical changes in frying and baking applications of olestra are that changes are similar to triglycerides. The fatty acid chains oxidize in both cases. In baking, there is slower degrading of the fatty acids, but the same by-products are produced. Olestra has baking and frying applications and may be used in dairy-based or oil-based foods.

A special label statement is required for all Olean-containing products. Labels must state "This Product Contains Olestra. Olestra may cause abdominal cramping and loose stools. Olestra inhibits the absorption of some vitamins and other nutrients. Vitamins A, D, E, and K have been added." In three small test markets, the major user of Olean® has not observed nor has there been evidence of severe abdominal cramps and loose stools resulting from the consumption of products containing Olean® (Frito Lay).

Health concerns regarding the use of olestra have been addressed in part by over 150 Procter and Gamble studies. Some concerns are that 1) olestra is an additive with very high use in food products compared to other additives, 2) olestra may cause a loss of fat-soluble vitamins from the body, 3) it may leak and not be held by the final sphincter of the body in elimination—the anal sphincter, and 4) it may negatively impact the environment and water quality through wastewater treatment. But in answer to these concerns, 1) very few products contain olestra, and it is not carcinogenic, 2) vitamins A, D, E, and K are added to olestra-containing foods, 3) a reformulation has created longer-chain fatty acids that do not leak from the digestive tract, and 4) adverse environmental effects to the environment are not expected (12).

Nabisco Foods has developed a proprietary family of low calorie **SALATRIM** fats–named for **s**hort **a**nd **l**ong **a**cyl**tri**glyceride **m**olecule. Salatrim is a patented ingredient of conventional glycerol backbones to which long-chain fatty acids and short-chain fatty acids are added. The long-chain stearic acid is combined with the short-chain acetic, propionic, and butyric acids on a glycerol molecule (13). Nabisco states that SALATRIM is different from other fat replacers because it is made from real fat, whereas other fat substitutes are made from protein and carbohydrates, which "don't give you the flavor and taste you need for baking" (14, 15). SALATRIM received GRAS status by the FDA in 1994. It was approved for use in baked products, chocolates and confections, dairy products, and snacks, but it cannot be used successfully in frying applications.

A nutritional advantage of using these fat replacers is that they contain 5 cal/g, instead of the normal fat amount of 9 cal/g. This calorie reduction may be due to hydrolysis of short-chain fatty acids that are rapidly hydrolyzed to carbon dioxide and long-chain fatty acids that are incompletely absorbed.

Caprenin (Procter and Gamble) is another fat replacement that contains 5 cal/g. It contains a glycerol backbone with three fatty acids. Two of the fatty acids are medium chain—caprylic and capric—which are metabolized similarly to carbohydrates, and the other chain consists of a long fatty acid—behenic acid (22 C)—that is incompletely absorbed. These fatty acids are selected on the basis of their specific, desired properties.

Carbohydrate-Derived Fat Replacements

Fat replacements may also be derived from carbohydrates. *Starches* work well as fat replacements in high-moisture systems and have been utilized in the bakery industry for many years. An example is a pregelatinized dull waxy cornstarch that is used to reduce fat in bakery products (16). Starch hydrolysis derivatives known as **maltodextrins** (classified as hydrocolloids) may be used to replace fats, as they are bland in flavor and have a smooth mouthfeel. They may assist in maintaining product moisture.

Some FDA approved fat replacements, and kcalories per gram (kcal/g), available in the United States, include the following:

- Avicel[®] (FMC Corp.)—microcrystalline cellulose from purified wood pulp (0 kcal/g), may replace all of the fat in frozen desserts and salad dressings.

- Caprenin[®] (Proctor & Gamble)—a triglyceride with capric, caprylic, and behenic fatty acids (5 kcal/g), used in candies.

- Maltrin M040[®] (Grain Processing Corp.)—a cornstarch maltodextrin (4 kcal/g), for cold food applications, cereals, and snacks.

- N-Oil[®] (National Starch and Chemical Corp.)—tapioca maltodextrin (1 kcal/g), for cold food applications.

- Nutri-fat PC[®]—dextrin and soluble fiber (1.2 kcal/g), fat replacer in cold foods, and cakes.

- Oatrim[®] (USDA)—β-glucan amylodextrin from oat fiber [1 kcal/g, cholesterol lowering benefit; in cold food applications, and baked products.

- Olestra[®] (Procter & Gamble Co.) Sucrose polyester (0 kcal/g), used in fying and baking applications.

- Paselli SA2[®] (Avebe America, Inc.)—potato starch dextrin (4 kcal/g), used in cold food applications and confections.

- Polydextrose (Pfizer Inc.)—starch polymer made from dextrose, sorbitol, and citric acid (1 kcal/g), a bulking agent, and fat replacer in diverse foods.

- Salatrim (Nabisco)—fat and acids from fruit and vinegar (5 kcal/g).

- Simplesse[®] (Nutrasweet Co.) MPP (egg white and milk protein, water, pectin, and citric acid) (1–2 kcal/g), useful in cold food applications.

- STA-SLIM 143[®] (A. E. Staley Manufacturing. Co.)—potato starch dextrin (4 kcal/g), diverse uses.

- STELLAR (A.E. Staley Manufacturing Co.)—acid-modified corn starch (1 kcal/g), providing mouthfeel of fat, used in diverse products.

- Xanthan gum, Algin—kelp (negligible kcal/g), stabilizer, emulsifier in salad dressings.

The plant root, *tapioca*, and the tuber, *potato*, as well as the cereal starches *corn* and *rice* are also used as fat replacers. An *oat*-based fat replacement is made by partial hydrolysis of oat starch using a food-grade enzyme, and *barley* is being investigated for use as a possible fat substitute.

Polydextrose (Chapter 17) may be used as a 1-cal/g substitute for either fat or sucrose. Polydextrose is a bulking agent created by the random polymerization of glucose, sorbitol, and citric acid, 89:10:1. It may be used in a variety of products such as baked goods, chewing gum, salad dressings, and puddings.

Several dried-fruit-based substances are available for replacement of fat in recipes. Raisin, plum, and other fruit mixtures are available for consumer use at this time. Applesauce is also used to replace fat in formulations. Many additional fat replacers is being explored, including the use of encapsulated technologies (USDA).

NUTRITIVE VALUE OF FATS AND OILS

Food guides such as the Food Guide Pyramid suggest that fat be used sparingly. Most health authorities in the United States agree with this recommendation. Yet, fats are needed for numerous functions in the human body, and two polyunsaturated fatty acids are essential—linoleic and linolenic acid are required for human growth. In addition to the many roles fat plays in functionality of foods, fats are a very concentrated energy source—providing 9 cal/g. This is $2\frac{1}{4}$ times as many calories per gram as either carbohydrates or protein. Labeling studies have indicated that fat and calories are the two most frequently read items on food labels (17).

Whereas the *food technologist* looks at industrial "processing methods to enhance the quality of existing fats and oils" such as hydrogenation and interesterification, *plant breeders* work "to produce new vegetable oils with altered fatty acid composition" (17). In combination, the more conventional methods and biotechnology can be used to facilitate breeding and create more healthful fats. Breeders look at new crops containing selected fatty acids from which fats can be designed (18). Biotechnology, such as genetic engineering and enzyme techniques, has potential in enhancing quality of vegetable oils because of the time reduction (possibly 50% shorter) and targeting gene manipulation (18).

The food industry has had a major impact in reducing heart disease, as they have changed formulations containing lard and tallow to vegetable oil such as corn and soybean oil, which contain essential fatty acids. They have also replaced fat in formulations. Both of these steps have major impact on reducing heart disease (20). The health-conscious consumer may make choices of reducing certain foods that are major contributors of less desirable fatty acids, and, as well, substitute foods, possibly increasing fats that are major contributors of the fatty acids that are desired (22). Consumers' switch in use of cooking oils, the health aspects of a variety of foods containing fats and oils, familiarity with fat and health terminology, and eating trends are reported elsewhere (17, 20, 21).

In 1998, the first high-oleic, low polyunsaturated fatty acid line of soybean oil became commercially available. A nutritional advantage is that it contains approximately 83% monounsaturates, 5% polyunsaturates, and 11% saturated fatty acids. The use of this oil may decrease the risks of heart disease. With its inclusion in food products, a reduction of the *trans* fatty acid level from the partially hydrogenated fat is also possible.

Similar to the role of cholesterol in animal cell membranes, phytosterols perform the same role in plants. The structures are alike, differing only in the side chain (Figure 4). Plant sterols are commercially available in margarines and salad dressings, and although there are several theories suggested, and the precise mechanism is unknown, phytonutrients have been shown for many decades to significantly reduce low-density lipoprotein (LDL) or "bad" cholesterol. They inhibit the uptake of endogenous and dietary cholesterol. Due to the knowledge of their health benefits, more phytosterols are expected to be included in margarines and other foods as a cholesterol-lowering functional food ingredient (Chapter 20). The cost factor continues to be a challenge, as is the marketing of any "healthy food" that incorporates new ingredients.

CONCLUSION

Fats and oils add or modify flavor, aerate batters and doughs, contribute flakiness and tenderness, emulsify, transfer heat, and provide satiety. They are composed of a glycerol molecule with one, two, or three fatty acids attached creating mono-, di-, or triglycerides, respectively. Minor components of fats and oils include phospholipids, sterols, tocopherols, and pigments. Fatty acid chains of even number may exist as geometric or positional isomers. Nomenclature may be according to a common name, systemic or Geneva name, or omega system.

Fats and oils exist in several crystalline forms and have different melting points. Solid fats have higher melting points than oils. Fats and oils may be processed by being deodorized or rendered. They are modified by hydrogenation, interesterification, acetylation, or winterization.

The deterioration of fats and oils occurs as they absorb odors or become rancid. Hydrolytic rancidity releases free fatty acids, oxidative rancidity produces shorter, off-odor free radicals catalyzed by heat, light, metals, or enzymes. Prevention of oxidation by avoiding catalysts in the environment or by the addition of sequestering agents or antioxidants may be useful in extending shelf life.

Monoglycerides and diglycerides have uses as emulsifiers, permitting fats and liquids to mix. Fats and oils are useful as shorteners; they tenderize and produce flakes in baked products. They may also be used in the preparation of salad dressings and for frying applications. Foods may contain reduced-fat, low-fat, or no-fat formulations using a variety of fat replacers derived from carbohydrates, proteins, or fats.

Plant breeders are researching the development of healthier fats. A variety of vegetable oils continue to be available to food processors and, to a lesser extent, to the consumer. Stability without increased saturation is the goal of processors. Advanced hybridization of vegetable sources of oil may reduce saturated fatty acids, and thus improve nutritional value. Fats and oils should be used moderaltely in the daily diet.

GLOSSARY

Acetin fat: A triglyceride with one or two fatty acids on a triglyceride replaced by acetic acid; this decreases the melting point.

Acetoglyceride: Acetin fat.

Antioxidant: Prevents, delays, or minimizes the oxidation of unsaturated bonds by donating a H atom to the double bond in a fatty acid.

Autoxidation: Progressive oxidative rancidity in an unsaturated fatty acid promoted by heat, light, the metals iron and copper, and lipoxygenases.

BHA: Butylated hydroxyanisole; an antioxidant.

BHT: Butylated hydroxytoluene; an antioxidant.

Cis configuration: A double-bond formation when H atoms attach to the C atoms of the double bond on the same side of the double bond.

Continuous phase: The phase or medium in which the dispersed phase is suspended in an emulsion.

Deodorized oils: Oils that have undergone the process of removing odors by heat and vacuum or by adsorption onto charcoal.

Dispersed phase: A phase that is disrupted or finely divided in the continuous phase of an emulsion.

Emulsifier: Bipolar substance with a hydrophilic and hydrophobic end, which reduces surface tension and allows the ordinarily immiscible phases of a mixture to combine.

Fat replacement: A substance used to replace fat in a formulation; these may be protein, carbohydrate or fat-based.

Flakiness: Thin, flat layers formed in some dough products desirable in biscuits or pie crusts.

Hydrocolloid: Long-chain polymers; colloidal material that binds and holds water.

Hydrogenation: Process of adding H to unsaturated fatty acids to reduce the number of double bonds; an oil becomes more solid and more stable in storage.

Hydrolytic rancidity: Reaction of fats with water to liberate free fatty acids.

Hydrophilic: Water-loving substance attracted to water.

Hydrophobic: Water-fearing substance attracted to fat.

Interesterification: Rearrangement as fatty acids migrate and recombine with glycerol in a more random manner.

Interfacial tension: See surface tension.

Isomer: Fatty acids have the same number of carbons, hydrogens, oxygens, but form different arrangements that create different chemical and physical properties.

Lecithin: Phospholipid of two fatty acids esterified to glycerol and a third group of phosphoric acid and choline as the N group, useful as an emulsifier.

Maltodextrin: Hydrocolloid; starch derivative of tapioca, potato, corn, rice, oats, or barley that may be used to replace fat in a formulation.

Oxidative rancidity: Fat is oxidized and decomposes into off-odor compounds with shorter-chain fatty acids, aldehydes, or ketones.

Plastic fat: Able to be molded and hold shape; contains both liquid and solid triglycerides in various ratios.

Phospholipid: A lipid containing two fatty acids and a phosphoric acid group esterified to glycerol.

Polymorphism: Fats existing in different crystalline forms: α, β′ intermediate, β.

Rearrangement: Interesterification of fatty acids on glycerol, i.e., modified lard.

Rendered: Fat freed from connective tissue and reduced, converted, or melted down by heating; for example, lard is rendered hog fat.

Sequestering agent: Binds metals, thus preventing them from catalyzing autoxidation; for example, EDTA, citric acid.

Sterols: A lipid containing a steroid nucleus with an 8–10 C side chain and an alcohol group; cholesterol is the most well known.

Surface tension: (interfacial tension) force that tends to pull molecules at the surface into the bulk of a liquid, and prevent a liquid from spreading. Reduction of surface tension enables a liquid to spread more easily.

Tenderization: Easily crushed or chewed, soft, fragile, baked dough.

TBHQ: Tertiary butylated hydroquinone; an antioxidant.

Tocopherols: Minor component of most vegetable fats; antioxidant; source of vitamin E.

Trans configuration: A double-bond formation in fatty acids where the H atoms attach to the C atoms of the double bond on opposite sides of the double bond.

Winterized: Salad oil that is pretreated prior to holding, to control undesirable cloudiness from large, high-melting-point triglyceride crystals.

REFERENCES

1. Erickson MD, Frey N. Property-enhanced oils in food applications. *Food Technology.* 1994; 48(11): 63–68.
2. Central Soya Company, Inc. Ft. Wayne, IN.
3. Huffman M. "Trans fat" labeling? *J Am Diet Assoc.* 2001; 101: 28.
4. Giese J. Fats, oils, and fat replacers. *Food Technology.* 1996; 50(4): 78–84.
5. Morris CE. Value-added vegetable oils. *Food Engineering.* 1994; 66(5): 132–135.
6. Federation of American Societies for Experimental Biology (FASEB), Bethesda, MD.
7. Dorko C. Antioxidants used in foods. *Food Technology.* 1994; 48(4): 33.
8. Saguy IS, Pinthus EJ. Oil uptake during deep-fat frying: Factors and mechanism. *Food Technology.* 1995; 49(4): 142–152.
9. Hatchwell LC. Overcoming flavor challenges in low-fat frozen desserts. *Food Technology.* 1994; 48(2): 98–102.
10. Glicksman M. Hydrocolloids and the search for the "Oily Grail." *Food Technology.* 1991; 45(10): 94–99.
11. Staff Report. Blends reduce fat in bakery products. *Food Technology.* 1994; 48(6): 168–170.
12. Giese J. Olestra. Properties, regulatory concerns and applications. *Food Technology.* 1996; 50(3): 130–132.
13. Nabisco develops family of structured fats. *Food Technology.* 1994; 48(8): 24.
14. Kosmark R. Salatrim. Properties and applications. *Food Technology.* 1996; 50(4): 98–101.
15. Brooks E. IFT Newsmakers. *Food Technology.* 1994; 48(9): 28.
16. Hippleheuser AL, Landberg LA, Turnak FL. A System approach to formulating a low-fat muffin. *Food Technology.* 1995; 49(3): 92–96.
17. Sloan, A.E. Fats and oils slip and slide. *Food Technology.* 1997; 51(1): 30.

18. Liu K, Brown EA. Enhancing vegetable oil quality through plant breeding and genetic engineering. *Food Technology.* 1996; 50(11): 67–71.

19. McGrady J. More-healthful fats and oils. *Food Technology.* 1994; 48(11): 148.

20. Giese J. Fats and fat replacers: Balancing the health benefits. *Food Technology.* 1996; 50 (9): 76.

21. Hollingsworth, P. Jack Sprat revisited. *Food Technology.* 1997; 51(1): 28.

22. Pszczola DE. Putting fat back into foods. *Food Technology.* 2000; 54(12): 58–60.

BIBLIOGRAPHY

American Soybean Association. St. Louis, MO.

Cargill Foods—Vegetable Oils. Minneapolis, MN.

Central Soya Co. Inc. Ft. Wayne, IN.

Charley H. *Food Science,* 2nd ed. New York: Macmillan, 1982.

Code of Federal Regulations (CFR), Title 21 Section 101.25(c)(2)(ii)(a & b).

Dallas Fort Worth Hospital Council, Irving, TX. *Manual of Nutritional Therapy,* 1997.

Gurr MI. *Role of Fats in Food and Nutrition.* New York: Chapman & Hall, 1992.

Hicks KB, Moreau RA. Phytoosterols and phytostanols: Functional food cholesterol busters. *Food Technology.* 2001; 55(1): 63–67.

Institute of Shortening and Edible Oils. *Food Fats and Oils.* Washington, DC. 1994.

Izzo M, Stahl C, Tuazon M. Using cellulose gel and carrageenan to lower fat and calories in confections. *Food Technology.* 1995; 49(7): 45–46.

Lawson HW. *Food Oils and Fats: Technology, Utilization and Nutrition.* New York: Chapman & Hall, 1994.

Lawson HW. *Standards for Fats and Oils.* Westport, CT: AVI, 1985.

Moreira RG, Palan JE, Sun X. Deep-fat frying of tortilla chips: An engineering approach. *Food Technology.* 1995; 49(4): 146–148.

Product Update. *Food Technology.* 1994; 48(11): 140–192.

Understanding Fat Substitutes. Atlanta, GA: Meta Media. Calorie Control Council, 1990.

CHAPTER 13

Food Emulsions and Foams

INTRODUCTION

Many convenience foods, such as frozen desserts, meat products, margarine, and some natural foods, such as milk and butter, are emulsions. That is, they contain either water dispersed in oil, or oil dispersed in water. These liquids do not normally mix, and so when present together, they exist as two separate layers. However, when an emulsion is formed, the liquids are mixed in such a way that a single layer is formed with droplets of one liquid dispersed within the another. Food emulsions need to be stable; if they are not, the oil and water will separate out. Stability is usually achieved by adding a suitable emulsifier. In some cases, a stabilizing agent is also required.

Food foams, such as beaten egg white, are similar to emulsions except that instead of containing two liquids, they contain a gas (usually air or carbon dioxide) dispersed within a liquid. The factors affecting stability of emulsions also apply to foams. Some foods, such as ice cream and whipped cream, are highly complex being both an emulsion and a foam.

Understanding of food emulsions and foams is complex, but is important if progress is to be made in maintaining and improving the stability, and hence the quality of these types of foods. This chapter will discuss the principles of formation and stability of emulsions and foams, and the characteristics of the ingredients necessary to stabilize them.

EMULSIONS

Definition

An **emulsion** is a **colloidal system** containing droplets of one liquid dispersed in another, the two liquids being immiscible. The droplets are termed the **dispersed** *phase*, and the liquid that contains them is termed the ***continuous phase***. In food emulsions, the two liquids are oil and water. If water is the continuous phase, the emulsion is said to be an ***oil-in-water*** or ***o/w emulsion***, whereas if oil is the continuous phase the emulsion is termed a ***water-in-oil*** or ***w/o emulsion.*** Oil-in-water emulsions are more common and include salad dressings, mayonnaise, cake batter, and frozen desserts. Butter, margarine, and some icings are examples of water-in-oil emulsions.

An emulsion must also contain an ***emulsifier***, which coats the emulsion droplets and prevents them from ***coalescing*** or recombining with each other. Emulsions are colloidal systems because of the size and surface area of the droplets (in general, around 1 μm, although droplet size varies considerably, and some droplets may be a lot larger than this). Emulsions are similar to colloidal dispersions or sols, except that the dispersed phase is liquid and not solid. Colloidal dispersions are mentioned in chapter 2.

Surface Tension

To form an emulsion, two liquids that do not normally mix must be forced to do so. To understand how this is achieved, we must first consider the forces between the molecules of a liquid. Imagine a beaker of water placed on a desk (Figure 13.1).

The water molecules are attracted to one another other by hydrogen bonds as described in Chapter 2. A molecule in the center of the beaker has forces acting on it in all directions, because water molecules surround it. The net force on this molecule due to attraction by other water molecules is zero, because these forces are acting in all directions. However, this is not the case for a water molecule on the surface. Since

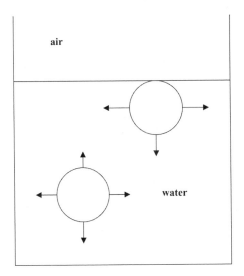

FIGURE 13.1 Schematic diagram of the forces acting on water molecules in the bulk and at the surface of the liquid.

there are no water molecules above it, there is a net downward pull on the molecule. This results in the molecule being pulled in towards the bulk of the liquid. This can be seen when one fills a narrow tube such as a pipette or a burette with water. The surface of the liquid curves downward at the center, and the curve is called the meniscus. The greater the attractive forces between the liquid molecules, the greater the depth of the meniscus. Water molecules have strong attractive forces among them, and so it is relatively hard to penetrate the surface, or to get the water to spread. Try placing a needle gently on the surface of clean or distilled water. It will float, because the attractive forces between the water molecules keep it on the surface. (To make it sink, see below.)

If there are strong attractive forces among the molecules of a liquid, the force required to pull the molecules apart to expand the surface or to spread the liquid will be high. This force is known as **surface tension**. A liquid such as water, with strong attractive forces among the molecules, has a high surface tension. This makes it hard to spread. You can see this if you put water on a clean surface. It will tend to form droplets rather than spreading evenly as a thin film across the surface. (A droplet has minimal surface area and maximal internal volume, and so is the most energetically favorable shape for liquids with a high surface tension, where the molecules are being pulled into the interior.)

The term surface tension is normally used when a *gas* (usually air) surrounds the *liquid* surface. When the surface is between two *liquids*, such as water and oil, the term **interfacial tension** is used.

A high surface or interfacial tension makes it hard to mix the liquid either with another liquid or with a gas. This is a drawback when making an emulsion or foam, and needs to be overcome. So how can surface tension be reduced?

Surface-Active Molecules

To reduce the surface or interfacial tension, something must be done to decrease the attractive forces between the liquid molecules, so that it is easier to spread them. This can be achieved by adding a **surface-active** molecule, or a **surfactant**. As their name suggests, surface-active molecules are active at the *surface* of a liquid, rather than at the bulk of it. Surfactant molecules prefer to exist at the surface of a liquid rather than at the bulk, because of their structure. In all cases, a section of the molecule is water-loving or **hydrophilic**, because it is polar or charged, and a section is water-hating or **hydrophobic**, because it is apolar. In other words, the molecules are **amphiphilic**.

The apolar section has little or no affinity for water, and so it is energetically favorable for this section to be as far away from the water as possible. However, the polar section is attracted to the water and has little or no affinity for the oil. Therefore, the molecule orients at the surface with the polar section in the water, but the apolar section either in the air or in the oil (see Figure 13.2).

Because the molecule **adsorbs** at the surface, it reduces the attractive forces of the water molecules for themselves, and makes it easier to expand or spread the surface. In other words, it reduces the surface or interfacial tension.

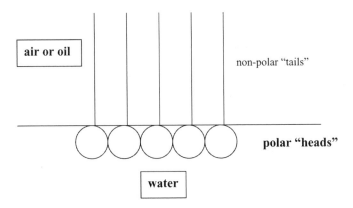

FIGURE 13.2 Orientation of amphiphilic molecules at an interface.

Detergent is an example of a surfactant. When detergent is added to water, it enables the water molecules to spread much more easily, so that they wet a surface more readily. After adding detergent, water will flow over a surface, forming a thin sheet, instead of tending to gather into droplets. Going back to the example of the needle floating on water (see above), if a small drop of detergent is added, the needle will sink. The surface tension is reduced allowing the water molecules to spread more easily, and so the needle no longer stays on the surface.

Obviously, detergents are not used as food ingredients! (However, they are used when washing dishes, because they enable the water to spread across the surface and remove food particles more easily.) There are many food ingredients that are surfactants. Polar lipids such as lecithin, which has a polar "head" and an apolar "tail," are surfactants, and may be used as food additives to increase the wettability and aid in mixing of products like hot chocolate mix.

Proteins are surface-active because they contain both hydrophilic and hydrophobic sections. The nature and extent of these sections depend on the specific amino acid sequence of each protein, and some proteins orient at the surface more readily than others do (Proteins are discussed in Chapter 8).

Some spices, such as dry mustard and paprika, are also used as surface-active ingredients. These finely divided powders tend to gather at the surface rather than the bulk of the liquid.

Molecules that are either hydrophilic or hydrophobic do not orient at an interface, but remain in the bulk of the liquid. For example, sugars, which are hydrophilic, or salt, which dissociates into ions, will be located in the bulk water phase. These types of molecules are not surface-active and will not decrease the interfacial tension. In fact, they may increase it, depending on their ability to bind the water molecules, hence increasing molecular attraction.

Emulsion Formation

An emulsion is formed when oil, water, and an emulsifier are mixed together. Although there are different food emulsions, they *all* contain these three components. To form an emulsion, it is necessary to break up either the oil or the water phase into small droplets that remain dispersed throughout the other liquid. This requires energy, and is usually carried out using a mixer or a homogenizer. As the oil and water are mixed, droplets are formed. (They may be oil or water, but are usually oil droplets.) An emulsifier is adsorbed at the surface of new droplets, decreasing the interfacial tension and allowing formation of more and smaller droplets. The lower the surface or interfacial tension of the oil and water, the more easily one liquid can be disrupted to form droplets, and the more easily the other liquid will flow around the droplets. The liquid with the higher interfacial tension will tend to form droplets, and the other liquid will flow around the droplets to

---

PRINCIPLES OF FORMATION OF A STABLE OIL-IN-WATER EMULSION:

- Emulsifier is dispersed in the aqueous phase.
- Oil is added and the interfacial tension of each liquid is reduced by the emulsifier.
- Energy is supplied by beating or homogenizing the mixture.
- The oil phase is broken up into droplets, surrounded by water.
- Emulsifier adsorbs at the freshly created oil droplet surfaces.
- Small droplets are formed, protected by an interfacial layer of emulsifer.
- The interfacial area of the oil becomes very large.
- The aqueous phase spreads to surround each oil droplet.
- The emulsion may become thick due to many small oil droplets surrounded by a thin continuous phase.
- If the interfacial film is strong, the emulsion will be stable.

---

form the continuous phase. The emulsifier generally determines the liquid that would from the continuous phase. Emulsifiers that are more easily dispersed in water (and therefore are more hydrophilic overall) tend to reduce the interfacial tension of the water more than that of the oil, promoting formation of o/w emulsions. Emulsifiers that disperse more readily in the oil phase tend to form w/o emulsions. The emulsifier is usually dispersed in the preferred phase before the oil and water are mixed together.

An emulsifier does not simply reduce interfacial tension. It must also form a stable film that protects the emulsion droplets and prevents separation of the emulsion. The droplets are continually moving through the continuous phase, and so they constantly encounter or collide with each other. When two droplets collide, one of the three things happens, as shown in Figure 13.3:

(a) The emulsifier film stretches or breaks, and the droplets combine to form one larger droplet (or in other words, they coalesce). This ultimately leads to separation of the emulsion.

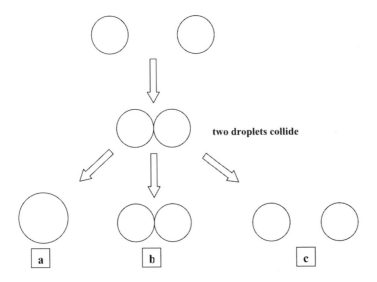

two droplets collide

FIGURE 13.3 Diagram to illustrate what may happen after two droplets collide: (a) coalescence, (b) aggregation, and (c) droplets move apart again.

(b) The two emulsifier layers surrounding the droplets interact and an aggregate is formed. This occurs when a cream layer develops on top of fresh milk.

(c) The droplets move apart again.

Which of these three events occurs depends on the nature of the emulsifier molecules, and on their ability to completely coat all the emulsion droplets with a stable, cohesive, **viscoelastic** film. A viscoelastic film tends to flow to coat any temporarily bare sections of the surface, and is also able to stretch instead of breaking when, for example, another droplet bumps into it. Therefore, it is less likely to break when droplet collisions occur. As the droplets are formed, their surface or interfacial area increases dramatically, and sufficient emulsifier must be present to completely coat all the droplet surfaces. Incompletely coated droplets will coalesce resulting in larger droplets, and ultimately in separation of the emulsion.

Emulsifiers

Emulsifiers must be able to:

- Adsorb at the interface between two liquids such as oil and water.
- Reduce the interfacial tension of each liquid, enabling one liquid to spread more easily around the other.
- Form a stable, coherent, viscoelastic interfacial film.
- Prevent or delay coalescence of the emulsion droplets.

Reduction of the interfacial tension facilitates emulsion formation, because it reduces the amount of energy needed to break up one liquid into droplets and to spread the other liquid around them. Formation of a film that prevents coalescence promotes emulsion stability.

All emulsifiers are surfactants, because all emulsifiers adsorb at the surface and reduce interfacial tension. However, all surfactants do *not* make good emulsifiers, because not all surfactants are able to form a stable film at the interface and prevent coalescence. The stability of the film is important in determining the stability and shelf life of the emulsion. Some emulsifiers work better than others do, in terms of forming a stable emulsion. In general, large macromolecules such as proteins form stronger surface films than smaller surfactant molecules such as lecithin, because of their greater ability to extend over the droplet surface. They also have a greater ability to interact with other groups within the same molecule or on different molecules, and are able to form viscoelastic surface films. Small molecules are not usually able to form stable interfacial films by themselves, and their role is normally that of a surfactant rather than an emulsifier, in that they lower interfacial or surface tension and promote spreading or wettability. Although they do not make good emulsifiers, they are often called emulsifiers. Many food scientists do not differentiate between surfactants and emulsifiers, and so the words may be used interchangeably in some cases. However, in the world of a colloid scientist, there is a clear distinction between the two!

Characteristics of an emulsifier:
- Contains hydrophilic and hydrophobic sections (amphiphilic)

Functions of an emulsifier:
- Adsorbs at the oil/water interface ⎫
- Reduces interfacial tension   ⎭ facilitates emulsion formation
- Forms a stable interfacial film   ⎫
- Prevents coalescence   ⎭ promotes emulsion stability

Natural Emulsifiers

The best emulsifiers are proteins, which uncoil or denature and adsorb at the interface, and interact to form a stable interfacial film. Proteins tend to uncoil such that their hydrophobic sections are oriented in oil, and their hydrophilic sections are oriented in water. Hence, a series of loops, trains, and tails, may be envisioned at the interface, as shown in Figure 13.4.

The loops and tails are able to interact with each other, thus forming a stable film that resists rupture. The proteins of *egg yolk* tend to be the best emulsifiers, as exemplified by their use in mayonnaise. These proteins are lipoproteins, and are associated with each other and with phospholipids such as lecithin, in structures known as micelles. These micellar structures appear to be responsible for the excellent emulsifying properties of egg yolk proteins.

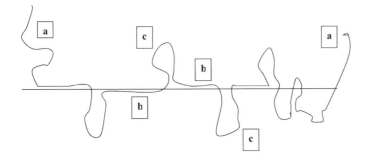

FIGURE 13.4 Schematic diagram of a protein adsorbed at an interface: (a) tails, (b) trains, and (c) loops.

The *caseins* of milk are also excellent emulsifying agents. They are important emulsifiers in homogenized milk, and in dairy desserts. In fresh (unhomogenized) milk, the caseins are associated with each other in structures known as casein micelles. Electron micrographs have shown that after homogenization, intact micelles are present at the fat globule surfaces, as well as individual protein molecules. It is thought that the micelles are responsible for the stability of homogenized milk, rather than the individual protein molecules.

Other food proteins used as emulsifiers include *meat* proteins and *soy* proteins. Lecithin is often considered to be an emulsifier. Lecithin is a surfactant, and is useful for promoting wettability and aiding mixing of products such as hot drink mixes. However, it does not usually form strong interfacial films by itself, and so would not be the emulsifier of choice unless other emulsifiers or stabilizers were added.

Synthetic Emulsifiers or Surfactants

Most synthetic emulsifiers would more correctly be termed *surfactants*, because they are relatively small molecules compared with proteins, and they are used mainly to aid in dispersion of fat, rather than to stabilize emulsions.

Surfactants such as *mono-* and *diglycerides* are added to shortening and to cake mixes, to aid in dispersion of the shortening. Cakes are complex, in that they contain fat droplets and air bubbles, and so are both emulsions and foams. (Foams are discussed later in this Chapter.) The mono- and diglycerides enable the shortening to be dispersed into smaller particles, and this promotes incorporation of a large number of air cells, which increases cake volume and promotes a more even grain in baked products (Chapter 15).

Glycerol monostearate is an example of a monoglyceride that is commonly used in foods. Acids may be esterified with monoglycerides to give another group of surfactants, including sodium stearoyl-2-lactylate, which is often used in baked products. Two other groups of manufactured surfactants include the *SPANS*, which are fatty acid esters of sorbitan, and the *TWEENS,* which are fatty acid esters of polyoxyethylene sorbitan. Although all surfactants are amphiphilic, they have different degrees of hydrophobic (**lipophilic**) and hydrophilic character. This can be expressed as the **hydrophilic/lipophilic balance**, or **HLB.** An HLB scale has been developed, which goes from 1 to 20. Surfactants with a low HLB (3–6) have more hydrophobic or lipophilic character. These would be used to form a w/o emulsion. Examples include glycerol monostearate and sorbitan monostearate (SPANS 60). Surfactants with a high HLB (8–18) have more hydrophilic character, and form w/o emulsions. Examples would be polyoxyethylene sorbitan monostearate (TWEENS 60) or sodium stearoyl-2-lactylate. SPANS usually have a low HLB and form w/o emulsions, whereas TWEENS have a high HLB and form o/w emulsions. The HLB scale is useful to food scientists to help them in determining which emulsifier is most suited to their needs.

Examples of Emulsions

French dressing is an example of a **temporary emulsion**, or in other words, an unstable emulsion that separates fairly soon after formation. The basic ingredients of French dressing are oil (the dispersed phase), vinegar (the continuous phase), dry mustard, and paprika. Other ingredients may be added for flavor. The "emulsifiers" used here are the mustard and paprika. Combining the ingredients and shaking them vigorously forms the emulsion. The mustard and paprika adsorb at the interface and reduce interfacial tension as the dressing is shaken, thus facilitating formation of an emulsion, but they do not interact at the interface to form a stable film. Hence, when shaking is stopped, the oil droplets are not protected, and so they soon coalesce,and the oil and vinegar layers separate.

Mayonnaise is an example of a **permanent emulsion**, since it is stable and does not separate under normal handling conditions. The main ingredients of mayonnaise are oil (the dispersed phase), vinegar (the continuous phase), and egg yolk. The egg yolk proteins, being excellent emulsifiers, protect the oil droplets against coalescence. Mayonnaise usually contains about 75% oil, which exists as stable droplets surrounded by a thin aqueous film. It is unusual in that it contains so much more dispersed phase than continuous phase. Generally, the continuous phase is present in greater quantity. Mayonnaise is made by slowly pouring small amounts of oil at a time into the vinegar and egg yolk mixture, and continuing to beat to break up the oil into droplets and form the emulsion. As more oil is added, more droplets are formed, and the surface area increases dramatically. The continuous phase spreads out to surround the oil droplets, and becomes a thin film. It is hard for the droplets to move around, since they are packed tightly together, and separated only by a thin film of aqueous phase, and so the mayonnaise becomes very thick, and may even be stiff enough to cut. Some salad dressings may be similar to mayonnaise, except that they contain less oil and have a thinner consistency. Adding stabilizers such as gums or starches often enhances the stability of the emulsion.

Milk is an example of an emulsion that occurs in nature (Chapter 11). Milk contains about 3.5% fat in emulsified form. In fresh (unhomogenized) milk, the fat droplets are stabilized by a complex protein membrane known as the milk fat globule membrane. Fresh milk is a stable emulsion, but will cream fairly quickly if left to stand. The fat droplets vary in size from about 0.1 to 10 μm. There are many more small droplets than large ones, but because of their size, the larger ones account for most of the fat. Because of the density difference between the milk fat and the aqueous phase, the fat droplets tend to rise though the milk. This is especially true for the larger droplets. Milk fat globules are unique in that as they rise, they tend to cluster together. This results in larger fat particles, which rise even faster. Hence, after a few hours, a cream layer can be seen at the top of the milk. This is not a true separation of oil and water, since the cream layer is still an emulsion and the interfacial film is still intact. The milk has separated into a concentrated emulsion and a dilute one. The cream can be removed, and either used as cream or made into butter. Homogenizing the milk, which breaks up the fat globules into much smaller ones, prevents this creaming effect.

Factors Affecting Emulsion Stability

Obviously, the main factor affecting emulsion stability is the *emulsifier* itself. As has been discussed, emulsifiers that form stable interfacial films produce stable emulsions. There must also be sufficient emulsifier to completely coat the surface of all the droplets in order to ensure stability. *Droplet size* is also important because larger droplets are more likely to coalesce. Also, because of the density difference between oil and water, large oil droplets will tend to rise through the emulsion more quickly, creating a more concentrated emulsion closer to the surface, as is seen in milk. This may cause the emulsion to break.

Changing the *pH* by adding acid, or changing the *ionic strength* by adding salts may reduce the stability of the interfacial film, especially if it is made of protein. Such changes may denature the protein, as explained in Chapter 8, and cause the emulsion to separate.

Another factor affecting emulsion stability is the *viscosity* of the emulsion. The thicker the emulsion, the lesser the movement of the molecules within the system, and the longer it will take for the two phases to separate. Emulsions can be made thicker by adding ingredients such as gums, pectin, or gelatin. If gums are added to French dressing, a permanent emulsion may be formed without the need for egg yolk as the emulsifier. Gums are often added to emulsions as stabilizers. They are not emulsifiers themselves, and they do not normally adsorb at an interface, because they are hydrophilic. However, they act by increasing the viscosity of the system, which slows movement, and hence reduces the number of collisions between droplets. This slows down, and may prevent separation of emulsions.

Storage and *handling* affect emulsion stability. Although some emulsions are termed permanent, it should be noted that all emulsions are delicate systems that are inherently unstable, because they contain two immiscible liquids, and the wrong handling conditions can cause emulsion breakage.

Temperature also affects emulsion stability. When emulsions are warmed, the oil droplets become more fluid, and coalescence is more likely. On the other hand, cooling an emulsion to refrigeration temperatures may cause some solidification of the oil droplets, depending on the composition of the oil. This may enhance stability. Most emulsions do not survive freezing conditions. This is usually because the proteins at the interface become denatured, or because the interfacial film is physically disrupted by the formation of ice crystals. *Gums* are often added to emulsions that are to be frozen to enhance stability.

Heat and *violent shaking* are also likely to disrupt emulsions. For example, cream is converted to butter by churning the warm emulsion. The emulsion breaks, the aqueous phase is drained off, and a water-in-oil emulsion is formed, with water droplets (approximately 18%) dispersed throughout the butterfat.

FACTORS AFFECTING EMULSION STABILITY:

- Type of emulsifier
- Concentration of emulsifier
- Droplet size
- Changing pH or ionic strength
- Viscosity
- Addition of stabilizers
- Heating, cooling, freezing, and/or shaking

FOAMS

Foams make a vital contribution to the volume and texture of many common food products. They give volume and a distinctive mouthfeel to products such as whipped cream and ice cream, and they give a light, airy texture to baked goods. Improperly formed or unstable foams result in dense products with a low volume, which are unacceptable to consumers. Foams are inherently unstable, and it is imperative that food scientists increase their knowledge of the factors affecting foam stability, in order to enhance the quality and shelf life of these products.

A foam contains gas bubbles dispersed in a liquid continuous phase. The liquid phase may be a simple dispersion, as in egg white, which is a dilute protein dispersion, or it may be complex, containing emulsified fat droplets, ice crystals, and/or solid matter. Examples of complex food foams include ice cream, angel food cake, marshmallows, and yeast-leavened breads. Foams such as meringue and baked goods are heat set, which denatures the protein and converts the liquid phase to a solid phase. This gives permanence to the foam structure.

Comparison between Foams and Emulsions

Foams are similar to emulsions, in that the gas bubbles must be protected by a stable interfacial film otherwise they will burst. Therefore, the factors affecting emulsion formation and stability also apply to foams, and, in general, good emulsifying agents also make good foaming agents. However, there are some important differences between emulsions and foams. The bubbles in foams are generally much bigger than the droplets in emulsions, and the continuous phase surrounding the gas bubbles is very thin. In fact, it is the continuous phase that has colloidal dimensions, rather than the dispersed phase. The density difference between the two phases is much greater in a foam, and there is a tendency for the liquid continuous phase to drain due to gravity, and for the gas bubbles to escape. The factors affecting formation are similar for both emulsions and foams. However, there are additional factors involved in foam stability.

Foam Formation

In order to produce a foam, energy must be supplied (by whipping) to incorporate gas into the liquid, to break up large bubbles into smaller ones, and to spread the liquid phase around the gas bubbles as they form. The foaming agent, which is contained in the liquid phase, adsorbs at the surface of the liquid, reducing surface tension, and also forming a film around the gas bubbles. It is important that the surface tension is low, so that the liquid will spread rapidly around the gas bubbles during whipping. If newly formed gas bubbles are not immediately coated with foaming agent, they will burst or coalesce, and be lost. The amount of energy supplied during whipping is also important; the higher the energy, the smaller the bubbles and the greater the foam volume, provided that sufficient foaming agent is present to completely coat and stabilize the bubbles.

Foam Stability

The stability of a foam may be measured in terms of loss of foam volume over a period of time. When a liquid is whipped to form a foam, the volume of the liquid increases due to incorporation of air. If the foam is stable, the volume does not change very much. However, loss of air from an unstable foam may cause a considerable reduction in volume.

Foam stability may be *reduced* due to the following factors:

- The tendency of the liquid film to drain due to gravity. As it drains, a pool of liquid gathers at the bottom of the container, and the film surrounding the gas bubbles becomes very thin. This may allow the gas to escape, and the volume of the foam to shrink.

- The tendency for the film to rupture and allow coalescence or escape of gas bubbles.

- Diffusion of gas from small bubbles to larger ones. This results in fewer bubbles, and the foam shrinks.

- Evaporation of the continuous phase also affects foam stability, but to a lesser extent. If the liquid evaporates, gas bubbles burst and foam volume is reduced.

If gas bubbles are lost due to any of these factors, a more dense, low-volume foam is produced, which is not usually desirable, especially in foods such as angel food cake or ice cream.

To produce a *stable* foam with a high volume, film rupture, liquid drainage, and evaporation must be prevented or atleast minimized. As with emulsions, the gas bubbles must be stabilized by the presence of a stable interfacial layer, which resists rupture. However, the composition of the continuous phase is also very important in determining foam stability. The liquid phase must have a low vapor pressure, so that it does not evaporate readily at storage and handling temperatures. More importantly, drainage of the continuous phase must be minimized. Thick liquids drain more slowly than thin ones, and so increasing the viscosity of the continuous phase will reduce drainage. A high viscosity is essential if a stable foam is to be produced.

Foaming Agents

The two most important characteristics of a foam are foam *volume* and foam *stability*. Foam volume depends on the ability of the foaming agent to adsorb at the interface and rapidly reduce interfacial tension, and on the level of energy input during whipping. Foam stability depends on the ability of the foaming agent to produce a stable interfacial film, and a viscous continuous phase. Although all surfactants are able to reduce surface tension and produce foams, not all are able to form stable foams. In fact, some may act as foam suppressants!

A good foaming agent has the same characteristics as an emulsifier, in that it is able to adsorb at the interface, reduce interfacial tension and form a stable interfacial film that resists rupture. As might be expected, the best foaming agents used in foods are proteins. Although many proteins are able to produce foams, egg white proteins are superior foaming agents, and are used in food foams such as meringues, angel, cake and other baked goods. Other proteins used as good foaming agents include gelatin and milk proteins.

When egg white is whipped (Chapter 10), the proteins denature at the interface and interact with one another to form a stable, viscoelastic, interfacial film. Some of the egg white proteins are glycoproteins, containing carbohydrate. When these proteins adsorb at the interface, the carbohydrate sections orient toward the aqueous phase. Being hydrophilic, they bind water, and increase the viscosity of the liquid. This helps to reduce drainage, thereby contributing to foam stability.

Gelatin is a good foaming agent, and a warm gelatin sol can be whipped to three times its original volume. When cooled, the gelatin solidifies or forms a gel, which traps the air bubbles and stabilizes the foam; Marshmallows are gelatin foams.

The Effect of Added Ingredients on Foam Stability

Many food foams have additional ingredients added to *enhance stability*. For example, egg white foams, such as meringue or angel food cake, also have sugar added. The *sugar* increases the viscosity of the liquid, aiding stability. It also protects the proteins

FACTORS AFFECTING FOAM STABILITY

- Drainage of the liquid film between gas bubbles
- Rupture of the interfacial film around gas bubbles
- Diffusion of gas from small to large bubbles
- Evaporation of the continuous phase

FACTORS PROMOTING FOAM STABILITY

- Stable viscoelastic surface film
- Very viscous continuous phase
- Low vapor pressure liquid

EFFECTS OF ADDED INGREDIENTS

Foam Stabilizers	Foam Destabilizers
Gums	Lipids
Thickeners	Phospholipids
Sugar	Small molecule surfactants
Acid	Salts
Solid particles	

from excessive denaturation and aggregation at the interface. Too much interaction results in an inelastic film which is not resistant to rupture, and in reduced foam volume. Therefore it is important to guard against this when making egg white foams.

Acid, such as cream of tartar or lemon juice, may also be used to increase foam stability. Addition of acid reduces the pH, which reduces the charge on the protein molecules and usually brings them closer to their isoelectric point. This generally results in a stronger, more stable interfacial film. When added to egg whites, acid prevents excessive aggregation at the interface. However, acid delays foam formation. It may therefore be added towards the end of the whipping process. In the case of egg whites, it is often added at the "foamy" stage. Whipping is not complete until the egg whites have formed soft peaks. (Egg white foams are discussed in more detail in Chapter 10.)

Other ways to increase viscosity of the continuous phase include addition of *gums* and other *thickening agents*. Also, addition of *solid matter* may promote stability. Whipped cream, for example, is stabilized by solidified fat globules that are oriented in the continuous liquid film. The emulsified fat increases viscosity and is responsible for the stability of whipped cream. To form a stable foam, cream to be whipped must contain at least 30% fat. Creams with lower fat contents may be whipped successfully if thickening agents such as carrageenan are added. If the cream is warm, and too much of the butterfat is liquid, then whipping will not produce a stable foam. Instead, the emulsion will break and the cream will be converted to butter.

Ice cream is another example of a complex foam, which is stabilized by emulsified fat droplets and small ice crystals oriented within the continuous phase. Angel food cake contains solid particles, in the form of flour, which are folded into the egg white/sugar foam. The flour contributes to stability by increasing the viscosity of the liquid, which minimizes film drainage. The increased viscosity and presence of solid particles also reduces breakage of the interfacial film, hence minimizing loss of foam volume.

Anti-Foaming Agents and Foam Suppressants

As all cooks know, egg whites will not whip to a stable foam if there is any egg yolk present (Chapter 10). This is because the phospholipids and lipoproteins in the yolk adsorb at the surface, in competition with the egg white proteins, and interfere with formation of a stable egg white protein film. Unlike the egg white glycoproteins, which are hydrophilic, the phospholipids and lipoproteins are unable to increase the viscosity of the continuous phase, because they are hydrophobic, and so orient away from the water. This prevents formation of a stable foam.

Such molecules are termed *foam suppressants*. They suppress foam volume because they adsorb at the interface, thus suppressing adsorption of the desired foaming agent, and preventing it from forming a stable foam. They do not have the properties required to form a stable film or to sufficiently increase the viscosity of the continuous phase. Hence, their presence makes formation of a stable foam impossible. Typical foam suppressants include fats, phospholipids, and other small amphiphilic molecules.

Salts also tend to act as foam suppressants, because they weaken interactions between the protein molecules at the surface, thus weakening the interfacial film around the gas bubbles. However, their effect is not as important as surfactant molecules, because they do not adsorb at the interface.

Anti-foaming agents are able to break up foams or prevent them from forming. Anti-foaming agents are added to fats and oils used in frying, to prevent foaming during the frying process. Like foam suppressants, they act by adsorbing at the air/liquid interface in place of the foaming agents, and because they do not have the characteristics of a foaming agent, they prevent foam formation.

CONCLUSION

Food emulsions and foams are complex colloidal systems, and understanding of their formation and stability is important if the quality and shelf life of these products is to be improved.

Emulsions contain liquid droplets stabilized by an interfacial layer of emulsifier and dispersed throughout a liquid continuous phase. Foams are similar, but the dispersed phase consists of large gas bubbles surrounded by a very thin, continuous, liquid film. The nature of the emulsifier or foaming agent is crucial in determining stability. It must adsorb at the interface, reduce surface tension and form a stable, viscoelastic interfacial layer that resists rupture, so that coalescence of liquid droplets or loss of gas bubbles is avoided. Additional factors are important in foam stability; it is important that the liquid film between the gas bubbles is very viscous, so that drainage due to gravity is minimized. Evaporation of the liquid must also be prevented during normal storage and handling conditions.

Both natural and synthetic emulsifying agents are available to food companies. The best emulsifiers and foaming agents are proteins. Egg yolk proteins are known as the best emulsifiers, whereas egg white proteins are considered to be the best foaming agents used in food products.

GLOSSARY

Adsorb: To bind to a surface.

Amphiphilic: A molecule containing both hydrophobic and hydrophilic sections.

Coalescence: Two liquid (or gas) droplets merge to form one larger droplet.

Colloidal system: Emulsions, foams, dispersions (or sols) and gels are all colloidal systems. A colloidal system contains one phase (usually the dispersed phase) with dimensions ranging mainly from 0.1 to 10 μm. The dispersed phase contains large numbers of small droplets or particles, and so the surface or interfacial area of this phase is very large. This is an important characteristic of colloidal systems.

Continuous phase: The phase or substance that surrounds the liquid droplets or gas bubbles in an emulsion or foam.

Dispersed phase: The discrete bubbles (air, carbon dioxide or liquid) that are surrounded by liquid in an emulsion or foam.

Emulsifier: A substance that enables two normally immiscible liquids to be mixed together without separating on standing.

Emulsion: An emulsion contains liquid droplets stabilized by a layer of emulsifier and dispersed throughout a liquid continuous phase.

Foam: A foam contains gas bubbles coated with a stable interfacial layer, and surrounded by a thin, viscous liquid continuous phase. In food foams, the gas is usually air or carbon dioxide.

Foaming agent: A molecule that is able to promote foam formation. Useful foaming agents in foods are also able to promote foam stability by forming a stable interfacial layer, and also by increasing the viscosity of the continuous phase.

Foam suppressant: A molecule that prevents or hinders foaming, generally by adsorbing to the interface in place of the desired foaming agent and interfering with the action of the foaming agent.

Hydrophilic: Water-loving. Hydrophilic molecules are either charged or polar, and have an affinity for water.

Hydrophilic/lipophilic balance or HLB: A scale that goes from 1 to 20 and indicates the ratio of hydrophilic and hydrophobic groups on a molecule. It is used to determine the suitability of emulsifiers when formulating an emulsion. A high HLB indicates a molecule with more hydrophilic groups, which is suitable for o/w emulsions. A low HLB indicates that there are more lipophilic groups, and the molecule has a greater affinity for oil and is more suited for w/o emulsions.

Hydrophobic: Water-hating. Hydrophobic molecules are nonpolar, and have an affinity for apolar solvents.

Interfacial tension: The force required to increase the interfacial area of a liquid, or to spread it over a surface such as oil. See also, surface tension.

Lipophilic: Fat-loving, or water-hating. Lipophilic molecules are nonpolar, and have an affinity for lipids and other apolar solvents.

Oil-in-water or o/w emulsion: An emulsion containing oil droplets dispersed in water. Oil is the dispersed phase and water is the continuous phase.

Permanent emulsion: A stable emulsion that does not separate over time.

Surface tension: The force required to increase the surface area of a liquid, or to spread it over a surface. Surface and interfacial tension are often used interchangeably. Generally, surface tension applies at the surface of a liquid (i.e., when it is in contact with air), whereas interfacial tension applies when two liquids are in contact with each other.

Surface active: A molecule that adsorbs at the surface of a liquid. Surface active molecules contain both hydrophobic and hydrophilic sections, and it is energetically favorable for them to exist at the interface rather than in the bulk phase of a liquid.

Surfactant: A surface active molecule (see above).

Temporary emulsion: An unstable emulsion, which separates into two layers on standing.

Viscoelastic: Exhibits both viscous (liquid) and elastic (solid) properties. In other words, the material will flow if force is applied, but it will also stretch. When the force is removed, the material does not return completely to its original position. It is important for an emulsifier film to flow around droplets to cover temporary bare patches, and also to be able to stretch, so that when disrupted, it does not break.

Water-in-oil or w/o emulsion: An emulsion containing water droplets dispersed in oil. Water is the dispersed phase and oil is the continuous phase.

BIBLIOGRAPHY

1. Charley H, Weaver C. *Foods: A Scientific Approach*, 3rd ed. Upper Saddle River, NJ: Prentice-Hall, 1998.
2. Walstra P. Dispersed Systems—Basic Considerations. In: Fennema O. ed. *Food Chemistry*, 3rd ed. New York: Marcel Decker, 1996.
3. McWilliams M. *Foods: Experimental Perspectives*, 4th ed. Upper Saddle River, NJ: Prentice-Hall, 2001.
4. Setser CS. Water and Food Dispersions. In: Bowers J. ed. *Food Theory and Applications*, 2nd ed. NewYork: Macmillan, 1992, pp 7–68.

PART V

Sugars in the Food Guide Pyramid

CHAPTER 14

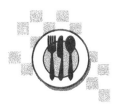

Sugars, Sweeteners, and Confections

INTRODUCTION

Sugars are simple carbohydrates that may be classified as monosaccharides or disaccharides (Chapter 3). The common granulated or table sugar is sucrose. This chapter on sugars, sweeteners, and confections examines the roles and properties of sugars, the various types of nutritive sweeteners, and sugar substitutes added to foods. Confections and factors influencing candy types are covered. The Food Guide Pyramid advises that sugar should be used sparingly in the diet, and depending on serum glucose and lipid goals (see Nutritive Value), nutritive sweetener intake should be individualized by consumers.

SOURCES OF SUGAR

Sugar naturally exists as syrup in the sugar cane or in sugar beet, both of which are identical in chemical composition. Raw *cane* is shredded, pressed, and heated, and the extracted juice is centrifuged to create raw sugar with its slightly brown color. As the juice is centrifuged, molasses separate from the crystals and become a by-product of sugar-cane sugar production. The crystals are then further refined for uses in various forms.

Roots of the *beet* are less frequently used to produce sugar. They are washed, shredded, treated with lime to remove impurities, and further refined to yield usable sugar.

ROLES OF SUGAR IN FOOD SYSTEMS

Sugar may be utilized in *trace* amounts or it may be the *primary* ingredient of a formulation. It imparts sweetness, tenderness, and browning, is hygroscopic (water retaining), and functions in various other ways in food systems, as may be seen in the following examples of sugar function.

Sweetness

Sugar provides flavor appeal to foods. It is incorporated into many foods and is a significant ingredient of baked goods and frostings as well as beverages and candies.

Tenderness

A batter/dough formula *with* sugar is more tender than one *without* sugar, because sugar provides tenderization when it limits gluten formation (Chapter 15). It also absorbs water that gliadin and glutenin proteins would otherwise absorb in forming gluten.

Browning

Sugar browns and imparts color to foods by two types of nonenzymatic browning: 1) the Maillard browning reaction (Chapter 3), and 2) caramelization. **Maillard browning** involves the reaction of the carbonyl group of sugar with the amine group of an amino acid and occurs with heat, a high pH, and low moisture. It is responsible for the color changes that occur in many baked breads, cakes, and pie crusts, as well as caramel candies (which, although the name is used, do *not* undergo caramelization).

Caramelization is another nonenzymatic browning process that occurs in sugars. As sugar is heated to temperatures above its melting point [338°F (170°C)], it dehydrates and decomposes. The sugar ring (either pyranose or furanose) opens and loses water. The sugar becomes brown, more concentrated, and develops a caramel flavor as it continues to increase in temperature. (Culinary use of the term caramelize refers to enhanced color and flavor upon reaching a high temperature, and does not refer to the burning of any sugars in food, Chapter 3.)

Other Roles of Sugar in Food Systems (not all-inclusive)

- Functions as a separating agent to prevent lump formation in starch-thickened sauces (Chapter 4)
- Reduces starch gelatinization (Chapter 4)
- Dehydrates pectin and permits gel formation in jelly-making (Chapter 5)
- Stabilizes egg white foams (Chapter 10)
- Raises the coagulation temperature of protein mixtures (Chapter 10)
- Adds bulk and body to foods such as yogurt (Chapter 11)
- Slows/prevents crystallization in candies if invert sugar is used in place of sucrose
- Helps aerate batters and doughs (Chapter 15)
- Reduces gluten structure by competing with gliadin and glutenin for water, thus increasing tenderness (Chapter 15)
- Acts as the substrate that ferments to yield CO_2 and alcohol (Chapter 15)
- Adds moisture retention properties to baked products

TYPES OF SUGARS AND SUGAR SYRUPS*

Sucrose. The *disaccharide* consisting of the monosaccharides glucose and fructose. Commonly referred to as "sugar".

Fructose. Fructose is the *monosaccharide* that combines with glucose to form sucrose. It is known as fruit sugar, as it is contained in many fruits. Fructose is 1.2–1.8 times as sweet as sucrose.

Glucose. Glucose is the *monosaccharide* that combines with fructose to form sucrose, with galactose to form lactose, and with another glucose to form the disaccharide maltose.

Galactose. Galactose is the *monosaccharide* that combines with glucose to form lactose.

Lactose. Lactose is a *disaccharide* (a glucose and galactose molecule) known as milk sugar. It is less sweeter than sucrose.

Maltose. Maltose is a *disaccharide* (two glucose molecules) formed by the hydrolysis of starch.

Invert sugar. Invert sugar is created when sucrose is treated by acid or enzyme to form an equal amount of fructose and glucose. It is more soluble and sweeter than sucrose.

Raw sugar. Raw sugar has a larger grain than ordinary granulated sugar. It is 97–98% sucrose. It is not approved by the FDA, for sale in the U.S. since impurities, and contaminants remain in the granule.

Turbinado sugar. Turbinado sugar is raw sugar with 99% of the impurities and most of the by-product of sugar crystal formation (molasses) removed.

Brown sugar. Brown sugar has a molasses film on the sugar crystals, which imparts the brown color and characteristic flavor of this sugar. It contains approximately 2% moisture and requires storage protection against moisture loss.

Confectioners' sugar. Confectioners sugar (confectionery sugar) is also called powdered sugar and is derived from either sugar cane or the sugar beet. Sugar grains are pulverized by machine to change the sugar grain to a powdered substance and form such sugars as "6 × sugar" (pulverized 6 times to create "Very Fine"), "10 × sugar" (pulverized 10 times to form "Ultra fine"), and so on. Confectioners' sugar typically contains 3% cornstarch to prevent caking.

Granulated sugar. Granulated sugar is typically sucrose and is commonly known as white sugar or table sugar. It is derived from concentrated sugar cane or sugar beet juice.

Syrups (liquids)

The starch conversion to dextrose (glucose) is measured as D.E., or dextrose equivalents. Syrups may have a D.E. of 36–55. More pure glucose yield is 96–99 D.E.

Corn Syrup: Corn syrup is a mixture of carbohydrates (glucose, maltose, and other oligosaccharides) formed from the hydrolysis of cornstarch by the use of acid or enzymes (HCl, or α and β amylases).

---

*All monosaccharides contain a free carbonyl group and are reducing sugars, as is the disaccharide maltose.

$$\text{Starch} + \text{Water} \xrightarrow[\text{enzymes}]{\text{acid+heat}} \text{Dextrins} + \text{Maltose} + \text{Glucose}$$

Following hydrolysis, it is subsequently *refined* and *concentrated*. The sugar solution contains approximately 25% water and is viscous.

High-fructose corn syrup (HFCS): HFCS is a specialty syrup prepared by the same three steps as corn syrups—it is hydrolyzed, refined, and concentrated. In addition, isomerization occurs whereby the glucose is made into the more soluble fructose by the enzyme action of another enzyme, isomerase. The syrup contains approximately 42% fructose. Those corn syrups that contain 42% fructose may undergo a fractionation process to further remove glucose and create syrup that is 55 or 90% fructose. HFCS containing 42 and 55% fructose are Generally Recognized As Safe (GRAS). They are added to many beverages.

Honey: Honey is made from the nectar of various flowers and therefore differs in color, flavor, and composition. It contains approximately 20% water and a mixture that is 75% glucose and fructose (predominantly the latter), with no more than 8% sucrose. Darker colored honey is more acidic and more strongly flavored than light colored honey, and the strains of alfalfa and clover honey (commonly sold in the United States) are mild-flavored honey. "Strained honey" is honey from a crushed honeycomb that is strained. The addition of honey to a formulation increases moisture, as the fructose is hygroscopic.

Maple syrup: Maple syrup is obtained from the sap of the maple trees. The sap is boiled and evaporated, and the final product contains no more than 35% water (40 parts sap = 1 part maple syrup).

Molasses: Molasses is the syrup (plant juice) separated from raw sugar beet or sugar cane during its processing into sucrose, and it is thus a by-product of sugarmaking. The predominant sugar is sucrose, which becomes more invert sugar with further processing. Molasses provides very low levels of the minerals, calcium and iron, although *blackstrap molasses* is the product of further sugar crystallization and contains a slightly higher mineral content.

PROPERTIES OF SUCROSE

In addition to supplying sweetness and body to foods, other properties of sucrose important in food systems, such as confections, are discussed in the following subsections.

Solubility

Sucrose is *more* soluble than glucose and *less* soluble than fructose (fructose > sucrose > glucose). In its dried, granular form, sugar becomes increasingly soluble in water with an increase in temperature. For example, *room-temperature* water is capable of dissolving sucrose in a ratio of 2:1 (67% sucrose and 33% water). If that same water is *heated*, more sugar is dissolved, and as the sugar–water is brought to a *boil*, the sugar syrup gets increasingly concentrated.

Sugar may precipitate from solution, forming an undesirable grainy, crystalline product. Therefore, in order to increase the solubility of sucrose and reduce possible crystallization, sucrose may be treated by inversion to become invert sugar.

Types of Solutions

Solutions are the homogeneous mixtures of **solute**, dissolved in **solvent**. Solutions may be dilute (unsaturated), saturated, or supersaturated, depending on the amount of dissolved solute that the water is holding at any specific temperature (see Sugar Concentration).

Elevation of Boiling Point

Increasing concentrations of sucrose increase the boiling point, as shown in Table 14.1. Therefore, temperature may be used as an indication of sucrose concentration, but the addition of sugars other than sucrose, as well as the addition of interfering agents also elevates the boiling point.

The boiling point rises as more sugar is added to water or liquid evaporates from a boiling solution because more heat is needed to raise the reduced vapor pressure found in a more concentrated sugar solution. For every gram molecular weight of sucrose that is dissolved in water, there is a 0.94°F (0.52°C) increase in boiling point. [For each 500 ft in elevation above sea level, there is progressively less atmospheric pressure and the boiling point decreases 1°F. For example, at an elevation of 5,000 ft, the boiling point is lowered by 10°F, to

TABLE 14.1 Boiling Point of Sucrose–Water Syrups of Different Concentrations[a]

Percent of sucrose in syrup	Percent water	Boiling point in °F (°C)
0 (all water, no sugar)	100	212 (100)
20	80	213.1 (100.6)
40	60	214.7 (101.5)
60	40	217.4 (103)
80	20	233.6 (112)
90	10	253.1 (123)
95	5	284 (140)
99.5	0.5	330.8 (166)

[a]At sea level.

202°F (94°C). The boiling point is lowered 1°C (1.8°F) for each 960 ft above sea level.]

Formation of Invert Sugar

As mentioned, invert sugar is more soluble than sucrose and is formed by *sucrose hydrolysis* to yield equal amounts of the monosaccharides *glucose* and *fructose* in the process of **inversion**. Therefore, the use of invert sugar in confections is desirable, as it is more soluble, slows crystallization, and helps keep crystals small. Sucrose may be hydrolyzed into invert sugar by either *weak acids,* such as in cream of tartar, the acid salt of weak tartaric acid, or *enzymes* such as invertase.

$$C_{12}H_{22}O_{11} + H_2O \xrightarrow[\text{enzyme}]{\text{acid + heat}} C_6H_{12}O_6 + C_6H_{12}O_6$$

Sucrose   Water   Glucose   Fructose

In *acid hydrolysis,* it is both 1) the *amount* of acid, and 2) the rate and length of heating that determines the quantity of invert sugar that forms. *Too much* acid may cause too much hydrolysis, which forms a soft or runny sugar product. *Slow* attainment of the boiling point (thus, a longer heating time) increases inversion opportunity, whereas a *rapid* rate provides less inversion.

In *enzyme hydrolysis,* sucrose is treated with the *enzyme* invertase (also known as sucrase) to form glucose and fructose. Enzyme hydrolysis of sucrose is responsible for forming the liquid from the sugar mixture in chocolate-covered cherries.

The glucose that forms from inversion is *less* sweet than sucrose, and the fructose *more* sweet, with the overall reaction producing a sweeter, more soluble sugar than sucrose. Invert sugar is combined in a ratio of 1:1 with sucrose in many formulations to control crystal formation and achieve small crystals.

Hygroscopicity

Another property of sugar is **hygroscopicity,** or ability to readily absorb water. Sugars that are high in fructose, such as invert sugar, HFCS, honey, or molasses, retain moisture. They are more hygroscopic than sucrose. It is therefore important to control the degree of inversion that these sugars undergo, or they may exhibit runny characteristics in storage.

Sugar that is stored in a humid storeroom location, or candy that is prepared on a humid day are both situations that demonstrate this property of hygroscopicity in that the sugar is lumpy and the candy is soft. Moisture-proof containers are recommended for the storage of sugar and sugar products. Due to this hygroscopic property of sucrose, product developers may encapsulate or coat sugars, so that they are time-released, which prolongs the sweetness perception, and allows sucrose to withstand expected processing conditions (1).

Fermentable

Sugar is fermentable. It undergoes **fermentation** by the biological process in which bacteria, mold, yeast, and enzymes anaerobically convert complex organic substances, such as sucrose, glucose, fructose, or maltose, to carbon dioxide and alcohol.

SUGAR SUBSTITUTES

Sugar substitutes include the *two* categories of *sugar alcohols* (caloric, nutritive) and *artificial sweeteners* (noncaloric, non-nutritive) sweeteners. Sugar substitutes are used in small quantities, and they do not crystallize, so they do not produce satisfactory results in all candies, where real sugar may be necessary as a major recipe ingredient. Some examples of sugar substitutes are identified in the following subsections.

Sugar Alcohols (Polyols)

Sugar alcohols are caloric, chemically reduced carbohydrates that provide sweetness to foods. They are a distinct classification from artificial sweeteners. The sugar alcohols are similar in chemical structure to glucose, but an alcohol group replaces the aldehyde group of glucose. *Sorbitol* is commercially produced from glucose and contains 2.6 cal/g while *mannitol* contains 1.6 cal/g. Both of these naturally occurring sugar alcohols provide half the sweetness of sucrose and may be used as humectants (Chapter 18) because they increase the water-holding capacity of the food. Sorbitol is also used as a bulking agent. In combination with aspartame and saccharin, it provides the volume, texture, and thick consistency of sugar. Xylitol, isomalt, hydrogenated starch hydrolysate (HSH), and hydrogenated glucose syrup (HGS) are also sugar alcohols. Isomalt is 45–65% as sweet as sucrose and contains 2 cal/g HSH and HGS have 3 cal/g.

The body does not metabolize sugar alcohols and, therefore, when consumed, these sugars do not require insulin. Persons with diabetes may use sugar alcohols without a rise in their blood sugar. Large amounts of sugar alcohols may cause intestinal diarrhea; therefore, they are not recommended for use in significant amounts.

Artificial or High-Intensity Sweeteners

Artificial sweeteners are noncaloric, non-nutritive sugar substitutes, whose use has grown in response to increased consumer demand for noncaloric foods. Some examples of artificial sweeteners are as follows.

Acesulfame K.   Acesulfame potassium (Acesulfame K) is a noncaloric, synthetic derivative of acetoacetic acid that received FDA approval in 1988. It is an organic salt

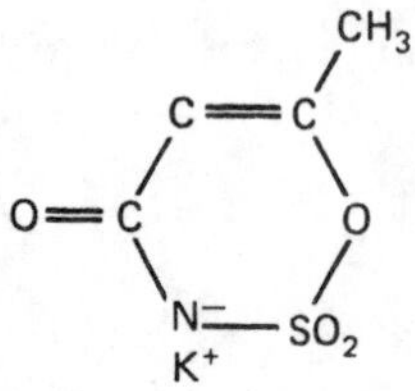

FIGURE 14.1 Chemical structure of acesulfame K.

consisting of carbon, hydrogen, nitrogen, oxygen, potassium, and sulfur, and is not metabolized by the body, but is rather, excreted unchanged. It is 200 times sweeter than sucrose and is heat stable, thus, it may be used for baking and cooking purposes in addition to use as a tabletop sweetener. Acesulfame K has no bitter aftertaste and may be used alone or in combination with the sweeteners saccharin or aspartame (Figure 14.1). Some brand name examples of acesulfame K are Sunette®, Sweet One®, Swiss Sweet®, and Nutra Taste®.

Aspartame.   Aspartame is a *nutritive* sweetener that contains the same number of calories per gram as sugar (4 cal/g), but because it is much sweeter and used in minute amounts, it is not a significant source of calories or carbohydrates and is often put in the category of *non-nutritive, noncaloric* sweeteners. It is a methyl ester comprising two amino acids: aspartic acid and phenylalanine; thus, it should not be consumed by those with the genetic disease phenylketonuria (PKU) because it contains phenylalanine, which is not metabolized (Figure 14.2).

Aspartame gained FDA approval in 1981, and is 180–200 times sweeter than sucrose. It is marketed under the trade name NutraSweet®, and Equal® is the tabletop low-calorie sweetener with NutraSweet®. Aspartame was not originally intended for use in heated products, but it may be encapsulated in hydrogenated cottonseed oil with a time–temperature release, which makes its inclusion in baked products acceptable.

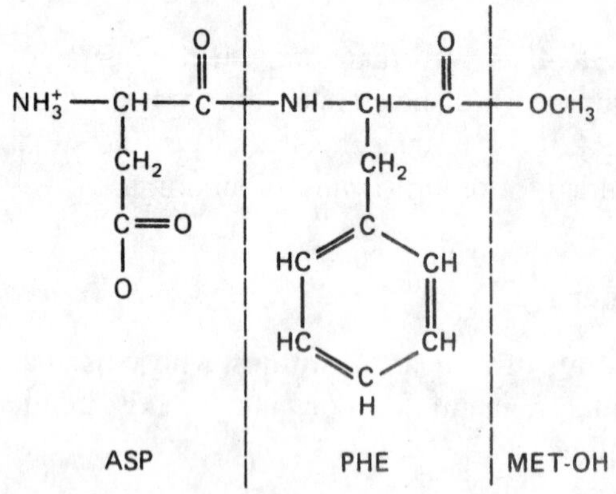

FIGURE 14.2 Chemical structure of aspartame. ASP = aspartic acid; PHE = phenylalanine; MET-OH = methyl alcohol.

Saccharin.   Saccharin is a noncaloric substance produced from methyl anthranilate, a substance naturally found in grapes. It has been used as a noncaloric sweetener since 1901 in the United States, and is 300–700 times sweeter than sucrose.

The use of saccharin was periodically reviewed as specified by U.S. Congress in the Saccharin Study and Labeling Act. The ruling required that foods containing saccharin must be labeled to read as follows: "Use of this product may be hazardous to your health. This product contains saccharin which has been determined to cause cancer in laboratory animals." Yet, following a moratorium on banning saccharin, which was extended by Congress several times, pending further safety studies, it was shown that saccharin has not demonstrated any carcinogenicity applicable to humans.

Therefore, after several decades with this moratorium, the safety of saccharin has been shown, and the use of a warning label is no longer required. The use of saccharin has been reported to be acceptable by the American Medical Association, the American Cancer Society, and the American Dietetic Association. In December 2000, Congress passed H.R. 5668—the **S**accharin **W**arning **E**limination via **E**nvironmental **T**esting **E**mploying **S**cience and **T**echnology (SWEETEST) Act. It is approved for use in more than 100 countries.

Calcium or sodium saccharin, combined with dextrose (nutritive, glucose) and an anticaking agent may be used in tabletop sweeteners. Saccharin may be used in combination with aspartame. Brand-name examples include Sweet'nLow®, Sugar Twin®, Necta Sweet®, and Sweet-10®.

Sucralose.   Sucralose gained FDA approval in 1998 for use in 15 food and beverage categories, including baked goods and baking mixes; beverages and beverage mixes; chewing gum; coffee and tea; confections and frostings; dairy product analogs; fats and oils (salad dressings); frozen dairy desserts and mixes; fruit and water ices; gelatins, puddings, and fillings; jams and jellies; milk products; processed fruit and fruit juices; sweet sauces, toppings, and syrups; and sugar substitutes. It is a noncaloric trichloro derivative of sucrose [three hydroxyl (hydrogen–oxygen) groups on a sugar molecule are selectively replaced by three atoms of chlorine], plus maltodextrin, which gives it bulk and allows it measure cup-for-cup, like table sugar. It is 400–800 times sweeter than sucrose.

Several advantages to its approval are that 1) it is the only noncaloric sweetener made from sugar, 2) it is stable under a wide range of pH, processing and temperature scenarios, for example, it is water- and ethanol-soluble, and heat stable in baking and cooking, and 3) it carries no health warnings. Splenda® is the brand-name under which sucralose is marketed (Figure 14.3).

Cyclamate.   Cyclamate does not have FDA approval. It was in use in 1960s, but banned in the U.S. in 1970. Currently, the FDA is considering a petition for reapproval, as evidence of its connection with bladder cancer is not verified. It is noncaloric and 30 times sweeter than sucrose.

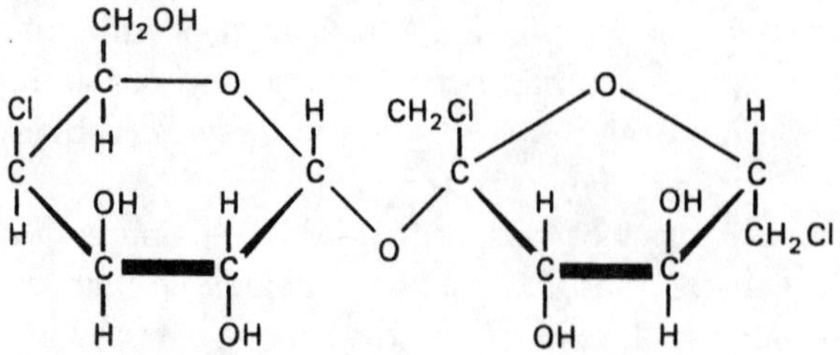

FIGURE 14.3   Chemical structure of sucralose.

CONFECTIONS

Sweet food products may utilize the terms confections or candy. For example, chocolates may be known as "chocolate confectionery," cakes and pastries may be referred to as "flour confectionery," and the term "sugar confectionery" may signify any sugar-based products. In the United States, however, both chocolates and the various sugar-based confections are simply referred to as candy.

Candy-making is primarily dependent on the concentration of sugar in boiled sugar syrups, and controlling or preventing crystal formation. Various ingredients, such as gelatin, fruit, nuts, milk and so forth, in addition to sugar, may be added to produce specific candies. In the preparation of candies, the sugar solution must be *saturated*—holding the *maximum* amount of dissolved sugar it is capable of holding at the given temperature needed for the specific candy type. Upon cooling, the solution becomes **supersaturated**—holding *more* dissolved sugar that it can theoretically hold at a given temperature. Next, the sugar mixture for crystalline candies must be left undisturbed to cool.

Several cautions must be adhered to in candy making. For example, high humidity during candy preparation results in excess moisture retention and less than desirable results because sugar is hygroscopic. Another caution is that sugar syrups have a very high temperature and can cause severe skin burns.

Major Candy Types—Crystalline and Amorphous Candies

Two distinct types of candies are crystalline and amorphous candies. **Crystalline** candies are formed in the process of **crystallization** as heat is given off—**Heat of crystallization**—and have crystals suspended in a saturated sugar solution. They have a highly structured crystalline pattern of molecules that forms around a nuclei or seed. Crystals may be *large* and glasslike, as in rock candy, or they may be *small* and smooth textured, breaking easily in the mouth, as in fondant or fudge candies.

Amorphous or *noncrystalline* candies are those *without* a crystalline pattern and include caramel and taffies, which are *chewy* amorphous candies, brittles, which are *hard* amorphous candies, and marshmallows and gumdrops, which are aerated, *gummy* amorphous candies. In general, amorphous candies contain a high sucrose concentration (Table 14.2) and a large amount of interfering agents (see Interfering

TABLE 14.2 Major Candy Types

Candy Type	Final temperature in °F (°C)	Percent sucrose
Crystalline		
Fudge	234 (112)	80
Fondant	237 (114)	81
Amorphous		
Caramel	248 (118)	83
Taffy	265 (127)	89
Peanut brittle	289 (143)	93

Agents) to prevent crystal formation. They have a low moisture level (the ring opened and water was lost) and are more viscous as syrup than crystalline candies.

Factors Influencing Degree of Crystallization and Candy Type

Crystals are closely packed molecules that form definite patterns around nuclei as a sugar solution is cooled. Their development is dependent on factors discussed in the following text, such as the *temperature, type and concentration* of *sugar, cooling method,* and *use of added substances* that interfere with crystal development. For example, *large crystals* and a grainy texture form in the sugar mixture, if the mix is disturbed prior to cooling to the proper temperature. The same occurs due to **seeding**, or the introduction of existing sugar crystals into the sugar, such as when undissolved sugar on the sides of the cooking pot, falls into the mixture. On the other hand, *small crystal nuclei*, and a smooth textured candy result from the addition of an acid (usually cream of tartar), or corn syrup to the solution.

Some factors that influence the degree of crystallization and, thus, candy type, are as follows.

Temperature. Temperature of a sucrose solution is an indication of its concentration and specific temperature requirements must be met for cooking each type of candy (Table 14.2). If the designated temperature needed for a preparation of some candies has been exceeded, water may be added to the sugar solution in order to dilute its concentration and, thus, lower the temperature. This is possible only as long as the sugar solution has not reached the caramelization stage wherein sugars yield their characteristic flavor and color.

A *slow rate* of achieving the boiling point of a sucrose and water solution increases the time available for inversion of sucrose; thus *slow* heating increases the solubility of the sugars and produces a softer final product compared to *rapid* heating.

Candy-making temperatures exceed the boiling point of water, and as water evaporates, the sugar syrup becomes viscous, causing more severe burns than boiling water if it contacts the skin.

Sugar Type. *Sucrose* molecules are able to align and form large lattice arrangements of crystals. Other sugars, such as the monosaccharides *glucose* and *fructose* (or invert sugar), possess shapes that interfere with aggregation and crystal development; thus, a candy with too much invert sugar will fail to harden and is deemed unsatisfactory. High-fructose corn syrup, honey, and invert sugar are examples of sugars that are added to syrup in candy-making in order to *prevent* the formation of large crystals.

Sugar Concentration. As previously mentioned, candy making is dependent upon the sugar concentration. A sugar solution is *dilute* (*unsaturated*) if the concentration of a solute is less than maximum at a given temperature. Then, as the sugar solution boils, water evaporates, it contains an increased concentration of sucrose, and the solution becomes *saturated*. When the saturated solution is cooled, it becomes *supersaturated*. It is only a supersaturated solution that may easily precipitate sugar.

Amorphous candies have a higher sugar concentration (Table 14.2) than crystalline candy, and the candy mixture is so viscous that crystals cannot form.

Cooling Method and Agitation. The premature crystalline formation in a sugar solution may be the result of stray sugar that remains on the side of the pan after stirring and causes seeding. To prevent this, it is recommended that the pan lid initially remain on the sugar mix for a few minutes so that steam can cause the sugar to dissolve and fall into the sugar solution.

Crystalline candy must not be disturbed by the addition of nuclei or by premature beating during cooling, or the crystallization process will begin prematurely, occur rapidly, and form large crystals. *Crystalline* candy is formed by *slowly* cooling the sugar solution to approximately 100–104°F (38–40°C) *before* stirring or beating occurs. Agitation produces many, small nuclei with which the solute may have contact in the supersaturated solution. Agitation must be sufficient to prevent excess sugar molecules in the solution from attaching to already developed crystals, which would enlarge the crystal size.

Amorphous candy is formed from a very supersaturated solution (Table 14.2) such that it is too viscous to allow aggregation of solute molecules and crystal formation. An undisturbed cooling method is not crucial for success of amorphous candies.

Interfering Agents. In crystalline products, **interfering agents** reduce the speed of crystallization and help to prevent undesirable growth of crystal structures that result in the formation of large, crystalline, gritty candies. *Chemical* interfering agents, including corn syrup or cream of tartar, reduce the quantity of excess sucrose (the solute) available for formation of the crystalline lattice. Corn syrup contains nonsucrose molecules (glucose), and cream of tartar inverts sucrose to its component monosaccharides, glucose, and fructose which produces small crystals that do not aggregate to form large-sized crystals. These nonsucrose molecules do not fit properly (are not able to join) onto existing sucrose lattice structures, thereby keeping sucrose crystals small.

Mechanical interfering agents used in candy-making *adsorb* to the crystal surface and physically prevent additional sucrose from attaching to the crystalline mass; thus, crystals are many and small. Some examples of mechanical interfering agents are fat, the fat in milk or cream, and the proteins in milk and egg whites. In *amorphous* products such as caramel, taffy and peanut brittle, interfering agents prevent crystallization and add flavor.

Other Ingredients. Moisture, air, and other added ingredients affect candy hardness or softness. A hard candy has 2% moisture; gummy candy, such as gumdrops, contain 15–22% moisture and are aerated by whipping.

Ripening

Crystalline candies must ripen in order to produce an acceptable candy. Ripening occurs in the initial period of storage, following the cooking, cooling, and crystallization of a sugar solution, as the moisture level (sugar is hygroscopic) increases, and small crystals are redissolved in the syrup, preventing unwanted crystallization. Smoothness of the finished candy is observed.

NUTRITIVE VALUE OF SUGARS AND SWEETENERS

Sucrose is a carbohydrate that contains 4 cal/g. It supplies energy, but no nutrients to the body. "Guidelines for use of nutritive sweeteners as a part of a well-balanced diet should be individualized based on a patient's eating habits along with serum glucose and lipid goals" (1). For example, the diabetic must manage *blood glucose* levels, and those individuals concerned with levels of *serum lipids* are adversely affected by large amounts of fructose.

Non-nutritive (artificial) sweeteners and sugar substitutes, such as sugar alcohols, may pose adverse health effects for some individuals, in which case, intake of that product should be limited or eliminated from the diet. For example, aspartame contains phenylalanine, a substance phenylketonurics are unable to properly rid from their bodies.

A healthful diet uses sugars sparingly, as high consumption equates to a diet with low nutrient density. "Sugars" that appear on the Nutrition Facts label include: 1) the total sugars found *naturally* in foods, and 2) *added* sugars. Labeling criteria require that all monosaccharides and disaccharides be listed as "sugars" on the Nutrition Facts label, regardless of whether they are a natural part of the food or added to the product. Clarification of natural and added sugars may be determined by reading the food's *ingredients* list. Sugars have a recommended intake of 10% of calories, but no % Daily Value. "Sample dietary patterns recommend limiting total added sweeteners, on a carbohydrate-content basis to no more than 6 tsp/day at 1,600 kcal, 12 tsp/day at 2,200 kcal, and 18 tsp/day at 2,800 kcal ... 6–10% of energy" (USDA).

The designation "Sugar free" signifies that there is less than 0.5 g of sugar per serving. "Reduced sugar" indicates that the food contains 25% less sugar per serving than the regular product. "No added sugar" signifies that the product has no sugar added. Product labels may state that the product is a reduced- or low-*calorie* food, if the food meets other necessary requirements (Chapter 20).

The American Dietetic Association Position Statement with regard to sweeteners is as follows: "It is the position of The American Dietetic Association that consumers can safely enjoy a range of nutritive and non-nutritive sweeteners when consumed in moderation and within the context of a diet consistent with the Dietary Guidelines for Americans."

CONCLUSION

Sugar comes from sugar cane or sugar beets, both of which have the same chemical structure. The roles of sugar are many and include providing flavor, color, and tenderness. Sugars elevate boiling point, are soluble in water, hygroscopic, and fermentable. A variety of sweeteners, including sugar substitutes, and syrups are incorporated into food systems to provide sweetness.

In order to control the rate of crystallization and the formation of small crystals and to ensure a smooth texture, interfering agents are incorporated into a sugar formulation. *Chemical* interfering agents produce invert sugar (glucose and fructose), thereby slowing crystallization and reducing the solubility of solute. *Mechanical* interfering agents such as fat and protein help to keep crystals small by preventing the adherence of additional sugar crystals onto the nuclei. According to the USDA Food Guide Pyramid, a healthful diet uses sugars sparingly.

GLOSSARY

Amorphous: Noncrystalline candies without a crystalline pattern; may be hard candies and brittles, chewy caramel and taffies, gummy marshmallows and gumdrops.

Artificial sweetener: Noncaloric, non-nutritive sugar substitute; examples are acesulfame K, aspartame, saccharin.

Caramelization: Sucrose dehydrates and decomposes when the temperature exceeds the melting point; it becomes brown and develops a caramel flavor, nonenzymatic browning.

Crystalline: A repeating crystal structure; solute forms a highly structured pattern of molecules around a nuclei or seed; includes large crystal, glasslike rock candy, or small crystal fondant and fudge.

Crystallization: Process whereby a solute comes out of solution and forms a definite lattice or crystalline structure.

Fermentation: The anaerobic conversion of carbohydrates (complex organic substances), such as sucrose, glucose, fructose or maltose, to carbon dioxide and alcohol by bacteria, mold, yeast, or enzymes.

Heat of crystallization: The heat given off by a sugar solution during crystallization.

Hygroscopicity: The ability of sugar to readily absorb water; sugars high in fructose such as invert sugar, HFCS, honey or molasses retain moisture more than sucrose.

Interfering agent: Used in crystalline products to reduce the speed of crystallization and help prevent undesirable growth of large crystal structures; interference by mechanical or chemical means.

Inversion: The formation of equal amounts of glucose and fructose from sucrose; by acid and heat, or enzymes; invert sugar is more soluble than sucrose.

Maillard browning: Browning as a result of reaction between the amino group of an amino acid and a reducing sugar.

Nuclei: An atomic arrangement of a seed needed for crystalline formation; fat is a barrier to seeding of the nuclei.

Saturated: A sugar solution holding the maximum amount of dissolved sugar it is capable of holding at the given temperature.

Seeding: To precipitate sugar from a supersaturated solution by adding new sugar crystals (the seed may originate from sugar adhering to the sides of the cooking utensil).

Solute: That which is dissolved in solution; the amount of solute held in solution depends on its solubility and the temperature.

Solution: Homogeneous mixture of solute and solvent; it may be dilute, saturated, or supersaturated.

Solvent: Medium for dissolving solute; i.e., water dissolves sugar.

Sugar alcohol: Caloric sugar substitute; chemically reduced carbohydrates that provide sweetening; examples are mannitol and sorbitol.

Supersaturated: Solution contains more solute than a solution can hold at a specified temperature; formed by heating and slow, undisturbed cooling.

REFERENCES

1. Pszczola D. Encapsulated ingredients: Providing the right fit. *Food Technology*. 1998; 52 (12): 70–76.

BIBLIOGRAPHY

ADA Position of the American Dietetic Association: Use of nutritive and non-nutritive sweeteners. *Journal of the American Dietetic Association*. 1993; 93: 816–821.

Alikonis TJ. *Candy Technology*. Westport, CT: AVI, 1979.

Bakal AT. Saccharin functionality and safety. *Food Technology*. 1987; 41(1): 17.

Calorie Control Council, Atlanta, GA.

FASEB, Life Sciences Research Office. *Evaluation of the Health Aspects of Sucrose as a Food Ingredient*. Bethesda, MD: USFDA, 1976.

FruitSource Associates. Santa Cruz, CA.

Fruitrim/LSI. Santa Cruz, CA.

Institute of Food Technologists' Expert Panel on Food Safety and Nutrition. Sweeteners: Nutritive and non-nutritive. *Food Technology*. 1986; 40(8): 195.

Iverson C, Schwartzberg HG. Developments in beet and cane sugar extraction. *Food Technology.* 1984; 38(1): 40.

Liquid Sugars, Emeryville, CA.

Nutra-Sweet Company, Deerfield, IL.

Pancoast H, Junk WR. *Handbook of Sugars,* 2nd ed. Westport, CT: AVI, 1980.

Pennington N, Baker CW. *Sugar: Users Guide to Sucrose.* New York: Chapman & Hall, 1990.

Pfizer Food Science Group. New York, NY.

Staff. Crystalline fructose: A breakthrough in corn sweetener process technology. *Food Technology.* 1987; 41(1): 66.

Staff. Future ingredients. *Food Technology.* 1988; 42(1): 60.

Stegink LD. Aspartame: A review of the safety issues. *Food Technology.* 1987; 41(1): 119.

Sugar Association. Washington, DC.

PART VI

Baked Products in the Food Guide Pyramid

CHAPTER 15

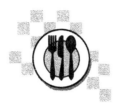

Baked Products—Batters and Doughs

INTRODUCTION

This chapter on baked products requires knowledge of the functional properties of carbohydrates, fats, and proteins. Specific batter and dough ingredients that are discussed include previously studied commodities, such as flour, eggs, milk, fats and oils, and sweeteners.

Many baked products contain flour, especially *wheat* flour, as the *primary* ingredient, which classifies them as "Hard-to-Place" foods (1) that fit in the Bread, Cereal, Rice and Pasta Group of the Food Guide Pyramid (Figure 15.1). This flour may also include *non-wheat* flours. Although flour may be the primary ingredient, baked products vary significantly in their fat and sugar content, which are constituents that are classified at the top of the Pyramid as foods that should be used sparingly.

Batters and *doughs* each contain different proportions of liquid and flour and are therefore, manipulated differently–by stirring, kneading, and so forth. They consist of a *gluten* network from flour that holds many additional substances, such as starch or sugar, often a leavening agents such as yeast, baking powder, or baking soda to produce CO_2, a liquid, and perhaps eggs and fats and/or oils. Other items, including salts or acids are also found in baked products.

The gas cell size and shape as well its surrounding ingredients create the "grain" and texture of a baked product. Most batters and doughs are "foams" of coagulated proteins around air cells; for example, angel food cakes and sponge cakes form definite foam structures. Pastries are *high* in fat and shortened cakes contain fat, whereas other cakes such as angel food cake may be *fat-free*.

A *quick bread* is one that is relatively quick to mix before baking, and leavened primarily by added *chemical* agents, such as baking powder, or baking soda, *not* by yeast. It may be leavened by steam or air. *Yeast breads,* leavened *biologically* by yeast,

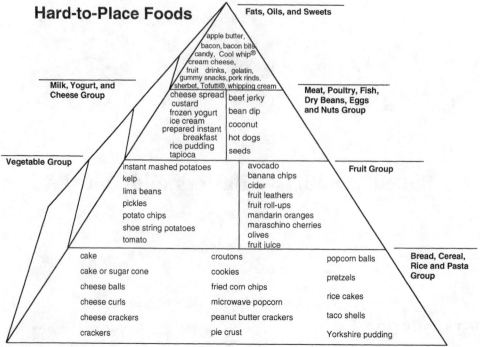

FIGURE 15.1 Hard-to-Place Foods Pyramid
(*Source:* Penn State Nutrition Center).

are more time-consuming to prepare. Ready-to-eat, and ready-for-baking products continue to replace some baking "from scratch."

Among other important points, this chapter will view the functions of various ingredients in a *general* manner, and the role of those ingredients in *specific* baked products.

CLASSES OF BATTERS AND DOUGHS

Batters and doughs are classified according to their ratio of liquid to flour (Table 15.1), and they utilize various mixing methods. Exact ingredient proportions of both batters and doughs vary by recipe, but for use as a planning guide or in recipe analysis, the ratios in Table 15.1 provide useful guidelines.

Batters are flour–liquid mixtures that are *beaten* or *stirred*, and incorporate a considerable amount of liquid as the continuous medium. Batters are classified as either pour batters or drop batters. *Pour* batters, such as those batters used in the preparation of pancakes and popovers, are thin and have a 1:1 ratio of liquid to flour, while *drop* batter contains more flour than a pour batter and has a ratio of 1:2 of liquid to flour. Muffins and some cookies are examples of products prepared with drop batter.

TABLE 15.1

TABLE 15.1

Type	Liquid	Flour
Batter		
Pour batter	1 part	1 part
Drop batter	1 part	2 parts
Dough		
Soft dough	1 part	3 parts
Stiff dough	1 part	6–8 parts

Doughs are thicker than batters. They are *kneaded*, not beaten or stirred, and the *gluten matrix* is the continuous medium. The flour mixtures are classified as soft or stiff doughs. For example, *soft* doughs, such as that used in biscuit preparation, or yeast bread have a liquid-to-flour ratio of 1:3, and *stiff* doughs may have a ratio of 1:6 or higher, and might be used for cookies or pastry dough, such as pie crust.

GLUTEN

Various flours differ in their protein composition. *Wheat* flour is frequently used for baking, as it contains both gliadin and glutenin, the two insoluble proteins, which when hydrated by liquid ingredients and mixed/manipulated, form **gluten**. The proteins aggregate and form disulfide bridges producing a gluten protein matrix that is *denatured* and, subsequently *coagulated* upon baking. This *gluten* provides the framework for many batters and doughs, although *starch* from non-gluten-forming flours provides some structure too.

Gluten, or the gluten matrix, is noted for the *strong*, three-dimensional, viscoelastic structure that is created as the hydrophobic gliadin proteins contribute sticky, fluid properties to the dough, and the insoluble glutenins contribute **elastic** properties to the dough. This three-dimensional structure that forms is capable of stretching without breaking and is important in determining the texture and volume of the finished product. Yeast breads, for example, require extensive **gluten development** in order to create a strong, stretchable structure.

If the manipulated dough is washed in *cold* water (*hot* water will gelatinize starch) to remove the nonprotein components of the flour, only the gummy gluten component of flour remains. It resembles already chewed chewing gum! When this gluten ball is subsequently baked, the entrapped water becomes steam and leavens the structure. Figure 15.2 shows the size of raw and baked gluten balls, which indicates the relative amount of gluten in the various types of flour.

Many baked products contain flour that is derived from *wheat*, and *especially hard wheat*, or *oat*, *rye* or *barley*. These have greater gluten-forming potential than corn, rice, and soy, which do not have **gluten-forming potential** due to inherent

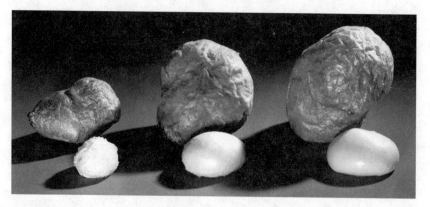

FIGURE 15.2 Unbaked and baked gluten balls. *Left to right*: gluten balls prepared from cake flour, all-purpose flour and bread flour
(*Source*: Wheat Flour Institute).

differences in protein composition. The latter do not have a dough structure capable of expansion without breaking when CO_2 is generated from yeast.

The gluten structure in the batter/dough mixture is embedded with other recipe ingredients such as the starch in the flour, added fat or sugar, or leavening in the formulation. These added ingredients (see Functions of Various Ingredients in Batters and Doughs) influence the development of the gluten structure, the dough strength, and the finished baked product. For example, dough does not reach its maximum strength when the recipe includes high levels of 1) sugar, which *competes* with gliadins and glutenins for available water, or 2) fat, which *covers* flour particles and prevents water absorption needed for gluten development.

Doughs such as biscuit dough, have a *low* liquid-to-flour ratio, and are more likely than batters to become tough due to the extensive development of gluten. *Batters*, particularly *pour* batters (with considerable liquid and less flour), do not exhibit a significant difference in gluten development between *adequately mixed* and *overmixed batters*. An overmixed *drop* batter, such as a muffin batter, has a greater chance of developing gluten, and may exhibit obvious internal holes in a tunnel formation (see Mixing Methods for Various Batters and Doughs).

Less flour produces less gluten. So, therefore, *sifting* flour for use in a recipe incorporates less flour, and there is less gluten-forming potential compared to an equal measure of *unsifted* flour. Sifting also incorporates air that provides leavening.

Gluten in a dried form may be added to other flours, providing extra strength and several times the gluten forming potential of bread flour. Extracted gluten is used to fortify protein content of some breakfast cereal, for binding breading on meat, poultry or fish, and as an extender for fish and meat products. As well, nonfood uses of gluten may be as a constituent of mascara and pharmaceutical tablets.

A look at the Codex Standard for gluten-free food, daily gliadin consumption, and studies on the safety of wheat starch-based gluten-free foods is found in other literature (2, 3, 4)

FUNCTION OF VARIOUS INGREDIENTS IN BATTERS AND DOUGHS

Not intended to be redundant, the following discussion will view the principle items that might be included in the preparation of batter and doughs—flour, liquid, leavening, fat, eggs, sugar, and salt. They create a watery mixture of substances that bakes around gas cells and subsequently, determines texture, flavor, and appearance of baked products.

Flour

Flour provides structure to baked goods because of its *protein*, and to a lesser degree, its *starch* components. For example, to the extent that the gluten forming proteins are present in flours, there is dough elasticity and structure (see Gluten) due to formation of a gluten matrix. Starch in flour is also capable of contributing some structure to a batter or dough, as it gelatinizes and makes the crumb more rigid. Additionally, it is also a source of fermentable sugar that is acted upon by yeast in producing CO_2 for leavening.

Many types of flour (Chapter 6) are used in the preparation of baked goods.

Wheat flour, derived from the endosperm of *milled wheat* is the most common. **All-purpose flour** is produced by blending hard and soft wheat during milling and has applications in all baked products. Consumers refer to it simply as "flour."

Hard wheat flour, such as bread flour has high gluten potential important for the expansion of yeast dough, such as bread dough, and it absorbs more water than soft wheat flour. *Soft wheat flour,* such as cake flour, contains less gluten-forming proteins and is effectively used in the preparation of the more tender (due to less gluten) cakes and pastries. (At the household level, 1 cup of all-purpose flour minus 2 tablespoons is used to replace 1 cup of cake flour in a formulation.)

Whole-wheat flour contains *all* of the three kernel parts, including the endosperm, germ, and bran (Chapter 6). Bran has sharp edges that cut through the developing protein structure and results in a lower-volume baked product, especially when a recipe replaces *all* of the flour with *whole-wheat* flour. Although if *finely ground,* whole-wheat flours have less sharp edges, and therefore exhibit less of a volume and texture difference. Generally, when a whole grain flour is desired in a baked product, the recipe should replace the flour with no more than *half* whole grain flour, used in combination with *half* bread flour. Due to the presence of *bran*, the percentage of protein is lower in whole-wheat flour than refined flour. (At the household level, 1 cup of whole-wheat flour plus 2 tablespoons may be used as a substitute for all-purpose flour.)

Although *wheat* flours are the most common types of flour used in baked products, *non-wheat* flours such as corn, rice, and soy are popular in many types of bread. Unless a *gluten-free* product is desired, the formulation typically combines the rice, corn, or soy with wheat flour for more desirable baking results.

Regardless of the type of flour incorporated into a formulation, it is typically *sifted* prior to measurement, as it standardizes the amount of flour added to a formulation and assures consistency in product preparation. Consistency is also more likely when ingredients are *weighed,* not *measured.* In general, recipe recommendations specifying a particular type and amount of flour, should first be analyzed, and then followed precisely, in order to yield a successful product, as flours do differ. There is even variance in the same brand of flour milled in *different milling locations* throughout the country. Consequently, the same recipe may yield a slightly different finished product.

Liquids

Liquids are necessary to hydrate flour *proteins* required in *gluten* formation, and the flour *starch* needed for subsequent gelatinization that assists in forming the *texture* of the baked crumb. Additionally, liquids are the solvent for dissolving many recipe ingredients such as the leavening agents baking powder and baking soda, as well as salt and sugar. Liquids are a leaven that produces steam, and expands air cells during baking.

Some liquids contribute more than water. For example, *milk* contains protein, milk salts, and the milk sugar, lactose that is important in Maillard browning. Although lactose is not fermentable, it softens the crumb, and contributes both flavor and color. The near-neutral pH of milk causes it to act as a buffer, preventing an acid environment that would be unacceptable to the growth of bakers yeast. Nonfat milk solids (NFMS) may be added to baked products for some of these same purposes, or to increase nutritive value. If *juice* is the liquid that is included in a formulation, the addition of alkali *may* be required to balance the increase in acidity that juice imparts.

According to federal regulations, the water level of a finished commercially prepared bread loaf may not exceed 38%.

Leavening Agents

Leavening agents raise or "make light and porous." They include *air, steam*, and *carbon dioxide* (CO_2), discussed briefly below. Virtually, *all* baked products are leavened to some extent, if not solely, by *air*. The mixing method and treatment of various added ingredients, such as sifting flour prior to addition, beating, or creaming, greatly influences the amount of air that is incorporated into a batter or dough mixture.

Carbon dioxide gas is a leavening agent produced by baking soda, baking powder, and yeast. As air cells are filled and expand with the CO_2, *steam* may then work in combination to further expand cell size, making batters and doughs light and porous.

Leavening agents make foam out of batters as they create air pockets or cells, contributing to the "**grain**" of the product. Holes in the crumb may be large or small; they may be intact or exploded.

Examples of these leavening agents and how they function in batters and doughs are discussed in The Leavening Process of Baked Products later in this chapter.

TABLE 15.2 Effects of Fats and Oils on Baked Products

Coating and mechanical tenderizing effect—Fats and oils shield gluten protein from water, thus physically interfering with the hydration needed for gluten development. Both fats and oils tenderize baked products by coating, although oil (liquid at room temperature) coats more completely and yields a more tender product than solid fats; if coating is extreme, the texture of the product will be mealy, and the dough will show reduced gluten formation.

Fats containing emulsifiers help water and fat to mix and may promote the stretching of gluten strands, yielding a higher volume of the baked product.

Shortening—Fats and oils minimize the length of developing gluten protein platelets; that is, they keep them short.

Flakiness—Plastic fat that is cut into pea-sized chunks in pie crust doughs (or smaller in biscuits) contributes the characteristic of flakiness to baked products as it melts in the dough, forming layers in the dough. Fats contribute *flakiness,* oil provides *tenderness.*

Leavening—Plastic fats may be creamed in order to incorporate air and aerate batters and doughs.

Less staling—Fats with monoglyceride addition, such as hydrogenated shortenings and commercially available lard, soften the crumb and function to retain moisture. It is primarily the amylopectin component of starch that forms a dry crumb.

Fat

Fats and oils are discussed in Chapter 12, and the reader is referred to that chapter for more specific information. Fat functions in various ways in batters and doughs as is seen in Table 15.2. This illustrates effects of fats and oils on baked products. Fats and oils *tenderize* baked products by *coating* flour proteins in the batter or dough and physically interfering with the development of protein structure. They *"shorten"* by controlling gluten strand length, *create flakes* or *dough layers* (such as in biscuits or pie crust), and they *leaven* by incorporating air (by creaming solid fats with sugar). Fats and oils help *prevent the staling* process of baked products.

"Plastic" fats, such as hydrogenated shortening or other solid fats, may be spread or molded to shape; they do not pour. Both hydrogenated vegetable shortenings and lard may contain a small percentage of emulsifier, such as monoglyceride or diglyceride, to increase fat distribution and promote greater volume of the developed protein matrix, as it is able to stretch more easily.

Polyunsaturated oils yield a more ***tender***, mealy and crumbly product than saturated fats because the oil covers a larger surface area of flour particles than *saturated fat* and helps control absorption of water (Chapter 12). Saturated fat, such as lard produces a less tender, but ***flaky*** pie crust with many layers in the dough. *Chilled* oils or fats exhibit slightly more flakiness in the baked product compared to room-temperature versions, as the *covering potential* is reduced.

Oils, hydrogenated vegetable oils, or animal fat (such as lard) are 100% fat. Other fats such as margarine and butter contain approximately 20% water, and reduced-fat "spreads" have an even higher percentage of water. Those fats containing water in the mix are less effective in their shortening ability than 100% fats. Often, specially modified recipes are required to assure success in baking with reduced-fat replacements. Cup for cup, the various fats and oils *cannot* be substituted for one another and produce the same quality of baked product. For example, 1 cup of margarine or butter may be substituted with 7/8 cup of oil.

Whole milk introduces more fat into batters and doughs than *low-fat* milk. This inclusion increases tenderness.

Baked products such as angel food cake *do not* contain added fat in the formulation, whereas other products such as shortened cake and pastries are high in fat content. With a low-fat modification, products may be missing some of the flavor, tenderness, or flakiness that fat provided in the original version.

Eggs

Eggs function in various manners in the batter or dough. They provide nutritive value, color, flavor, structure, leavening, and more. In addition to the structure provided by *flour* proteins that form a gluten matrix, *egg* proteins contribute to the structure as well, as they *coagulate* by heat, beating, or a change in pH. As eggs are beaten, for example, the egg *whites* incorporate air, which helps leaven a batter or dough due to extension of the air cells from steam production. Egg white may be a substitute for a portion of the whole egg in a formulation, thus reducing cholesterol levels, and producing a lighter, drier finished product.

Eggs are also binders, which hold ingredients together. The whole eggs and yolks contain emulsifiers that distribute fat in the batter, which explains why greater percentages of egg are necessary in a *high*-fat formulation compared to a low-fat or *high*-liquid formulation. Eggs contribute elasticity to products such as popovers and cream puffs, and when omitted from a formulation, the baked product is significantly (and unacceptably) lower in volume. *Large* size eggs are generally used in a formulation that requires the addition of eggs. More information on eggs is contained in Chapter 10.

Sugar

In addition to contributing *flavor*, sugar functions in many additional ways in batters and doughs, particularly related to gluten and starch. As the sugar in a recipe absorbs water, *instead of flour proteins and starch*, there is less water available for *gluten formation* and *starch gelatinization*, and consequently, the product is tender.

Sugar functions to *elevate the temperature* at which the *starch* gelatinizes, and it elevates the temperature required for *protein* coagulation, thus extending the time for CO_2 to expand the baking dough. Since it exhibits *hygroscopic* (water-retaining) tendencies, baked products may become overly moist, gummy, or runny, especially if the formulation is high in fructose (i.e., honey). Reducing sugars, such as the lactose in milk, provide *browning* due to the Maillard browning reaction, and sugars also caramelize.

A *small* amount of sugar is helpful to include in yeast bread formulations because it is fermented by yeast to produce CO_2, while *large* amounts (more than 10% by weight) dehydrate yeast cells and *reduce dough volume*. Additionally, sweetened dough requires more kneading and rising time due to this osmotic effect of sugar. High levels of sugar are more easily tolerated in breads and cakes leavened by *baking soda* or *baking powder* than by *yeast*, since yeast cells are dehydrated by sugar.

Granulated white sugar, brown sugar, corn syrup, and as discussed below, honey, and molasses, are substrates for yeast, whereas *artificial sweeteners* are *not* suitable for fermentation. When *honey* is used as a baking ingredient, it makes a sweeter and moister baked product because it contains fructose, which is sweeter and more hygroscopic than sucrose. (One cup of sugar in a recipe may be replaced by 3/4 cup of honey plus 1 tablespoon of sugar, if liquid is reduced by 2 tablespoonfuls.)

Molasses may be used as the sweetener in baked products, yet, because it is more acidic than sugar, it should *not* be used to replace more than *half* of the total amount of sugar in a recipe. In order to control acidity, it may be necessary to add a small quantity of baking soda. As is the case with honey, when molasses is substituted for sugar, there needs to be a reduction in the amount of liquid in the recipe.

Sugar substitutes provide sweetness but do not provide the *functional* properties of sugar, including browning, fermenting, tenderizing, and hygroscopic properties of sugars. Among sugar substitutes, an equal replacement of one sugar substitute for another, by weight, is *not* possible due to inherent differences in bulk and sweetness. Acesulfame K, aspartame (if encapsulated) and saccharin are examples of heat-stable sugar substitutes successfully incorporated into baked products.

Salt

Salt contributes flavor to baked products, and is a necessary component of *yeast* breads because it dehydrates yeast cells and controls the growth of yeast and its CO_2 production. The *absence* of salt in yeast bread dough allows *rapid* yeast development and rapid rising. This produces a *collapsible*, extremely porous structure, as gluten is overstretched and breaks.

In a typical yeast dough containing salt, the salt exerts an osmotic effect on the dough, competing with other substances for water absorption. Therefore, there is less gluten development and less starch gelatinization in salted yeast dough due to the fact that water is unavailable for hydration.

THE LEAVENING PROCESS OF BAKED PRODUCTS

After gluten has formed in dough and the dough has subsequently been fermented, the gluten structure is extensible by the leaven. **Leavening** agents incorporate air, steam, or CO_2, the latter either biologically or chemically produced into the gluten structure. As dough is *proofed*, or rises in its final rising (usually two times), it increases in volume and makes a product light and porous.

Air as a Leavening Agent

Air, which is incorporated to some extent into almost every batter and dough, expands upon heating and increases the volume of the product. It may be the *only* leavening agent in "*unleavened*" baked products such as some breads, crackers or pie crusts. Air may be incorporated into the batter or dough by *creaming* fat and sugar for a cake, by *beating* egg whites/whole eggs for angel food or sponge cake, by *sifting* ingredients, or by *folding* (lifting and turning) the mixture to incorporate air. After its introduction into the food, air cells expand with heat in baking, and another leaven, such as steam or CO_2, diffuses into the air space.

Steam as a Leaven

Steam is water vapor and it, too, partially leavens almost everything. One part of water creates 1600 parts of steam vapor and is produced from liquid ingredients, including water, juices, milk, or eggs. Products such as cream puffs or popovers are dependent on steam formation for leavening. They obtain their characteristic high volume and hollow interior as dough expands due to steam development, and as the egg protein denatures and coagulates. A *high* liquid-to-flour ratio and a *high* oven temperature are needed for water vaporization and dough expansion in products leavened mainly by steam.

Carbon Dioxide as a Leaven

Carbon dioxide is a major leavening agent in batters and doughs. The amount required in a formulation is proportional to the amount of flour. For example, a formulation that is high in flour requires *more* CO_2 production for leavening than does a high-liquid product; therefore, the recipe must contain *more* of the ingredient responsible for forming CO_2.

Chemical Production of CO_2

CO_2 may be produced *chemically* (5, 6) by the reaction of sodium bicarbonate with an acid (wet or dry), or it may be produced *biologically*, through bacteria or yeast fermenting sugar (7). CO_2 is easily released into a batter and may escape, becoming unavailable for leavening, if a batter or dough is left *unbaked* for an extended time period.

One means of chemical leavening is by *baking soda*, or sodium bicarbonate, which chemically produces CO_2 as follows:

$$2NaHCO_3 + heat \rightarrow Na_2CO_3 + CO_2 + H_2O$$

| Sodium bicarbonate | Sodium carbonate | Carbon dioxide | Water |

When used *alone,* baking soda reacts quickly with heat and CO_2 may escape from the raw batter. Therefore, baking soda must be *combined* with either 1) *liquid* acid, or 2) *dry* acid, plus liquid, in order to produce sufficient CO_2 in a mixture. Examples of *liquid acid* are applesauce, buttermilk, citrus juices, honey, molasses, and vinegar. An example of a *dry acid* is cream of tartar. In the case of a recipe with a mildly acidic juice, 1/2 teaspoon of baking soda may be used to neutralize 1 cup of the juice.

Baking soda (perhaps 1/4 teaspoon per cup of flour) is added to the recipe ingredient mixture along with the *dry* ingredients. If it is added with the *liquid* ingredients, CO_2 may be prematurely released into the liquid and escape from the mixture during manipulation.

Cream of tartar (potassium acid tartrate, a weak acid) may be combined with baking soda for leavening, as it is an acid salt. The reaction is represented as

$$HKC_4H_4O_6 \ + \ NaHCO_3 \ \rightarrow \ NaKC_4H_4O_6 \ + \ CO_2 \ + \ H_2O$$

Cream of tarter	Sodium bicarbonate	Sodium potassium tartrate	Carbon dioxide	Water

If a batter or dough is made *too* alkaline, sodium carbonate is produced in the food product, and it forms a soapy flavor, spotty brown color, and *yellowing* of the flavonoid pigment. This may occur in buttermilk (soda—acid) biscuits, if *soda* is present in greater amounts than the *acid* with which it reacts, although, these *soda–acid* biscuits may be tenderer than *baking powder* biscuits because the soda softens the gluten. If the pH is *acidic*, biscuits exhibit *whitening* in color.

A *second* means of supplying CO_2 chemically is via the use of *baking powder*. It was first produced in the United States in the early 1850s and quickly provided consumers with the convenience of a premixed leaven. It contains *three* substances: *sodium bicarbonate* (baking soda), a *dry acid*, and inert *cornstarch filler*. The starch filler keeps the soda and acid from reacting with each other prematurely and standardizes the weight in the baking powder canister. Commercial baking powder must yield at least 12% available CO_2 gas by weight (each 100 g of baking powder must yield 12 g of CO_2), and home-use powders must yield 14% CO_2.

Baking powders are classified in several manners. One method is according to the *acid* component that differs in strength and determines the rate of CO_2 release. While in the past, *tartrate* and *phosphate* were used as the dry acid, now consumers use the more common *SAS (sodium aluminum sulfate) phosphate* (in the amount if $1–1\frac{1}{2}$ teaspoons per cup of flour.)

In addition to classification based on the type of acid, baking powders are also classified according to their *action* rate, or how quickly they react with water and heat to form CO_2. The SAS phosphate contains two acids with varying speeds of action, 1) SAS, which is *slow*-acting, acid ingredient, and 2) monocalcium phosphate, the *fast*-acting, acid ingredient. The SAS phosphate is a *slow-acting* baking powder, *double-acting* powder that releases CO_2 two times. The first release of CO_2 occurs as the mixture is *moistened;* the second occurs as the mixture is *heated.* A *fast-acting* baking powder, such as the monocalcium phosphate, is a *single-acting* powder whose soluble acids release CO_2 almost *immediately* upon moistening/mixing with liquid at room temperature.

The role of baking powder is to leaven, but cell walls may be stretched and break if an excessive quantity is added to a formulation. If this breakage occurs, CO_2 bubbles are released resulting in a lower-volume product with a soapy taste. SAS phosphate baking powder used in biscuits may form cracks because of attempted leavening with insufficient dough stretching.

A distinction between the use of baking *soda* and baking *powder* is seen when baking powder is used for *baking powder biscuits,* and buttermilk (liquid acid) is combined with baking soda to produce *buttermilk biscuits.* The use of *excessive* baking powder may result in a soapy flavor, yellow crumb, excessively browned, and coarse-textured product, the latter due to an overstretched and collapsed structure. If too *little* baking powder is used, the product is not sufficiently leavened, has a low volume, and is soggy with a compact grain of small air cells in the batter or dough.

The occasional inclusion of *both* baking powder and baking soda may be necessary if the amount of soda and liquid acid would not amply supply the CO_2 that is needed to leaven the mixture. It may also be that these are added to highly sweetened yeast dough at the second rise, in order to provide extra leavening power.

If baking powder is not available for use, substitution may be made. One teaspoon of baking powder is equal to 1/4 teaspoon baking soda and 1/2 teaspoon of cream of tartar.

Biological Production of CO_2

Leavening may occur by the above-mentioned nonfermentation methods, using air, steam, or chemical CO_2 production, or by **fermentation,** the *biological* process in which the microorganisms bacteria or yeast, function to metabolize fermentable organic substances. Starch hydrolyzing enzymes in flour such as amylase are important in commercial breadmaking because they produce such fermentable sugars upon which yeast acts. (Alpha-amylase breaks off one glucose unit, at a time, immediately yielding glucose, and β-amylase breaks off two glucose units—maltose)

Bacteria, such as *Lactobacillus sanfrancisco,* are responsible (along with a nonbakers' yeast *Saccharomyces exiguus*) for forming sourdough bread. The *bacteria* function to degrade maltose, yielding acetic and lactic acid, and producing CO_2. Starters or sponges of dough containing the bacteria, along with yeast, may be saved from one baking and used in a subsequent baking.

Yeast leavens by fermentation in the presence of water and a substrate. The most common strain of yeast used in breadmaking is *Saccharomyces cerevisiae.* It is a microscopic, one-celled fungi, a plant without stems or chlorophyll that grows by a process known as budding—a new cell grows and comes from an existing cell. It releases zymase, which metabolizes *fermentable sugars* in an anaerobic process, yielding *ethanol* and CO_2 (with more yeast cells, the more CO_2 is produced.) The alcohol is volatized in baking and the CO_2 provides leavening. The three main forms of yeast used in food include those listed in Table 15.3.

TABLE 15.3   Forms of Yeast

Active dry yeast (ADY)
  1 teaspoon ADY = 1 cake of compressed yeast (CY)
  Contains approximately 2–1/4 teaspoons per envelope
  Leavens 6–8 cups of flour
  Has a longer shelf life than CY
  Less moisture than CY

Cake or compressed yeast (CY)
  Moist yeast with starch filler
  Short shelf life—must be refrigerated or yeast cells die

***Quick* rising dry yeast**
  Is rapidly rehydrated
  Raises a mixture rapidly
  Is formed by protoplast fusion of cells

In the presence of liquid and temperatures of 105–115°F (41–46°C), each yeast cell rehydrates and buds, producing a new cell; temperatures greater than 130°F (54°C) have a negative effect (thermal death) on yeast development. Due to the osmotic pressure that sugar exerts, more time is necessary to leaven sweetened yeast dough.

Yeast dough must undergo sufficient *time* for fermentation after kneading. As well, the *temperature* is important in fermentation. The dough should not reach high temperatures, or be chilled. In home testing for adequate fermentation, fingertip impressions should leave a slight indentation in sufficiently risen dough. Following the CO_2 production and a *preliminary* rise, dough is punched down (Figure 15.3) and left to rise a *second time* for desirable texture and grain-size formation.

If dough is allowed to rise *too much*, gluten is *over*stretched and the dough is no longer as elastic and extensible as desired. As the stretched gluten structure collapses, volume decreases, and the texture is noticeably coarse, open, and dense instead of fine and even. In the case of *over*risen dough, it should be punched down again, and allowed to rise a third time, so that it is not baked in a condition where the overstretched structure will collapse.

It is possible that leavening may utilize baking soda or baking powder along with the yeast, especially if the recipe uses a high level of sugar that inhibits gluten development and the subsequent rise. Either may be added to the dough (at the second rise of the dough) to provide extra leavening.

Commonly shared among friends in their home kitchens, or used for repeated baking, a starter culture or "sponge" may be used in breadmaking. The starter is retained from a previous baking, and therefore fresh yeast is not required each time bread is prepared.

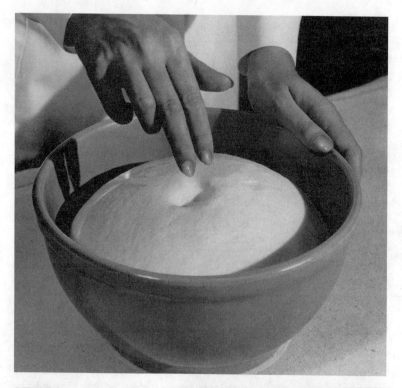

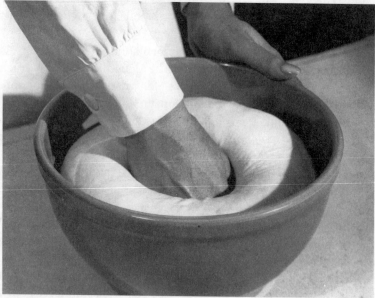

FIGURE 15.3 Testing and punching down yeast dough
(*Source:* USDA).

INGREDIENTS IN SPECIFIC BAKED PRODUCTS

Through an application of previously presented concepts, the role of ingredients in some specific baked products will be examined.

Yeast Bread Ingredients

Yeast breads (Figure 15.4) are prepared from *soft doughs* (1:3 to 1:4 ratio of liquid to flour) using *hard wheat* flours to form a gluten structure that is strong and elastic. The structure may also contains starch and sugar or other ingredients such as fat and eggs (see Function of Various Ingredients in Batters and Doughs). The yeast is responsible for the production of CO_2 within the gluten structure, and in turn, the CO_2 is responsible for the reduction of pH from 6.0 to 5.0.

Mandatory yeast bread ingredients in the United States are flour, yeast, liquid, and salt. Additionally, sugar, and the commercial enzyme α-amylase may be added during the commercial preparation of bread loaves. (The enzyme is naturally present in flour and may cause unwanted hydrolysis of the starch; *however*, it may be added in order to form desirable structure and texture in breadmaking and in creating food for yeast.)

The *general* function of various added ingredients has been addressed previously in this chapter. Now, the specific role of *yeast dough* ingredients (in addition to yeast) is highlighted in the following subsections.

Flour.   Yeast breads are made with *hard* flour, such as bread flour, that 1) contains sufficient gliadins and glutenins for the development of a coagulated gluten structure,

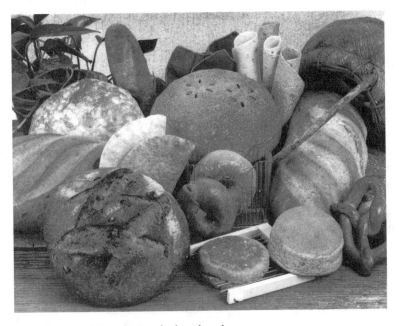

FIGURE 15.4   Yeast-leavened wheat breads
(*Source:* Wheat Foods Council).

and 2) holds more water than soft flour. Adequate gluten development and viscoelasticity are required for the entrapment of the CO_2 evolved from yeast fermentation. Therefore, some flours are not suitable for breadmaking, as they do not have gluten potential.

The starch component of flour contributes to structure as it is gelatinized, and it is converted to sugar, which provides food for yeast. Isolated gluten may also be added to flour to yield high-gluten flour.

Liquid. Liquid is necessary to hydrate flour proteins, starch, and yeast cells. Hydration of the gliadins and glutenins is necessary for gluten formation; hydration of starch is needed for gelatinization. Milk or water allows yeast cells to begin development (to bud) and should be warmed to approximately 105–115°F (41–46°C) for yeast to begin development. Milk that is not scalded may contain whey protein that results in diminished volume.

Sugar. The initial incorporation of a *small* amount of sugar with yeast promotes yeast growth. Sugar also functions to *brown* the crust of yeast breads by the Maillard browning reaction and it *tenderizes* doughs if added in large amounts. *High amounts* of sugar *inhibit* yeast development. Thus, sweet dough interferes with water uptake and gluten development; dough is slower to rise, and achieves less volume compared to an *unsweetened* dough. With high amounts of sugar, *less* salt or *more* yeast may be added.

Salt. Salt is a required ingredient in yeast formulas. It is added for flavor and to control gluten development, so that it stretches sufficiently without breaking. If omitted from a formulation, a collapsible structure would result from weak, overstretched gluten.

Optional Ingredients Used in Yeast Breads. *Optional* ingredients in yeast breadmaking include *fat* and *eggs*. Fat may be added for flavor and tenderness; eggs may be added to provide emulsification, for nutritive value, flavor, color, or tenderness. Many *other* ingredients including fruits and vegetables, nuts, cheeses, dried beans, herbs and flavorings may be added. The incorporation of various spices, including ginger, cinnamon, cardamom, and thyme increase gas production in dough by chemically enhancing yeast fermentation. The addition of dry mustard exhibits an inhibitory effect on yeast development (8).

Quick Bread Ingredients

Quick breads, as their name implies, are relatively quick to mix before baking, and the leaven is typically *chemically* produced by baking powder, baking soda, or by steam and/or air. They include the biscuits, loaf breads, muffins, pancakes, popovers, and waffles that may appear among the variety of other baked products in Figure 15.5. The function of various ingredients that may be incorporated in the formulation of quick breads appears in the following subsections.

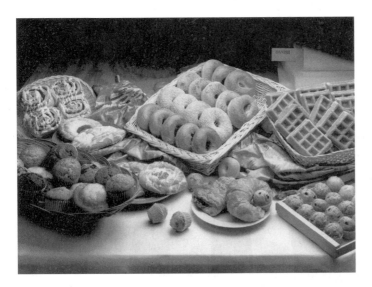

FIGURE 15.5   Various baked products (*Courtesy of SYSCO® Incorporated*).

Flour.   All-purpose flour is used to provide an adequate gluten structure for quick breads. The high liquid to flour proportion in a quick bread formulation limits gluten development and yields a tender product. The high proportion of liquid to flour *limits gluten* development.

Liquid.   Water, juice, or milk may be used as the dispersing medium for sugar, salt, and the leavening agent. As the liquid is heated, it forms steam, which leavens, gelatinizes starch, and contributes rigidity to the crumb.

Fat.   Various fats and oils are used in quick bread production. *Oils* coat flour granules, *covering* them to prevent water absorption, and chunks of *fat* form distinct layers in the product. For example, *oil* is used in pancakes and muffins, and *large-size* crumbs of *solid fat* are used in the preparation of biscuits to form flakes.

High levels of fat limit the development of gluten. When formulations are modified for health purposes, such as may occur with the substitution of oil for fat, there is a noticeable change of quality. For example, the absence of flakes becomes apparent. When a formulation is reduced-fat or fat-free, it produces a less tender crumb due to the increased development of gluten.

Sugar.   Sugar provides sweetness and tenderization. It also may assist in the Maillard browning reaction. High levels inhibit gluten development.

Eggs.   Eggs provide structure as they coagulate. They emulsify quick bread batters, allowing the *lipid* part to combine with *liquid* due to the presence of phospholipids in the yolk. Eggs also impart color.

Leaven. Typically, quick breads are leavened quickly by *baking powder*—e.g., *baking powder biscuits*, or by *baking soda* and a *liquid acid*—e.g., *buttermilk biscuits* (2 tsp. baking powder + 1 cup milk = 1/2 tsp. soda + 1 cup buttermilk).

Pastry Ingredients

Pastry is made with high-fat stiff dough, and produces a flaky product, as is seen in pie crusts or puff pastry. The *primary*, functional ingredient in pie crusts is flour; thus, pie crusts are classified as a "Hard-to-Place" food, placed at the bottom of the Food Guide Pyramid (Figure 15.1).

In addition to the flour, pastries are high in fat and, in fact, will not be as tender if the recipe is subject to fat reduction (Chapter 12). Two distinct features of a pastry are tenderness and flakiness, therefore, depending upon the specific product desired, the quantities of fat, flour, liquid, leavening, and so forth, will vary. The function of various ingredients in pastry is identified in the following subsections.

Flour. Pastry flour is *soft* wheat flour that is low in protein. It produces *less* gluten than both all-purpose and *hard* wheat flour, absorbs more liquid, and yields a more tender product. If a pastry depends upon steam to leaven, and it contains less egg, it may require the use of *hard* flour in order to provides a satisfactory structure in the pastry product. Examples of pastries include puff pastry, popovers, and streusel.

Liquid. The liquid in pastry doughs is chiefly water. Water hydrates flour and forms cohesiveness. As the liquid changes to steam, it leavens the mixture, i.e., cream puffs, popovers, puff pastry.

Fat. Solid pea-sized chunks of *fat* in pastries form many *flaky* layers in a crust, such as a pie crust. The use of *oil* in a recipe coats flour particles and permits less hydration of the flour particles, and *oil* will exhibit a crumbly mealiness and produce a pastry crust that is not flaky, but *tender*. On the other hand, *lard* and *hydrogenated shortenings* are solid shortenings that produce very flaky pastries, while *butter* and *margarine* are solid at room temperature but contain 80% fat and 20% liquid, thus reducing flakiness. Reduced fat and fat-free margarines do not contain sufficient levels of fat to function well in pastry.

Cake Ingredients

Cakes typically contain fat and may be high in sugar. Many of the ingredients affect the cake volume and texture. Some functions of cake ingredients are presented in the following subsections.

Flour. Soft wheat (7–8.5% protein) cake flour is desirable for cakes. The flour particles are small in size, and the cake is more lofty and tender with a finer grain than *hard* flour with its higher gluten-forming ability. Thinner walls, increased volume, and a less coarse cake result from using soft cake flour. If the flour is *bleached*, as is often the case with cake flour, the pigment is bleached and the baking performance is improved.

Liquid.   Liquid gelatinizes starch and develops minimal gluten. *Fluid* milk hydrates protein and starch providing structure and crumb texture, while *dry* milk adds protein. The milk sugar, lactose, and protein are valuable in determining the color of a finished cake. Milk proteins combine with sugars in nonenzymatic, Maillard browning.

Sugar.   Sugar imparts a sweet flavor to cakes and is often added to cake batters in large amounts. It competes with the protein and starch for water and inhibits both gluten development and starch gelatinization. Sugar also functions to incorporate air when plastic fats are creamed with sugar prior to inclusion in a batter, and even if not creamed, its addition increases the number of air cells in the batter, contributing to the tenderness of the grain.

Fat.   Fat functions in tenderizing cakes, since it shortens protein–starch strands. It provides increased volume, especially if creamed in a recipe or if monoglycerides and diglycerides are used as emulsifiers in the fat. *Butter* in a formulation may require more creaming than hydrogenated shortening because it is not as aerated and it has a narrow plastic range (Chapter 12). *Lard* has a large crystal size and therefore creams less well than most plastic fats. *Oils* produce tenderization. Fat in a recipe also functions to retain moisture in the mixture and it softens the crumb. Shortened cakes differ from sponge cakes in that the latter have no fat beside egg. Sponge cakes incorporate *whole* egg, and angel food cakes are prepared with beaten egg *whites* to create volume.

Eggs.   The protein of whole eggs or egg whites provides structure and may toughen the mixture as the protein coagulates. Eggs, especially egg whites, also leaven because they are beaten to incorporate air, and they provide liquid, which leavens as it becomes steam. Egg yolks, due to their lipoprotein content, function as emulsifiers. The addition of extra fat and sugar offset the toughness of egg in a formulation.

Leaven.   *Creaming* fat and sugar incorporates air as a leaven. The grain shows evidence of numerous air cells that may then hold other expanding gases released by baking soda as it reacts with acid. The use of chemical leavening by *baking soda* and *baking powder* is common, as is steam and air.

MIXING METHODS FOR VARIOUS BATTERS AND DOUGHS

The *function* of batter and dough ingredients, and *ingredients* in specific baked products have been addressed in former sections. This section covers specific *mixing methods* for various batters and doughs are discussed in the following subsections. The function of *mixing* is to distribute ingredients, including leavening agents, and to equalize the temperature throughout a mixture. Biscuits and pastries are manipulated by *kneading*; cakes, muffins, and pour batters are *stirred*.

Biscuits

Biscuits are quick breads made of soft doughs. The recommended mixing method is to cut a solid fat, pea size or smaller, into the sifted, dry mixture. Next, all of the liquid is added, a ball is formed, and the dough is kneaded. Kneading (see Yeast Doughs, Kneading)10–20 *times* develops gluten and orients the direction of gluten strands, necessary to create flakes. It mixes all ingredients, such as the *baking powder* or *soda and acid*, which leaven. *Under*kneading produces a biscuit that fails to rise sufficiently. *Over*kneading or re-rolling, overproduces gluten, and results in a smaller-volume, tougher biscuit, which will not rise evenly because CO_2 escapes through a weak location in the gluten structure.

Cakes

Cake batters may be prepared by several different methods, but, *conventionally*, they are mixed by first creaming a plastic fat with sugar, which provides aeration of the cake batter. Next, the egg is added, and the dry and wet ingredients are added alternately.

Muffins

Muffins are a quick bread prepared from drop batter. The optimal mixing method for muffins is to pour all of the liquid ingredients into all of the sifted, dry ingredients and mix *minimally*. *Overmixing* a high-gluten-potential batter develops long strands of gluten and results in the formation of tunnels or peaks. **Tunnels**, or hollow internal pathways, form long strands of gluten, allowing gases to escape from the interior.

Muffins may also take on this peaked appearance if the *oven temperature is too high* because at high oven temperatures, a top crust forms while the interior is still fluid and maximum expansion of the muffin has not occurred. Therefore, a *center* tunnel forms and gases escape, creating a ***peak***.

Pieces of the bran physically cut through the developing gluten strands during mixing, and thus, bran muffins do *not* rise as much as non-bran-containing muffins. If low or non-gluten flour is used in a formulation, it is best to mix them with an equal amount of wheat flour in order to obtain a desirable structure.

Pastries

The mixing method for pastry is similar to biscuit preparation. It involves cutting the large amount of fat into the sifted, dry ingredients, then adding all of the liquid. The mixture is stirred, then kneaded, and cut to desired shape. Croissant pastry dough must be repeatedly *folded*, not stirred or kneaded, numerous times over the course of several hours. This folding produces layers in the dough. *Well-chilled* oil restricts the covering potential of room-temperature oil and produces a slightly flaky product if pastry is prepared with oil.

Pour Batters

Items such as pancakes, popovers, and waffles contain a *high* proportion of liquid to flour and do not require a definite manner of mixing. Overmixing is unlikely to affect the shape or texture of the finished product due to the high level of water and low level of gluten development.

Yeast Doughs

The preparation of yeast dough includes kneading, fermenting, punching down the dough, resting, shaping, and proofing dough. Following these steps, the dough is baked (see Baking Batters and Doughs).

Kneading is the process of manipulating dough to develop gluten strands. It incorporates and subdivides air cells, promotes evenness of temperatures throughout the dough ($75-80° > F [27°C]$), removes the excess CO_2 (which may overstretch the gluten structure), and distributes yeast. The process comprises more than beating, or stirring. Rather, folding, pressing, and stretching dough is necessary for the development of yeast dough that is unable to be beaten or stirred.

In addition to the hand manipulation of yeast dough, kneading may be accomplished utilizing a heavy-duty mixer, bread machine or food processor, perhaps requiring 10, 5, and 1–2 minutes, respectively. *Underkneading*, or use of non-gluten forming flour, may produce less/no gluten strands and thus, breads with less volume. *Overkneading* is also possible, especially with the use of machine kneading. If this is the case, there may be a break of the gluten strands resulting in a less elastic mass of dough that fails to rise satisfactorily.

After kneading, the dough is left to rise as yeast cells convert fermentable sugar into ethanol and CO_2. Then, the dough is *punched down*. This is beneficial in that it allows the heat of fermentation, and CO_2 to escape, introduces more oxygen, controls the size of air cells, and prevents overstretching and collapse of gluten. As well, this punching down provides yeast contact with a fresh supply of food (the sugar), and oxygen.

Following this punching down step, the dough is left to *rest* for 15–20 minutes prior to shaping, so that gluten strands relax, and the starch absorbs water in the dough to make it less sticky. In this time period, fermentation continues and the gluten network becomes easier to manipulate.

Subsequent to the rest period, dough is *shaped* and allowed to rise a second time—it is **proofed**. The dough will have doubled in volume following the second rise, as many more yeast cells have budded and produced additional CO_2. It is ready to bake when a slight indentation mark remains in the dough when it is pressed lightly with the fingers.

BAKING BATTERS AND DOUGHS

Batters and doughs are foams of watery substance surrounding air cells. The surrounding mixture forms the *grain* of the finished product as it "sets" or coagulates around air cells. Major product changes that occur during baking involve protein, starch, gases, browning and importantly, a release of aroma.

Proteins in the flour, or added protein ingredients, harden or coagulate by heat. *Starch* granules swell and gelatinize as they imbibe moisture. *Gases* expand, and produce leavening. *Water* evaporates and a browning of the crust becomes evident due to the Maillard browning reaction. The alcohol waste product of yeast fermentation evaporates, albeit not completely.

The qualities of a finished baked product may be determined by oven temperature and degree of manipulation (stirring, kneading). The type of flour, the amount of liquid, and an almost unlimited list of possible added ingredients affect quality.

In the *oven*, yeast breads will exhibit an *initial* rising of the loaf known as "**oven spring**." This rise is due to heat, yeast's CO_2 and the steam from water. Subsequently, gases *expand the gluten* strands until they form a rigid structure. As well, the starch in the dough partially gelatinizes and loses its birefringence (Chapter 4). *Flavor* develops as the crust browns with water loss and aroma is released.

High-Altitude Baking

If a product is baked at *high altitude,* there is less atmospheric resistance and thus, increased dough expansion. As a result of this expansion, the product may break and, consequently, have low volume. Therefore, local instructions must be followed in manufacturing, foodservice, or home recipes. At high elevations (5000 ft or more above sea level), 1) a reduction in sugar is needed in order to provide a strong gluten structure, and 2) less leaven is needed for expansion. Additionally, an increase in the amount of liquid and in baking temperature is recommended. At still *higher* elevations, a greater reduction of sugar and the addition of a small amount of flour to the mixture are recommended.

SAFETY ISSUES IN BATTERS AND DOUGHS

Microbial Hazards

"*Rope*" is a condition attributed to bacilli *bacteria* that may be present in the field from which a crop was obtained to produce flour. Its presence causes a syrupy ropelike interior of bread, but an acid environment (pH < 4.5) prevents this growth of bacteria. *Mold* spoilage is also possible. Therefore, mold inhibitors such as *sodium* or *calcium propionate* or *sodium diacetate* are commonly added to commercially prepared bread to inhibit mold and bacteria.

Nonmicrobial Hazards

Nonmicrobial deterioration may occur due to rancidity or staling (Chapter 5). Staling is defined as all those changes occurring *after* batters and doughs are baked. It is thought that deterioration primarily involves the starch component *amylopectin*, and it includes a change in flavor, a harder, less elastic crumb, and less water-absorbing ability. In order to partially restore flavor, brief reheating is recommended. If heat is prolonged or too high, a dry crumb is evident.

Foreign substances also pose hazards if found in foods. Controls must be established and enforced to protect against deterioration and hazards.

NUTRITIVE VALUE OF BAKED PRODUCTS

The nutritive value of baked products varies according to the type and amount of ingredients used in the formulation. The primary ingredient of many baked products is flour; thus, as previously mentioned, cakes, crackers, cookies, and pie crusts may be classified as "Hard-to-Place" foods that belong to the Bread, Cereal, Rice, and Pasta Group of the Food Guide Pyramid (Figure 15.1). Those individuals following a gluten-free dietary regimen may avoid specific flours such as wheat, and instead, chose flour such as rice flour to bake. These items may also contribute fats and sugars as can be seen in the USDA's Food Guide Pyramid (the circles and triangles). Generally, food choices that provide less sugar and fat in the diet should be selected, as fats and sweets should be used sparingly.

Reduced-Fat and No-Fat Baked Products

Some baked products may be successfully prepared with a reduction in the fat content, and this modification may fit into many fat- or calorie-restricted diets; however, the baked good may be less tender and flavorful than the *unmodified* counterpart. The result of reducing or eliminating fat is altered flavor, more gluten development, and less tenderness than a product with the standard amount of fat. Such changes may not be acceptable to all individuals.

CONCLUSION

Batters and doughs are made with different proportions of liquids, flour, and other ingredients such as leavening agents, fat, eggs, sugar, and salt. Depending on the amount of flour, batter may be a pour type or drop batter, and dough may be soft or stiff. A formulation that includes wheat flour forms a protein network known as *gluten*, and liquid gelatinizes *starch* as the batter or dough bakes. Both gluten and gelatinized starch contribute to the structure of baked products. A quick bread is quick to prepare, whereas yeast breads require more lengthy time periods for the yeast to raise bread prior to baking.

Sugar and salt contribute flavor and exert an osmotic effect on dough as they compete with other added substances for water absorption. A small amount of sugar serves as the substrate for yeast in fermentation, whereas a large amount of sugar interferes with CO_2 development by dehydrating yeast cells. Salt is needed for control of yeast growth. Baked products may be leavened with air, steam, or CO_2 that enlarges air cells, and raises dough. Carbon dioxide may be produced biologically by yeast or chemically by baking powder or baking soda. Leavening is also accomplished by air or steam.

Fat is considered optional in some batters and doughs, and mandatory in other baked products. Liquid oil coats flour particles more thoroughly than solid fat, limiting gluten development and contributing tenderness. Solid fat, cut into pea-sized chunks or less, melts forming layers in pie crusts and biscuits, respectively. Eggs may be added to batter and dough formulation. Egg whites may be beaten to incorporate air; whole eggs or yolks contribute nutritive value, color, flavor, and emulsification. The nutritive value of baked products is dependent on the individual recipe ingredients.

GLOSSARY

All-purpose flour: The flour created by a blend of hard and soft wheat milling streams.
Batters: Thin flour mixtures that are beaten or stirred, with a 1:1 or 1:2 ratio of liquid to flour, for pour batters and drop batters, respectively.
Doughs: Thick flour mixtures that are kneaded, with a 1:3 or 1:6–8 ratio of liquid to flour for soft and stiff doughs, respectively.
Elastic: Flexible, stretchable gluten structure of dough.
Fermentation: A biological process where yeast or bacteria, as well as mold and enzymes metabolize complex organic substances such as sucrose, glucose, fructose, or maltose into relatively simple substances; the anaerobic conversion of sugar to carbon dioxide and alcohol by yeast or bacteria.
Flaky: Thin, flat layers of dough formed in some doughs such as biscuits or pie crusts; a property of some pastries that is inverse to tenderness.
Gluten: Three-dimensional viscoelastic structure of doughs, formed as gliadin, and glutenin in some flour, are hydrated and manipulated.
Gluten-forming potential: Presence of the proteins gliadin and glutenin that may potentially form the elastic gluten structure.
Gluten development: The hydration and manipulation of flour that has gluten potential.
Grain: The cell size, orientation, and overall structure formed by a pattern or structure of gelatinized starch and coagulated protein of flour particles appearing among air cells in batters and doughs.
Kneading: To mix dough into a uniform mass by folding, pressing, and stretching.
Leavening: To raise, make light and porous by fermentation or nonfermentation methods.
Oven spring: The initial rise of batters and doughs subject to oven heat.
Peak: A center tunnel where gases escape from a muffin.
Plastic fat: Solid fat able to be molded to shape, but does not pour.
Proofed: The second rise of shaped yeast dough.
Tender: Having a delicate, crumbly texture, a property of some pastries that is inverse to flakiness.
Tunnels: Elongated air pathway formed along gluten strands in batters and doughs, especially seen in overmanipulated muffins.
Wheat flour: Flour derived from the endosperm of milled wheat.

Whole wheat flour: Flour derived from the whole kernel of wheat—contains bran, endosperm, and germ of wheat.

REFERENCES

1. *Hard-to-Place Foods Pyramid*. University Park, PA: Penn State Nutrition Center, 1993.
2. Thompson T. Wheat starch, gliadin, and the gluten-free diet. *J Am Diet Assoc*. 2001; 101: 1456–1459.
3. Joint FAO/WHO Food Standards Program. Codex Committee on Nutrition and Foods for Special Dietary Uses. Draft revised standard for gluten-free foods. CX/NFSDU 98/4. July, 1998: 1–4.
4. Thompson T. Questionable foods and the gluten-free diet: Survey of current recommendations. *J Am Diet Assoc*. 2000; 100: 463–465.
5. La Baw GD. Chemical leavening agents and their use in baked products. *Bakers Digest*. 1982; 56(1): 16.
6. Reiman HM. Chemical leavening systems. *Bakers Digest*. 1983; 57(4): 37.
7. Dubois DK. What is fermentation? It's essential to bread quality. *Bakers Digest*. 1984; 58(1): 11.
8. Wright WJ, Bice CW, Fogelberg JM. The effect of spices on yeast fermentation. *Cereal Chemistry*. 1954; 31(3): 100–112.

BIBLIOGRAPHY

Allenson A. Refrigerated doughs. *Bakers Digest*. 1982; 56(5): 22.

American Yeast Sales. Derry, NH.

Clark JP. Bakery of the future. *Food Engineering*. 1994; 66(10): 109–114.

Dow Chemical. Midland, MI.

FruitSource. Santa Cruz, CA.

Fruitrim/LSI. Santa Cruz, CA.

Marston PE, Wannan TL. Bread baking. The transformation from dough to bread. *Bakers Digest*. 1983; 57(4): 59.

Pyler EJ. *Baking Science and Technology*, Vols I and II. Chicago, IL: Siebel, 1973.

Taranto MV. Structural and textural characteristics of baked goods. In: Peleg M, Bagley E, eds. *Physical Properties of Foods*. Westport, CT: AVI, 1983.

The Food Guide Pyramid: A Guide to Daily Food Choices. Home and Garden Bulletin No. 252. Washington, DC: US Dept of Agriculture, Human Nutrition Information Service, 1992.

Wheat Foods Council. Englewood, CO.

Wheat Flour Institute. Washington, DC.

Wheat Industry Council. Washington, DC.

Wheat Industry Council. Washington, DC.

PART VII

Aspects of Food Production

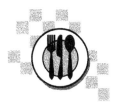

CHAPTER 16

Food Safety

INTRODUCTION

Food safety is an important issue of today as there are many demands on the food production system, and a variety of food handlers serving many immunocompromised individuals. Food safety, as applicable to specific food products, is discussed in chapters throughout this text.

Providing safe food is the responsibility of many individuals/groups. For example, federal agencies such as the U.S. Food and Drug Administration (FDA) and the U.S. Department of Agriculture (USDA), Centers for Disease Control and Prevention (CDC), as well as the state and local counterparts, numerous professional organizations, food processors, and consumers are all interested in preventing the occurrence of foodborne illness.

The FDA ranking of food safety concerns, according to risk includes *foodborne illness* as the *primary* concern, followed by nutritional adequacy of foods, environmental contaminants, naturally occurring toxicants, pesticide residues, and food additives (FDA).

Aspects of preservation and processing, additives, packaging, and government regulation that contribute to food safety are discussed in Chapters 17–20.

While it is important to educate the consumer regarding food safety at the home, hazards in the food supply may be controlled/prevented *before* foods reach the consumer. The effective use of The Hazard Analysis and Critical Control Point (HACCP) method of food safety, practiced in the food processing industry, has been shown to yield safer foods. Irradiation is also employed to reduce the incidence of disease.

FOODBORNE ILLNESS

Since the FDA ranks *foodborne illness* as the primary food safety concern, this chapter will focus on its causes and prevention (1,2). **Foodborne illness** represents disease carried to people by food, and is the result of various *biological, chemical,* or *physical hazards* to the food supply. Each of these hazards will be addressed in the following text. While *prevention* policies are the first line of defense against hazards, rapid *detection* of biological contaminants is imperative (3) as is proper *sanitation* (4,5). Disease must be controlled, as the *risk* may increase or decrease throughout the steps of processing, storage, and distribution of foods. Today, there is a high interest in improving the safety net of the food supply (6) and testing for bacteria such as *E. coli* O157:H7 (7).

Both feasting on fear (8) and panicking over pathogens (9) are unwanted actions in combating foodborne illness. Whereas the government must regulate the food supply considering scientific and societal forces (10), both the manufacturer and consumer play vital roles in food safety. Beyond the immediacy of illness, there is also increasing evidence that foodborne gastrointestinal (GI) pathogens may give rise to chronic joint disease such as arthritis (11).

Foodborne illness is typically due to ingestion of contaminated *animal* products, yet *plant* foods may be implicated as a result of airborne, water, soil, or insect contamination when they are grown or raised. The FDA classifies foods that support the growth of microorganisms as **potentially hazardous foods (phf)**, defined as follows:

(a) "Potentially hazardous food" means a FOOD that is natural or synthetic and that requires temperature control because it is in a form capable of supporting:

  (i) The rapid and progressive growth of infectious or toxigenic microorganisms;

  (ii) The growth and toxin production of *Clostridium botulinum,* or

  (iii) In shell eggs, the growth of *Salmonella enteritidis*

(b) "Potentially hazardous food" includes an animal FOOD (a FOOD of animal origin) that is raw or heat-treated; a FOOD of plant origin that is heat-treated or consists of raw seed sprouts; cut melons; and garlic and oil mixtures that are not acidified or otherwise modified

(c) "Potentially hazardous food" does not include:

  (i) An air-cooled hard boiled egg with shell intact;

  (ii) A FOOD with a WATER ACTIVITY (A_w) value of 0.85 or less;

  (iii) A FOOD with a pH level of 4.6 or below when measured at 75°F (24°C);

  (iv) A FOOD, in an unopened HERMETICALLY SEALED CONTAINER, that is commercially processed to achieve and maintain commercial sterility under conditions of nonrefrigerated storage and distribution; and

  (v) A FOOD for which laboratory evidence demonstrates that rapid and progressive growth of infectious and toxigenic microorganisms or the growth of *S. enteritidis* in eggs or *C. botulinum* cannot occur, such as a food that has an A_w and a pH that are above the levels specified above that may contain a preservative, or other barriers to growth

---

(vi) A FOOD that may contain an infectious or toxigenic microorganism or chemical, physical contaminant at a level sufficient to cause illness, but that does not support the growth of microorganisms as specified in the definition of potentially hazardous food.

Some examples of potentially hazardous foods are products that contain

- meat
- poultry
- eggs
- milk
- fish

- shellfish
- some synthetic ingredients
- tofu
- baked potatoes
- cut melon

BIOLOGICAL (MICROBIOLOGICAL) HAZARDS TO THE FOOD SUPPLY

Biological hazards that cause foodborne illness include microorganisms such as bacteria, viruses, fungi, and parasites. These may be small in size, but can cause serious foodborne illness or death. They are controlled by the following:

Temperature—adequate cooking, cooling, refrigeration, freezing, and handling of food

The avoidance of cross-contamination

Enforcement of *personal hygiene* among food handlers

Bacteria—The Major Biological Foodborne Illness

Of the microbiological hazards, *bacteria* are the primary organism implicated in foodborne disease and are, therefore, the primary microbial concern of many consumers, food processor microbiologists and others who are responsible for producing safe food. For example, microbiologists want to reduce the number of bacteria in a population, or the bacterial load in production environments, which can double in number every 20 min. Such reduction decreases the risk of foodborne illness and lengthens shelf life.

The bacteria cause foodborne illnesses by 1) *infection*, 2) *intoxication*, or 3) *toxin-mediated infection*. Some definitions of these types of illness appear as follows:

Foodborne **infection** results from ingesting *living*, pathogenic bacteria such as *Salmonella*, *Listeria monocytogenes*, or *Shigella* (see Figure 16.1).

> Foodborne **intoxication** results if a preformed *toxin* (poison) is ingested, such as that produced by *Staphylococcus aureus*, *Clostridium botulinum*, and *Bacillus cereus*, is present in the food (Figure 16.1).
>
> A **toxin-mediated infection** is caused by ingestion of *living*, infection-causing bacteria such as *C. perfringens* and *E. coli* O157:H7 that also produce a **toxin** in the intestine (Figures 16.1 and 16.3).

The Educational Foundation of the National Restaurant Association has compiled data on the most common **pathogenic**, or disease-causing bacteria in foods (12). In Figure 16.1, the bacteria name, incubation period, duration of illness, symptoms, reservoir, foods implicated, and means of prevention in foods are presented. An astute manager of a food manufacturing operation (as well as the consumer at home!) understands the benefit of having this knowledge, and applying this food safety information to their own food products. It promotes customer goodwill and prevents foodborne illness.

Major foodborne diseases of bacterial origin

	Salmonellosis Infection	Shigellosis Infection	Listeriosis Infection	Staphyloccal Intoxication	Clostridium Perfringens Toxin Mediated Infection	Bacillus Cereus Intoxication	Botulism Intoxication
Bacteria	*Salmonella* (facultative)	*Shigella* (facultative)	*Listeria monocytogenes* (reduced oxygen)	*Staphylococcus aureus* (facultative)	*Clostridium perfringens* (anaerobic)	*Bacillus cereus* (facultative)	*Clostiridium botulinum* (anaerobic)
Incubation Period	6–72 hours	1–7 days	1 day to 3 weeks	1–6 hours	8–22 hours	1/2–5 hours; 8–16 hours	12–36 hours + 72
Duration of Illness	2–3 days	Indefinite, depends on treatment	Indefinite, depends on treatment, but has high fatality in the immuno-compromised	24–48 hours	24 hours	6–24 hours; 12 hours	Several days to a year
Symptoms	Abdominal pain, headache, nausea, vomiting, fever, diarrhea	Diarrhea, fever, chills, lassitude, dehydration	Nausea, vomiting, headache, fever, chills, backache, meningitis	Nausea, vomiting, diarrhea, dehydration	Abdominal pain, diarrhea	Nausea and vomiting; diarrhea, abdominal cramps	Vertigo, visual disturbances, inability to swallow, respiratory paralysis
Reservoir	Domestic and wild animals; also humans, especially as carriers	Human feces, flies	Humans, domestic and wild animals, fowl, soil, water, mud	Humans (skin, nose, throat, infected sores); also, animals	Humans (intestinal tract), animals, and soil	Soil and dust	Soil, water
Foods Implicated	Poultry and poultry salads, meat and meat products, milk, shell eggs, egg custards and sauces, and other protein foods	Potato, tuna, shrimp, turkey and macaroni salads, lettuce, moist and mixed foods	Unpasteurized milk and cheese, vegetables, poultry and meats, seafood, and prepared, chilled, ready-to-eat foods	Warmed-over foods, ham and other meats, dairy products, custards, potato salad, cream-filled pastries, and other protein foods	Meat that has been boiled, steamed, braised, stewed or roasted at low temperature for a long period of time, or cooled slowly before serving	Rice and rice dishes, custards, seasonings, dry food mixes, spices, puddings, cereal products, sauces, vegetable dishes, meat loaf	Improperly processed canned goods of low-acid foods, garlic-in-oil products, grilled onions, stews, meat/poultry loaves
Spore Former	No	No	No	No	Yes	Yes	Yes
Prevention	Avoid cross-contamination, refrigerate food, cool cooked meats and meat products properly, avoid fecal contamination from foodhandlers by practicing good personal hygiene	Avoid cross-contamination, avoid fecal contamination from foodhandlers by practicing good personal hygiene, use sanitary food and water sources, control flies	Use only pasteurized milk and dairy products, cook foods to proper temperatures, avoid cross-contamination	Avoid contamination from bare hands, exclude sick foodhandlers from food preparation and serving, practice good personal hygiene, practice sanitary habits, proper heating and refrigeration of food	Use careful time and temperature control in cooling and reheating cooked meat dishes and products	Use careful time and temperature control and quick chilling methods to cool foods, hold hot foods above 140°F (60°C), reheat leftovers to 165°F (74°C)	Do not use home-canned products, use careful time and temperature control for sous-vide items and all large, bulky foods keep sous-vide packages refrigerated, purchase garlic-in-oil in small quantities for immediate use, cook onions only on request

FIGURE 16.1   Major foodborne diseases of bacterial origin
(*Source*: Reprinted with permission form *Applied Foodservice Sanitation: A Certification Coursebook, Fourth Edition*, © 1992, The Educational Foundation of the Naitonal Restaurant Association).

As is the case of bacteria in general, the bacteria causing foodborne illness need the following elements for growth:

- **protein** (or sufficient nutrients),

- **moisture** [water activity (A_w) above 0.85],

- **pH** (above pH of 4.5, generally neutral—pH 7),

- **oxygen** if aerobic, and

- a general **temperature** 40–140°F (4–60°C), the **temperature danger zone** (TDZ).

(Consult local jurisdiction for specific temperature requirements)

Bacterial growth is portrayed in Figure 16.2. Bacteria vary in their temperature requirements—e.g., they may be thermophiles (high temperatures needed for survival), mesophiles, or psychotrophs [cooler temperatures of 50–70°F (10–20°C) requirements]. They vary in their nutrient needs, and nutrient availablility. When bacteria are in the TDZ, they remain in the LAG phase of bacterial growth for approximately 4 hours, generally with no increase in number.

Bacterial growth curve

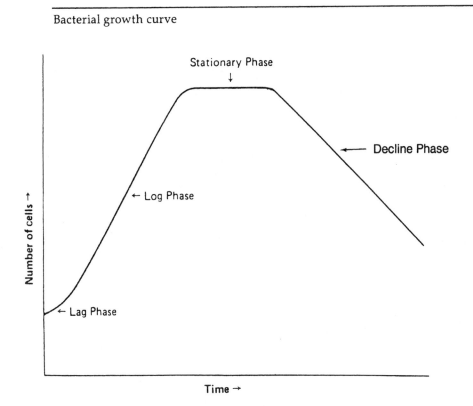

FIGURE 16.2   Bacterial growth curve
(*Source:* Reprinted with permission from *Applied Foodservice Sanitation: A Certification Coursebook,* 4th ed., © 1992, The Educational Foundation of the National Restaurant Association).

Then, after the LAG phase, the unicellular structure undergoes binary fission, and rapid growth in phfs. This rapid growth or multiplication of bacteria is termed the LOG (logarithmic) phase of bacterial growth. It is followed by the STATIONARY phase, where growth rates approximate death rates and there is no net change in the number of pathogens in the food, and, subsequently, by the DECLINE phase of bacterial growth, where the level of bacteria is reduced.

It is important to recognize the fact that although the end of the DECLINE phase may contain *less* than the original amount of bacteria that were present in the food, it may contain *more* harmful waste products or toxins that cannot be destroyed by cooking. In addition to toxins, the two *Clostridium* bacteria, and *Bacillus cereus* may contain **spores**, the highly resistant formations in bacterium that remain in food, even after vegetative cells are destroyed.

As mentioned, this makes *prevention* of food contamination the primary defense against foodborne illness. A careful time–temperature control of potentially hazardous food is required. Refrigeration, for example, slows growth while freezing halts growth. (Temperatures important to controlling foodborne illness in particular foods such as milk, eggs, and meats are found in appropriate chapters of this text.) The CDC reports that it is improper cooling that is the number one cause of foodborne illness.

Temperature control is better assured with the use of temperature indicators, including the pop-up type that is used for the traditional holiday turkey, and now present in a wide array of products. For example, The Food Temperature Indicator Association works with the USDA and food manufacturers to conduct studies

	Campylobacteriosis Infection	E. coli 0157: H7 Infection/Intoxication	Norwalk Virus Illness
Pathogen	*Campylobacter jejuni*	*Escherichia coli*	Norwalk and Norwalk-like viral agent
Incubation period	3–5 days	12–72 hours	24–48 hours
Duration of illness	1–4 days	1–3 days	24–48 hours
Symptoms	Diarrhea, fever, nausea, abdominal pain, headache	Bloody diarrhea; severe abdominal pain, nausea, vomiting, diarrhea, and occasionally fever	Nausea, vomiting, diarrhea, abdominal pain, headache, and low-grade fever
Reservoir	Domestic and wild animals	Humans (intestinal tract); animals, particularly cattle	Humans (intestinal tract)
Foods implicated	Raw vegetables, unpasteurized milk and dairy products, poultry, pork, beef, and lamb	Raw and undercooked beef and other red meats, imported cheeses, unpasteurized milk, raw finfish, cream pies, mashed potatoes, and other prepared foods	Raw vegetables, prepared salads, raw shellfish, and water contaminated from human feces
Spore former	No	No	No
Prevention	Avoid cross-contamination, cook foods thoroughly	Cook beef and red meats thoroughly, avoid cross-contamination, use safe food and water supplies, avoid fecal contamination from foodhandlers by practicing good personal hygiene	Use safe food and water supplies, avoid fecal contamination from foodhandlers by practicing good personal hygiene, thoroughly cook foods

FIGURE 16.3 Emerging pathogens that cause foodborne illness
(*Source:* Reprinted with permission from *Applied Foodservice Sanitation: A Certification Coursebook,* 4th ed., © 1992, The Educational Foundation of the National Restaurant Association).

regarding temperature and food safety. Specialized timers indicate doneness for a variety of meats and fish.

Today, the USDA's Food Safety and Inspection Service (FSIS) requires that establishments slaughtering cattle, chicken, swine and turkeys, test specifically for bacteria *Es. coli*. They must verify the adequacy of process controls for the prevention and removal of fecal contamination and associated bacteria. Additionally, the FSIS has extended such testing to establishments that slaughter species including ducks, equines, geese, goats, guineas, and sheep. The USDA also has an interest in reduction of the incidence of *Listeria*-related foodborne disease. The *Listeria monocytogenes* is an infectious bacterium that grows in a reduced oxygen environment. Significant legislation may require processors to test for this bacterium on areas (e.g., equipment, floors) near meat products in plants.

Understanding of the Listeria genome has been pursued by the USDA, Agricultural Research Service, who says research information is critical to regulatory their agencies such as FSIS. Regulations for safe processing and handling of ready-to-eat foods are created according to this research. Genome study and vaccines for culprits such as *Salmonella* and E. coli 0157:H7 are underway.

Viruses

In addition to bacteria, although with lesser incidence, *viruses* may also be responsible for an unsafe food supply and foodborne illness. A virus does not multiply in food, as do bacteria, but can remain in food if it is insufficiently cooked and, subsequently, infect individuals who ingest it. It is possible for spot contamination of food to occur, so that only those individuals consuming the contaminated portion of the food become ill.

A virus of concern to the consumer, or a food processing and handling operation, is the *Hepatitis A* virus. A person will become infected with the virus 15–50 days following ingestion of a contaminated product and will shed the virus, contaminating other people or food *prior* to displaying symptoms of illness. Although the actual infection may last several *weeks* or *months* and exhibit symptoms such as abdominal pain, jaundice, and nausea, there are possible *widespread* and *long-lasting* financial implications of this illness to the business that is responsible for its spread.

Two sources of the *Hepatitis A* virus are: 1) raw shellfish from polluted water where sewage is discarded, and 2) feces and urine of infected persons. Therefore, the growth and harvesting of raw shellfish (clams, oysters, mussels) is controlled by the FDA, which regulates the water-beds from which shellfish is harvested. Unreputable suppliers may obtain their shellfish supply from "off-limits" contaminated water, thus harvesting a contaminated product. Also, a tag must appear on commercial fresh shellfish to show its source, and it needs to be retained by the receiver for 90 days.

Feces and *urine* of infected persons who practice poor personal hygiene may also be a source of the *Hepatitis A* virus. Thus consumers at home, and food handlers in food processing or assembly operations, must practice good personal hygiene because even minute amounts of feces may spot contaminate food, causing foodborne illness. *Some* state or local health department jurisdictions require the use of disposable gloves by food handlers responsible for handling food that is not subject to further cooking.

This *Hepatitis A* is of major concern, but is controlled by harvesting from FDA-approved water-beds, by following Good Manufacturing Practices (GMPs) that include strict personal hygiene after using the restroom, and proper cooking. Another virus of concern to the consumer and food processing operation is *HIV*. The CDC states that there is no evidence that this can be transmitted by food.

Fungi

Mold and yeast are *fungi* that may be responsible for spoilage in the food supply.

Mold.   Mold is not known to cause gastrointestinal distress. Rather, it has been implicated in other long-term illness, such as liver cancer, in animals that have been fed moldy crops, and it obviously causes *food spoilage*. Mold is a multicellular fungus that reproduces by *spore* formation. After spores form they are then dispersed through the air, replicating when in contact with food. Mold is a common source of food spoilage. It is the unwanted blue, green, white, and black fuzzy growth on food but may be considered acceptable in medicine such as penicillin, or some cheeses such as blue cheese. A small percent of persons may fatally suffer from allergies to molds.

Yeast.   Yeast is a unicellular structure that grows by the budding process. It causes food *spoilage*, as is evidenced by the formation of pink patches on moist cheeses, or cloudy liquid in condiment (such as olives) jars. Foodborne yeast has *not* been shown to cause *illness*, but, nonetheless, undesirable growth must be controlled, or food is wasted. Yeast it is generally shown to have *beneficial* uses in the food industry such as when it leavens baked products or is used in fermentation to produce alcoholic beverages.

Parasites

Parasites are tiny organisms that depend on living hosts for their nourishment and life. Undercooked pork products may carry the parasite *Trichinella spiralis*, which causes the disease trichinosis. Two days to 28 days following ingestion of the *Trichinella* parasite, an individual may exhibit nausea, vomiting, abdominal pain, and swelling of tissue surrounding the eye. Fever and muscular stiffness then develop. Pork may be contaminated with this parasite; therefore, all pork products must be cooked to 155°F (68°C) [or 170°F (77°C) if cooked in a microwave oven], and all equipment used in its preparation should be sanitized.

Fish from unapproved sources may result in the parasitic disease, anisakiasis, caused by the parasite *Anisakis*. Reliable suppliers to processing plants are the best assurance that the product has been handled, or even frozen for the correct time and temperature needed to kill *Anisakis*. When fish is purchased with the intention of being served raw, the freezing process is important for parasite control.

Contamination, Spoilage

In reviewing illness that results from the microbiological hazards, it must be known that "bad" food is not always apparent to the eye. It is the ingestion of *unseen* microorganisms in **contaminated** food (which contains impure or harmful substances), moreso than the consumption of **spoiled** food, with *visible* damage to the eating quality of food, that is the primary cause of foodborne illness. Any chance of initial contamination should be prevented, and then subsequent growth controlled in order to maintain food safety. **Cross-contamination**, or the transfer of germs from one contaminated food or place to another by hands, equipment, or other foods should be avoided.

In addition to those pathogens mentioned, there is the possibility of contamination by **emerging pathogens**. Their incidence has increased within the last few years or they threaten to increase in the near future.

CHEMICAL HAZARDS TO THE FOOD SUPPLY

All food is made of chemicals and is expected to be safe for consumption (13). A **chemical hazard** to the food supply occurs when dosage levels of specific chemicals reach toxic levels. Chemical contamination includes *accidental* chemical contamination, such as when contents of a container, perhaps unlabeled, are mistakenly used in food. As well, excessive quantities of *additives* become problematic if an individual has a specific allergy. Also, included in the list of chemical hazards, are *toxic metals*. They may be used as a container for beverages, as a temporary working surface, or in shelving, and can contaminate food. *Naturally occurring toxins* in some foods such as the puffer fish may cause severe illness.

Control of chemical hazards prior to receipt or use, and control in inventory, storage, and handling are identified in Table 16.1. Care must be taken to avoid chemical hazards.

PHYSICAL HAZARDS TO THE FOOD SUPPLY

Physical hazards to the food supply are any foreign objects found in food that may contaminate it. Certainly, they are unwanted by the consumer! They may be present

TABLE 16.1 Control of Chemical Hazards

I. *Control before receipt*. Raw material specifications; vendor certification/guarantees; spot checks—verification

II. *Control before use*. Review purpose for use of chemical; ensure proper purity, formulation, and labeling; Control quantities used

III. *Control storage and handling conditions*. Prevent conditions conducive to production of naturally occurring toxicants

IV. *Inventory all chemicals in facility*. Review uses; records of use

Source: Ref. 14.

due to harvesting, or some phase of manufacturing, or they may be intrinsic to the food, such as bones in fish, pits in fruits, eggshells, and insects or insect parts. Animals or crops grown in open fields are subject to physical contamination, although, hazards may enter the food supply due to a variety of incidences that range from faulty machinery, to packaging wraps, to human error. An astute manager prevents the chance of physical contamination by following good manufacturing practices, and using his/her observational skills.

The main materials of concern as physical hazards include foreign objects such as glass, wood, metal, plastic, stones, insects and other filth, insulation, bones, and personal effects (14) (Table 16.2). Modern optical scanning technologies are capable of sorting difficult, potential problem products and are designed to minimize such contamination at the processing plant. Devices such as screen, filters, magnets, and metal detectors may be used on-line or throughout the manufacturing plant to search for foreign objects, and avert health disasters or product recalls. X-ray units are reliable in detecting a variety of objects (Figures 16.4 and 16.5).

Personal effects, such as jewelry, may not be worn in the production areas. Rules such as "no gum chewing" and "cover hair" need to be enforced in the workplace.

Physical hazards may harm a consumer's health, cause psychological trauma, or dissatisfaction. Ill, upset, or dissatisfied consumers may call or write to the responsible processor, contact the food-service establishment, or involve the local health department in investigating their complaint. Any chance of physical objects getting into the food supply should be prevented.

Foreign substance laboratories in food manufacturing companies as well as personnel in food service establishments need to look out for, and be informed of any

TABLE 16.2 Main Materials of Concern as Physical Hazards and Common Sources

Material	Injury Potential	Sources
Glass	Cuts, bleeding; may require surgery to find or remove	Bottles, jars, light fixtures, utensils, gauge covers
Wood	Cuts, infection, choking; may require surgery to remove	Fields, pallets, boxes, buildings
Stones	Choking, broken teeth	Fields, buildings
Metal	Cuts, infection; may require surgery to remove	Machinery, fields, wire, employees
Insects, other filth	Illness, trauma, choking	Fields, plant postprocess entry
Insulation	Choking, long-term if asbestos	Building materials
Bone	Choking, trauma	Fields, improper plant processing
Plastic	Choking, cuts, infection; may require surgery to remove	Fields, plant packaging materials, pallets, employees
Personal effects	Choking, cuts, broken teeth; may require surgery to remove	Employees

Source: Ref. 9. Adaptation from Corlett (1991).

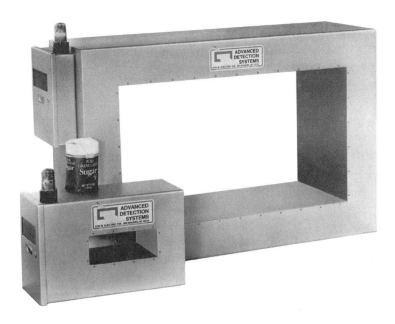

FIGURE 16.4 Metal detector
(*Source:* Advanced Detection Systems).

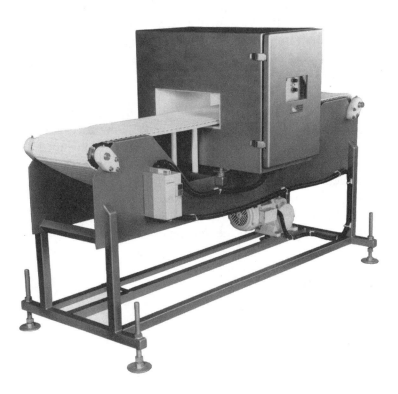

FIGURE 16.5 Metal detector
(*Source:* Advanced Detection Systems).

reported food safety problems—chemical or physical, so that they may investigate and prevent possible problems. Consumers benefit from this prevention and incidences of contamination are reduced.

FOOD PROTECTION SYSTEMS

Many agency names appear in this section of text addressing food protection systems. While the listing may be lengthy, the names actually represent only a portion of the many *groups* responsible for the United States' food safety—considered the safest in the world. As well, *individuals* such as you and I could be added to the list!

The CDC, FDA, the USDA's FSIS, and state and county health departments have regulatory authority for food protection, and they provide education to the public. There are also numerous trade associations and professional organizations involved in providing education and protecting the public from foodborne illness. Examples of these associations and organizations include The American Dietetic Association (ADA), National Center for Nutrition and Dietetics (NCND), American Public Health Association (APHA), Association of Food and Drug Officials (AFDO), Cooperative Extension Service (CES), Council for Agriculture Science and Technology (CAST), Food Marketing Institute (FMI), Institute of Food Technologists (IFT), International Association of Milk, Food, and Environmental Sanitarians (IAMFES), International Food Manufacturers Association (IFMA), International Council of Hotel and Restaurant Industry Educators (CHRIE), National Environmental Health Association (NEHA), National Sanitation Foundation (NSF), and The Educational Foundation of the National Restaurant Association (NRA).

In 1998, a federal, interagency group was created in the U.S. to improve the safety of the food supply. This President's Council on Food Safety (PCFS) was composed of departments such as The Department of Agriculture, Commerce, Health and Human Services, Management and Budget. It also included the Environmental Protection Agency. A coordination of inspection, enforcement, and research was made possible, as was food safety education.

Food companies also maintain extensive food protection systems. When food companies were asked to rank the areas of food science that they thought were most important, safety concerns were reported in the ranking as follows:

1. Developing healthy foods
2. Nutraceutical or medical foods
3. *Food safety* from a process standpoint
4. Developing "natural" foods
5. *Food safety* from an ingredient selection point of view
6. Organic food development
7. Reduced fat/altered lipids development
8. Methods development for quality control (14)

Eliminating or reducing the biological, chemical, and physical hazards to the food supply is the goal of food safety. In the quest to destroy pathogens, for example, the FDA approved irradiation of meat in 1997, as it was shown to yield safer meat than meat that is *not* irradiated (15). Irradiation, both *off-site* and *on-line* is also being utilized as a means of food safety for a wide array of food items (16). Such treatment of refrigerated or frozen raw meat and meat products (e.g., sausages, bologna) was approved in the year 2000. Additionally, high-pressure *processing* (e.g., 20,000–80,000 p.s.i and higher) is used for food products such as guacamole, meats, and seafood processing, including raw oysters. High-pressure *sterilization* is being considered (17) for added food safety.

Although they do not provide *real-time* information, processing plants may use *statistical analysis* to define acceptable upper and lower control limits, and then use this information to improve product quality. Statistical Process Control (SPC) provides advances in microbiological analyses that in turn, will allow the manufacturing process to integrate testing with quality improvement and productivity (18). SPC may also be integrated with the Hazard Analysis and Critical Control Point (HACCP) method of food safety (discussed below).

In addition to this *manufacturing* concern, many *food service operations* have sent at least one manager to local training in Food Protection Management. Many news shows and magazines have addressed the issue of food safety for consumers.

THE HACCP SYSTEM OF FOOD PROTECTION

In order to reduce foodborne illness risks from biological, chemical, or physical hazards, the Hazard Analysis and Critical Control Point—**HACCP** (pronounced hassip)—system of food safety may be required for use by food processors and foodservice operations (Table 16.3). The system depends upon *prevention*, rather than *inspection*. In fact, the "Mega-Reg" or *Pathogen Reduction: Hazard Analysis and Critical Control Point (HACCP) System regulation*, was signed by the U.S. President in 1996. It codified principles for the prevention and reduction of pathogens, and required both the development of Sanitation Standard Operating Procedures (SSOPs), and a written HACCP plan that is monitored and verified by inspectors of meat and poultry processing plants. Compliance deadlines were phased in, depending upon the size of the company.

In the plan, the FSIS tests raw livestock and poultry in the slaughtering processes for *Salmonella*, and plants are required to test for E. *coli*. Seafood HACCP became effective in 1997. Juice processors must have HACCP. Later, HACCP plans for protection against L. *monocytogenes* in ready-to-eat meat products were required by the FSIS. Currently, egg processors, as well as dairy plants, and additional industries where it is not required have implemented HACCP.

HACCP traces the flow of food from entry into an operation through customer purchase. It does more than *detect and correct* errors after they have occurred; it is a program that *prevents* errors regarding food safety. Thus, it more quality assurance than quality control.

TABLE 16.3 Steps of a Hazard Analysis and Critical Control Point (HACCP) Program

I. Assessing the hazards
Hazards are assessed at each step in the flow of food throughout an operation.

II. Identifying critical control points (CCPs)
Identify CCPs regarding hygiene, avoiding cross-contamination, and temperatures and procedures for cooking and cooling. A flowchart of preparation steps is developed, showing where monitoring is necessary to prevent, reduce, or eliminate hazards.

III. Setting up control procedures and standards for critical control points
Establish standards (criteria) for each CCP and measurable procedures such as specific times and temperatures, moisture and pH levels, and observable procedures such as hand washing.

IV. Monitoring critical control points
Checking to see if criteria are met is one of the most crucial steps in the process. Assigning an employee to monitoring temperatures of storage, cooking, holding, and cooling are necessary to see if controls against hazards are in place.

V. Taking corrective action
Observe if there is a deviation between actual and expected results. Correct the procedures by using an alternate plan if a deficiency or high-risk situation is identified in using the original procedure. This may be accomplished by a trained employee empowered to initiate corrective action without a supervisor being present.

VI. Develop a record-keeping system to document haccp
Time–temperature logs, flowcharts, and observations are used for record-keeping.

VII. Verify that the system is working
Make use of time and temperature logs completed during preparation, holding, or cooling. Observe.

HACCP was originally designed by the Pillsbury Company, in cooperation with Natick Laboratories of the U.S. Army, and the U.S. Air Force Space Laboratory Project Group. The system was designed for use by the National Aeronautics and Space Administration (NASA) Program. HACCP has been used as a food safety system in the food industry since 1971, and it offers practical food protection techniques that are needed anywhere food is prepared or served.

The National Advisory Committee for Microbiological Criteria for Foods (NACMCF) (20) has identified seven major steps involved in the HACCP system (Table 16.3). HACCP can be used in *multiple spots* within the food chain; for example, in growing, harvesting, processing, preparing, or serving of foods.

A written HACCP plan (21) is based on the principles of HACCP and delineates the procedures to be followed to assure the control of a specific process or procedure. A HACCP team (22) is responsible for developing an HACCP plan, and as a result of implementing the HACCP *plan*, the company has an HACCP *system* (Table 16.4).

Using the HACCP system, the HACCP team must first identify potentially hazardous foods that are prepared in their operation. Then, they must observe the flow

TABLE 16.4 Selected HACCP Definitions (Health and Human Service)

- *Control point:* Any point, step, or procedure at which biological, physical, or chemical factors can be controlled.
- *Corrective action:* Procedures to be followed when a deviation occurs.
- *Critical control point* (CCP): A point, step, or procedure at which control can be applied and a food safety hazard can be prevented, eliminated, or reduced to acceptable levels.
- *Critical limit:* A criterion that must be met for each preventive measure associated with a critical control point.
- *Deviation:* Failure to meet a critical limit.
- *HACCP Plan:* The written document which is based on the principles of HACCP and which delineates the procedures to be followed to assure the control of a specific process or procedure.
- *HACCP system:* The result of the implementation of the HACCP plan.
- *HACCP team:* The group of people who are responsible for developing an HACCP plan.
- *Hazard:* A biological, chemical, or physical property that may cause a food to be unsafe for consumption.
- *Monitor:* To conduct a planned sequence of observations or measurements to assess whether a CCP is under control and to produce an accurate record for future use in verification.
- *Risk:* An estimate of the likely occurrence of a hazard.
- *Sensitive ingredient:* An ingredient known to have been associated with a hazard and for which there is reason for concern.
- *Verification:* The use of methods, procedures, or tests in addition to those used in monitoring to determine if the HACCP system is in compliance with the HACCP plan and/or whether the HACCP plan is working.

of potentially hazardous foods from the acquisition of raw ingredients to completion of the finished product, especially studying the flow of sensitive ingredients known to have been associated with a hazard and for which there is a reason for concern. This observation leads to the development of a flowchart (Figures 16.6–16.9).

After identifying those foods that are potentially hazardous, and creating a flowchart, management needs to identify specific, measurable Critical Control Points (CCPs). In the absence of CCPs, food is subject to unacceptable risks or likelihood of a hazard. Next, control procedures and criteria for critical limits must be established and then monitored by individual assigned responsibility for tracking CCP procedures. The CCPs may include temperature of the food product and processing equipment; time of processing, package integrity, and more. Measurements and observational skills are employed in order to reveal any unacceptable *deviations* between *actual* and *expected* results that may require corrective action in order to prevent foodborne illness.

With the establishment of an HACCP Program, new terminology may be used; some selected HACCP definitions are given in Table 16.4.

Food *manufacturers* must ensure that food is safe, and in fact, only a small percentage of all foodborne illness cases is linked to poor processing practices.

HAZARD ANALYSIS CRITICAL CONTROL POINT FLOW PROCESS
FOOD: CHICKEN SALAD

FLOW PROCESS	CCP	CRITERIA FOR CONTROL	MONITOR & VERIFY	ACTION TO TAKE IF CRITERIA NOT MET
Receive refrigerated whole chickens		- Maximum 45°F internal temperature	- Take internal meat temperature with metal stem thermometer	- Reject product
Store in Walk-in-Cooler (WIC)		- Maximum 45°F internal temperature - Store chickens off floor - Prevent cross-contamination - Air temperature 40°F or less	- Observe proper storage practices - Monitor air temperature each shift-record on log	- Store chicken in approved manner - Lower air temperature
Boil chickens	CCP	- Minimum 165°F internal temperature of meat	- Take internal meat temperature - Observe cooking time	- Cook chicken until temperature is reached
Cool to debone (30 minutes in WIC)		- Do not cover chickens	- Observe storage in WIC	- Store chicken to allow rapid cooling to debone
Debone/dice chicken meat	CCP	- Clean hands or gloves used to handle meat - No infected wounds or bandages on hands - Wash and sanitize equipment used after completion	- Observe handling procedures - Inspect employee hands daily - Observe proper cleaning of equipment	- Instruct workers to wash hands or use gloves - Remove worker or require gloves - Have equipment rewashed
Mix ingredients (mayo, sour cream, relish, spices, meat)		- Use utensils for mixing - Limit time for preparation of meat salad - refrigerate when completed - Use refrigerated ingredients	- Observe use of utensils - Measure time to complete preparation process - Observe use	- Correct practice - Modify procedures to limit time at room temperature - Change practice
Store 1/3 of salad in prep cooler Store 2/3 of salad in WIC (Use 1/2 each day at prep cooler)	CCP	- Cool to 45°F within 4 hours after preparation - Maximum 45°F internal temperature in storage - Store salad 3 inches or less in pans - Air temperature 40°F or less	- Measure salad temperature periodically to determine cooling rate - Take internal temperature - Measure depth of salad stored in pans - Monitor air temperature each shift - record on log	- Remove excess salad from pan - Lower air temperature - Store in coolest part of cooler
Sell				
Discard after 3 days from preparation		- Old salad not mixed with fresh salad - Discard remaining salad	- Observe storage process - Observe salad discarded	- Correct practice - Discard salad

wssschickens.cur

FIGURE 16.6   HACCP Flow Process. Food: Chicken Salad
(Source: Alvin Black, R.S. City of Farmers Branch, Environmental Health Division. Farmers Branch, TX)

The greater number of cases are the result of faulty practices in *foodservice operations* and the *home*.

Many state and local health departments have adopted rules for *foodservice establishments*, requiring knowledge of foodborne illness and HACCP principles. These foodservice establishments include hospitals, restaurants, retail grocery stores, and schools. An example of HACCP plans for foodservice operations are shown for chicken salad and BBQ beef ribs in Figures 16.6 and 16.7. An example of HACCP programs appears in the literature for *supermarkets* (23) and the assessment of HACCP by meat and poultry companies (24).

A view of the headings on the chicken salad and ribs HACCP indicate several major concepts. First, the *flow process* of foods from the point of receiving food until it is discarded is drawn, secondly, the *CCPs* are identified, and then, *criteria for control* are established and briefly stated for ease of understanding. Criteria for control specify such factors as minimum and maximum temperatures that must be reached, correct storage procedures, instructions for personal hygiene and equipment sanitation, and discard rules.

Next, *monitoring and verifying* the HACCP program includes instructions to follow for assurance of compliance with criteria. It may be taking temperatures, measuring time to complete preparation, measuring depth of storage pans, or observing procedures that are used in preparation or storage. The entire HACCP process also states the *action to be taken if the criteria are not met*.

In *receiving* of chicken for chicken salad, for example, the corrective action to take if established criteria are not met, would be to reject the products upon delivery. In *storage,* the product may require a lower air temperature if the established criteria for maximum temperature were not met. A further criteria on requires that chicken reach a minimum temperature of 165°F (74°C) when boiled, and if it does not, it must be cooked until that temperature is reached. The HACCP continues with corresponding action to take for each criteria, if the criteria is not met, and includes corrective practices for handling, personal hygiene, equipment sanitation, food storage, and discarding.

In addition to the HACCP Flow Process charts in Figures 16.6 and 16.7, samples of two written *recipes* that incorporate the HACCP principles appear in Figures 16.8 and 16.9. These recipes demonstrate ways in which a foodservice operation may include CCPs in preparation steps and flowcharts. For example, an acceptable method of defrosting, cooking, and holding is stated after labeling the preparation step as a CCP, and CCPs are highlighted in the flowcharts.

HACCP systems require that a designated individual using reliable tools/instruments must monitor the CCPs. The reliability of instruments such as thermometers or thermocouples must be validated.

Identifying such items as the flow process of food, stating CCPs and criteria for control, monitoring and verifying, and specifying action to take if the criteria are not met, all function to assist management in controlling the spread of disease. Applying an HACCP system to food manufacturing or foodservice operation is an effective means of reducing the likelihood of foodborne illness.

HAZARD ANALYSIS CRITICAL CONTROL POINT FLOW PROCESS
FOOD: BBQ RIBS

FLOW PROCESS	CCP	CRITERIA FOR CONTROL	MONITOR & VERIFY	ACTION TO TAKE IF CRITERIA NOT MET
Frozen beef ribs		- Received frozen	- Feel if frozen upon delivery	- Reject if thawed
Thaw in walk-in-cooler (WIC)		- Meat thawed under refrigeration - Store meat off floor - Prevent cross-contamination	- Observe ribs stored in WIC - Observe proper storage practices	- Store ribs properly to prevent contamination or cross-contamination
Cook in oven (add BBQ sauce)	CCP	- Minimum 140°F internal temperature of ribs	- Take internal meat temperature with metal stem thermometer - Observe cooking time and oven temperature	- Cook ribs until temperature is reached
Hold at steam table with overhead heat lamp	CCP	- Minimum 140°F internal temperature	- Take temperature of meat every 2 hours - record on log	- Reheat ribs - Discard ribs if held below 130°F over 2 hours - Check equipment
Sell				
Leftover ribs cooled in WIC overnight	CCP	- Cool from 140° to 45°F within 4 hours - Store meat 3 inches or less in pans - No tight cover during cooling process - Do not stack pans - Store meat close to fans in WIC - Air temperature 40°F or less	- Measure meat temperature periodically to determine cooling rate in WIC - Measure depth of meat stored in pan - Monitor air temperature of WIC each shift-record on log - Observe meat uncovered during cooling process	- Remove excess ribs from pan - Lower air temperature - Remove covers - Eliminate stacking - Move ribs to coolest part of WIC - Discard inadequately cooled ribs
Reheat in convention oven next morning	CCP	- Minimum 165°F internal temperature within 2 hours - Leftovers not mixed with fresh ribs - Discard remaining ribs	- Take internal meat temperature with metal stem thermometer - Observe reheating time and oven temperature - Observe meat discarded	- Reheat meat until temperature is reached - Discard meat
Steam table		- Same instructions as above		
Sell				
Discard by 6:00 p.m.		- Leftovers not mixed with fresh ribs - Discard remaining ribs	- Observe storage process - Observe meat discarded	- Correct practice - Discard meat

FIGURE 16.7   HACCP Flow Process. Food: BBQ Ribs
(*Source:* Alvin Black, R.S. City of Farmers Branch, Environmental Health Division. Farmers Branch, TX)

Basic Beef Chili

Ingredients	Amount	25	50	100
Lean Ground Beef	Lbs	7	14	28
Canned Tomatoes	Qts	1½	3	6
Canned Kidney Beans	Qts	1¾	3½	7
Tomato Paste	Cups	1¾	3½	7
Water	Gals	½	1	2
Dehydrated Onions	Ozs	1	2	4
Chili Powder	Tbsp	3	6	12
Sugar	Tbsp	1¼	2½	5
Cumin	Tbsp	2	4	8
Garlic Powder	Tbsp	1	2	4
Onion Powder	Tbsp	1	2	4
Paprika	Tbsp	1	2	4
Black Pepper	Tbsp	½	1	2

Preparation

1. **CCP** Thaw ground beef under refrigeration (41°F, maximum 1 day).

2. Place ground beef in steam kettle or in large skillet on stove top. Cook meat using medium high heat until lightly browned (15 minutes). While cooking, break meat into crumbs of about ¼" to ¼" pieces.

3. Drain meat well, stirring while draining to remove as much fat as possible. If desired, pour hot water over beef and drain to remove additional fat.

4. Mash or grind canned tomatoes with juice. Add to kettle or stock pot with cooked ground beef. Add remaining ingredients to mixture and stir well.

5. **CCP** Simmer chili mixture for 1 hour, stirring occasionally. Temperature of cooked mixture must register 155°F or higher.

6. Remove from heat and portion into service pans.

7. **CCP** Cover and hold for service (140°F, maximum 1 hour).

8. Portion: 1 cup (8 ounces) per serving

Service:

1. **CCP** Maintain temperature of finished product above 140°F during entire service period. Keep covered whenever possible. Take and record temperature of unserved product every 30 minutes. Maximum holding time, 4 hours.

Storage:

1. **CCP** Transfer unserved product into clean, 2-inch deep pans. Quick-chill. Cooling temperature of product must be as follows: from 140° to 70°F within 2 hours and then from 70° to 41°F or below, within an additional 4 hour period. Take and record temperature every hour during chill-down.

2. **CCP** Cover, label, and date. Refrigerate at 41°F or lower for up to 10 days (based on quality maintained) or freeze at 0°F for up to 3 months.

Reheating:

1. **CCP** Thaw product under refrigeration, if frozen (41°F).

2. **CCP** Remove from refrigeration, transfer into shallow, 2-inch deep pans and immediately place in preheated 350°F oven, covered. Heat for 30 minutes or until internal temperature reaches 165°F or above.

Discard unused product.

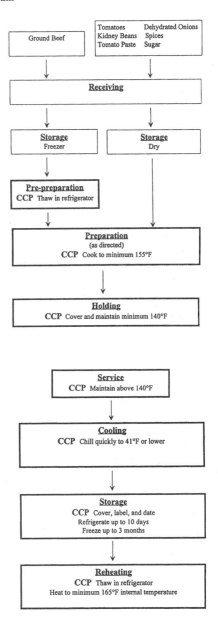

FIGURE 16.8 HACCP. Basic beef chili.
(*Source*: La Vella Food Specialists St. Louis, MO).

"In a nutshell, HACCP (pronounced hassip) is a preventive system that identifies, monitors, and controls to ensure food safety by preventing or reducing the likelihood of foodborne illness. To achieve this, every member of an organization in which food items are a factor must be informed and involved.

Chicken Stew

Ingredients	Amount	25	50	100
Chicken Pieces, 8 cut, frozen	Lbs	10	20	40
Carrots, fresh, peeled, cut in ¾ inch pieces	Lbs	2½	5	10
Onions, chopped	Qts	½	1	2
Potatoes, peeled, cut into ¾ inch pieces	Lbs	3¾	7½	15
Green Peas, frozen	Lbs	2	4	8
Margarine	Cups	½	1	2
Flour	Cups	1½	3	6
Chicken Stock	Qts	1	2	4
Salt	tsp	1	2	4
Pepper	tsp	1	2	4

Preparation

1. **CCP** Thaw raw chicken pieces under refrigeration (41°F, 1 day).

2. **CCP** Wash carrots, onions, and potatoes under cool running water. Cut as directed. Use immediately in recipe or cover and refrigerate until needed (41°F, maximum 1 day).

3. Place chicken pieces on sheet pans. Cover and bake in preheated 350°F conventional (325°F convection) oven for 30 minutes.

4. Cook potatoes, carrots, and peas separately in steamer or on stovetop, until tender (4–15 minutes).

5. Remove chicken from oven; drain off juices and fat. Place in 4-inch deep steamtable pans, cover, and return to heated oven (while preparing gravy).

6. In stockpot over medium heat, melt margarine and sauté onions until tender. Add flour and stir until smooth. Add chicken drippings, stirring well. Add chicken broth as needed for gravy-like consistency. Season with salt and pepper.

7. Add cooked vegetables and gravy to chicken pieces. Cover, place back in 350°F conventional (325°F convection) oven and bake for 30 minutes or until chicken pieces are tender and sauce is flavorful.

8. **CCP** Internal temperature of cooked stew must register 165°F for 15 seconds at end of cooking process.

9. **CCP** Cover and hold for service (140°F, maximum 1 hour).

10. Portion: 1–2 pieces of chicken, ½ cup vegetables with gravy (10 ounces) per serving

Service:

1. **CCP** Maintain temperature of finished product above 140°F during entire service period. Keep covered whenever possible. Take and record temperature of unserved product every 30 minutes. Maximum holding time, 4 hours.

Storage:

1. **CCP** Transfer unserved product into clean, 2-inch deep pans. Quick-chill. Cooling temperatures of product must be as follows: from 140° to 70°F within 2 hours and then from 70° to 41°F or below, within an additional 4 hours. Take and record temperature every hour during chill-down.

2. **CCP** Cover, label, and date. Refrigerate at 41°F or lower for up to 10 days (based on quality maintained) or freeze at 0°F for up to 3 months.

Reheating:

1. **CCP** Thaw product under refrigeration, if frozen (41°F).

2. **CCP** Remove from refrigeration, transfer into shallow, 2-inch deep pans and immediately place in preheated 350°F oven, covered. Heat for 30 minutes or until internal temperature reaches 165°F or above.

Discard unused product.

Flowchart:

- Carrots / Margarine | Chicken / Green Peas | Onions / Potatoes / Flour / Chicken Stock
- **Receiving**
- **Storage** Refrigerator | **Storage** Freezer | **Storage** Dry
- **Pre-preparation** CCP Clean vegetables under cool, running water; refrigerate | **Pre-preparation** CCP Thaw chicken in
- **Preparation** (as directed) CCP Cook to minimum 165°F internal temperature
- **Holding** CCP Cover and maintain minimum 140°F
- **Service** CCP Maintain above 140°F
- **Cooling** CCP Chill quickly to 41°F or lower
- **Storage** CCP Cover, label, and date Refrigerate up to 10 days Freeze up to 3 months
- **Reheating** CCP Thaw in refrigerator Heat to minimum 165°F internal temperature

FIGURE 16.9 HACCP. Chicken Stew
(*Source*: La Vella Food Specialists St. Louis, MO).

This includes awareness of the existence of pathogenic microorganisms and chemical residue, implementation of proper sanitation measures for physical objects and employee personal hygiene, and avoidance of food supply adulteration and cross contamination at all stages of the distribution, storage, and preparation process'' (25).

Many foods are processed in *manufacturing plants* (Table 16.5) and are distributed to operations such as retail grocery stores, hotels, restaurants, or institutional operations. These foods must provide assurance of food quality, including microbiological (M), chemical (C), and physical (P) safety, and have critical limits, including meeting all safety specifications prior to shipping, measuring temperatures of incoming and chilled ingredients with calibrated instruments, using microbiological tests for food contact surfaces and the environmental area, sanitizing equipment, storing, refrigerating palletizing products, distribution, and labeling.

As a result of testing in large plants over a two-year period, the FSIS reports that there are substantial reductions in the prevalence of *Salmonella* compared to pre-HACCP baseline figures in raw meat and poultry. A 50% decrease was shown in young chicken and swine carcasses, and more than 30% reduction was reported for ground turkey. One year of testing in small plants also showed decreases in *Salmonella*—40% in ground beef, approximately 20% in young chicken carcasses, 15% in cow and bull carcasses, but data showed an increased incidence in swine carcasses (USDA).

A revised HACCP model designed by the Food Safety and Inspection Service (FSIS) has shown improvements in food safety. Young chicken plants have demonstrated a greater achievement of performance standards in FSIS verfication checks over traditional slaughter inspection (FSIS).

SURVEILLANCE FOR FOODBORNE-DISEASE OUTBREAKS

The FDA *estimates* of foodborne diseases have been reported to be in the tens of millions, while the *actual* report of cases to the CDC is in the thousands. Since all illnesses are not reported, the true number is unknown. Below is the most current 5-year surveillance data (26).

Year	Number of outbreaks
1993	489
1994	653
1995	628
1996	477
1997	504

Since 1973, the CDC has maintained surveillance data regarding the occurrence and causes of foodborne-disease outbreaks (FBDOs). Now, the CDC *actively* surveys emerging foodborne diseases. The Foodborne Diseases Active Surveillance Network (FoodNet) is the primary foodborne disease component of the CDC's Emerging Infections Program (EIP). It began in the mid-1990s with five states, and now includes nine states, representing 25.4 million persons (10% of the United States population). FoodNet looks at seven bacteria and viral foodborne pathogens, including *Salmonella, Shigella, Campylobacter, E. coli 0157, L. monocytogenes, Yersinia*

TABLE 16.5 Ingredients of Refrigerated Chicken Salad (Pierson and Corlett)

CCP Number	CCP description	Critical limit(s) description
1-MPC	Hazard controlled: Microbiological, physical, and chemical Point or procedure: Incoming inspection	1.1 Sanitary condition 1.2 Refrig. material < = 45°F 1.3 Frozen material < = 32°F • 1.4 Vendor met all safety specifications before shipping
2-T	Hazard controlled: Microbiological Point or procedure: Refrigerated Ingredient Storage	2.1 Material internal temperature not to exceed 45°F 2.2 Calibrate temperature-measuring devices before shift
3-M	Hazard controlled: Microbiological Point or procedure: Sanitation requirements in • Preparation area • Staging area • Filling/packaging area Hazard controlled: Point or procedure: *Listeria*	3.1 Comply with USDA sanitation requirements 3.2 Sanitation crew trained 3.3 Each area must pass inspection before shift start-up 3.4 Food contact surface: Micro-biological test 3.5 Environmental area: Microbio-logical tests (USDA Methodology for 3.4 and 3.5)
4-M	Hazard controlled: Microbiological Point or procedure: Controlled treatment to reduce microbiological contamina-tion on raw celery and onions	Application of alternative approved treatments 4.1 Wash product with water containing • Chlorine, or • Iodine, or • Surfactants, or • No process additives 4.2 Hot water or steam blanch followed by chilling 4.3 Substitute processed celery or onions: • Blanched frozen • Blanched dehydrated • Blanched canned

(*continued*)

TABLE 16.5 *Continued*

CCP Number	CCP description	Critical limit(s) description
5-M	Hazard controlled: Microbiological Point or procedure: Chilled storage temperature of prepared celery, onions, and chicken	5.1 Not to exceed 45°F 5.2 Refrigerator not to exceed 45°F 5.3 Daily calibration of temperature measuring devices
6-MPC	Hazard controlled: Microbiological, physical, and chemical Point or procedure: Physical barrier to prevent cross-contamination from raw material preparation area	6.1 Physical barrier in place 6.2 Doors kept closed when not in use 6.3 Color-coded uniforms 6.4 Supervision in place
7-M	Hazard controlled: Microbiological Point or procedure: Cross-contami-nation prevention from transfer equipment from raw material area	7.1 Comply with USDA sanitation requirements 7.2 Prevent entry of soiled pallets cart wheels, totes, and other equipment
8-M	Hazard controlled: Microbiological Point or procedure: Time limit for in-process food materials	8.1 Time limit not to exceed 4 hours for any materials in staging area
9-M	Hazard controlled: Microbiological Point or procedure: Maximum pH limit on finished salad before packaging	9.1 Product pH must not exceed a pH of 5.5 9.2 pH meter must be calibrated with approved standards before each shift
10-M	Hazard controlled: Microbiological Point or procedure: Chilled product storage temperature and time before packaging	10.1 Internal temperature not to exceed 45°F 10.2 Product must not be held more than one shift before filling/packaging
11-P	Hazard controlled: Physical Point or procedure: Metal detector for packages	11.1 Ferrous metal detection device for individual packages 11.2 Calibration or inspection not to exceed every 4 hours

(continued)

TABLE 16.5 *Continued*

CCP Number	CCP description	Critical limit(s) description
12-M	Hazard controlled: Microbiological Point or procedure: Physical barrier to prevent cross-contamination from warehouse area	12.1 Physical barrier in place 12.2 Doors kept closed when not in use 12.3 Color-coded uniforms 12.4 Supervision in place
13-M	Hazard controlled: Microbiological Point or procedure: Refrigerated storage of cased/palleted finished product	13.1 Product internal temperature not to exceed 45°F in 4 hours 13.2 Temperature measuring devices calibrated before shift
14-M	Hazard controlled: Microbiological Point or procedure: Truck and shipping containers for distribution of finished product	14.1 Shipping compartments must be precooled to 45°F or less before loading product
15-M	Hazard controlled: Microbiological Point or procedure: Label instructions	15.1 Each package or bulk case shall have label instructions 15.2 Each label shall include: • Keep refrigerated • Code • Storage instructions

Source: Pierson MD, Corlett DA.
HACCP Principles and Applications;
M = microbiological hazard;
P = physical hazard;
C = chemical hazard.

enterocolitica, and *Vibio,* and parasites such as *Crytosporidium* and *Cyclospora.* The CDC program is designed to assist public health officials to better understand the epidemiology of foodborne diseases.

The goals of FoodNet are as follows:

• Describe the epidemiology of new and emerging bacterial, parasitic, and viral foodborne pathogens

• Estimate the frequency and severity of foodborne diseases that occur in the United States per year

• Determine how much foodborne illness results from eating specific foods, such as meat, poultry, and eggs

FoodNet is different from other foodborne disease surveillance systems in that it does not rely on current *"passive"* surveillance systems, with the complexities of reporting by clinical laboratories, to state health departments, to the CDC. Rather, as mentioned, it is an *"active"* reporting system where public health officials frequently contact laboratory directors for data that is then electronically transmitted to the CDC. It has five components:

- Active laboratory-based surveillance
- Survey of clinical laboratories
- Survey of physicians
- Survey of the population
- Epidemiologic Studies

Their *"Burden of Foodborne Disease Pyramid"* follows these hierarchical steps, beginning at the base with an initial report to the Health Department/CDC:

```
Exposures in the general population
Person becomes ill
Person seeks care
Specimen obtained
Lab tests for organism
Culture-confirmed case
Reported to Health Department/CDC
```

The reporting data appears several years after the occurrence of illness, and the *most current* data were reported in December 1997 for the years 1993–1997 (26). During this time period, there were 2,751 reported outbreaks involving 86,058 persons. Where the etiology was determined in outbreaks, it was as follows:

- **Bacterial** pathogens caused the largest percentage of outbreaks (75%) and the largest percentage of cases (86%). *Salmonella* accounted for the largest number of outbreaks, cases, and deaths, most of which were attributable to undercooked, infected eggs.
- **Viruses** caused 6% of outbreaks and 8% of cases.
- **Parasites** caused 2% of outbreaks and 5% of cases.
- **Chemical** agents caused 17% of outbreaks and 1% of cases.

Surveillance data for foodborne-disease outbreaks (FBDO) in the United States from the CDC for the most recent reporting year are shown in the Tables 16.6–16.8 and Figure 16.10.

The number of FBDOs is reported by state and territorial health departments to the CDC on a standard reporting form. The definition of FBDO is *"two or more cases of a similar illness resulting from the ingestion of a common food,"* whereas prior to

TABLE 16.6 Number of Reported Foodborne-Disease Outbreaks, Cases, and Deaths by Vehicle of Transmission—United States,[a] 1997[b]

Vehicle of transmission	Outbreaks No.	(%)	Cases No.	(%)	Deaths No.	(%)
Beef	7	(1.4)	302	(2.5)	0	(0.0)
Ham	4	(0.8)	85	(0.7)	0	(0.0)
Pork	2	(0.4)	50	(0.4)	0	(0.0)
Sausage	1	(0.2)	45	(0.4)	0	(0.0)
Chicken	9	(1.8)	256	(2.1)	0	(0.0)
Turkey	3	(0.6)	97	(0.8)	0	(0.0)
Other/unknown meat	5	(1.0)	137	(1.1)	0	(0.0)
Shellfish	11	(2.2)	49	(0.4)	0	(0.0)
Other fish	26	(5.2)	108	(0.9)	0	(0.0)
Milk	2	(0.4)	23	(0.2)	0	(0.0)
Eggs	3	(0.6)	91	(0.8)	0	(0.0)
Baked foods	4	(0.8)	69	(0.6)	0	(0.0)
Fruits and vegetables	15	(3.0)	719	(6.0)	1	(50.0)
Potato salad	3	(0.6)	242	(2.0)	0	(0.0)
Poultry, fish, and egg salads	1	(0.2)	143	(1.2)	0	(0.0)
Other salad	21	(4.2)	1,104	(9.2)	0	(0.0)
Chinese food	1	(0.2)	16	(0.1)	0	(0.0)
Mexican food	9	(1.8)	701	(5.9)	0	(0.0)
Nondairy beverage	3	(0.6)	63	(0.5)	0	(0.0)
Multiple vehicles	39	(7.7)	2,707	(22.7)	0	(0.0)
Known vehicle	169	(33.5)	7,007	(58.7)	1	(50.0)
Unknown vehicle	335	(66.5)	4,933	(41.3)	1	(50.0)
Total 1997	**504**	**(100.0)**	**11,940**	**(100.0)**	**2**	**(100.0)**

[a] Includes Guam, Puerto Rico, and the U.S. Virgin islands.
[b] Totals might vary by <1% from summed components because of rounding.

1991, it was *one* case of intoxication by chemical, marine toxin, or *C. botulinum* toxin as a result of the ingestion of food.

Many individuals who become ill do not relate it to food consumption, or report this incident to appropriate authorities. Therefore, perhaps only a small percentage of actual FBDOs are reported. Nonetheless, surveillance data provide "an indication of the etiologic agents, vehicles of transmission, and contributing factors associated with FBDO and help direct public health actions."

Persons most "at-risk" for, or likely to become ill with, a foodborne illness include the elderly (the largest risk segment of the U.S. population), pregnant and nursing women, school-age children, and infants. These are represented as "highly susceptible populations." As well, increasing numbers of persons testing positive for the human immunodeficiency virus (HIV), and persons with acquired

TABLE 16.7 Number of Reported Foodborne-Disease Outbreaks, Cases, and Deaths by etiology—United States,[a] 1997[b]

Etiology	Outbreaks No.	Outbreaks (%)	Cases No.	Cases (%)	Deaths No.	Deaths (%)
Bacterial						
Bacillus cereus	4	(0.8)	438	(3.7)	0	(0.0)
Campylobacter	2	(0.4)	104	(0.9)	1	(50.0)
Clostridium botulinum	1	(0.2)	2	(0.0)	0	(0.0)
Clostridium perfringens	6	(1.2)	255	(2.1)	0	(0.0)
Escherchia coli	8	(1.6)	300	(2.5)	1	(50.0)
Salmonella	60	(11.9)	1,731	(14.5)	0	(0.0)
Shigella	10	(2.0)	315	(2.6)	0	(0.0)
Staphylococcus aureus	9	(1.8)	393	(3.3)	0	(0.0)
Streptococcus, group A	1	(0.2)	122	(1.0)	0	(0.0)
Vibrio parahaemolyticus	4	(0.8)	36	(0.3)	0	(0.0)
Total bacterial	**105**	**(20.8)**	**3,696**	**(31.0)**	**2**	**(100.0)**
Chemical						
Ciguatoxin	17	(3.4)	48	(0.4)	0	(0.0)
Mushroom poisoning	3	(0.6)	9	(0.1)	0	(0.0)
Scombrotov in	15	(3.0)	65	(0.5)	0	(0.0)
Total chemical	**35**	**(6.9)**	**122**	**(1.0)**	**0**	**(0.0)**
Parasitic						
Giardia lamblia	1	(0.2)	17	(0.1)	0	(0.0)
Other parasitic	10	(2.0)	673	(5.6)	0	(0.0)
Total parasitic	**11**	**(2.2)**	**690**	**(5.8)**	**0**	**(0.0)**
Viral						
Hepatitis A	3	(0.6)	174	(1.5)	0	(0.0)
Other viral	14	(2.8)	591	(4.9)	0	(0.0)
Total viral	**17**	**(3.4)**	**765**	**(6.4)**	**0**	**(0.0)**
Confirmed etiology	168	(33.3)	5,273	(44.2)	2	(100.0)
Unknown etiology	336	(66.7)	6,667	(55.8)	0	(0.0)
Total 1997	**504**	**(100.0)**	**11,940**	**(100.0)**	**2**	**(100.0)**

[a] Includes Guam, Puerto Rico, and the U.S. Virgin Islands.
[b] Totals might vary by < 1% form summed components because of rounding.

immunodeficiency syndrome (AIDS), or persons with a weakened immune system due to pharmaceutical or radiological treatment are very susceptible to illness.

The growth of the number of persons at risk, coupled with a greater number of meals eaten away from home, provides increasing opportunities for the occurrence of foodborne illness. Controlling hazards and ensuring a safe food supply is possible through such methodologies as the use of an HACCP system and employee training. It is recommended that FSIS should seek authority to impose

TABLE 16.8 Number of Reported Foodborne-Disease Outbreaks by Etiology and Place Where Food Was Eaten—United States,[a] 1997

Etiology	Place where food was eaten							Known place	Unknown place	Total
	Private residence	Delicaessen cafeteria, or restaurant	School	Picnic	Church	Camp	Other			
Bacterial										
Bacillus cereus	2	–	–	–	1	–	1	4	–	4
Campylobacter	–	–	–	–	–	–	1	1	1	2
Clostridium botulinum	1	–	–	–	–	–	–	1	–	1
Clostridium perfringens	–	2	–	–	–	–	4	6	–	6
Escherchia coli	–	2	–	–	–	–	5	7	1	8
Salmonella	18	24	2	1	3	1	10	59	1	60
Shigella	3	5	–	–	–	–	2	10	–	10
Staphylococcus aureus	2	–	2	1	–	–	4	9	–	9
Streptococcus, group A	1	–	1	–	–	–	–	1	–	1
Vibrio parahaemolyticus	1	2	–	–	–	–	1	4	–	4
Total bacterial	**27**	**35**	**5**	**2**	**4**	**1**	**28**	**102**	**3**	**105**

Chemical								
Ciguatoxin	13	3	—	—	1	17	—	17
Mushroom poisoning	—	1	—	—	1	2	1	3
Scombrotoxin	5	8	—	—	2	15	—	15
Total chemical	**18**	**12**	—	—	**4**	**34**	**1**	**35**
Parasitic								
Giardia lamblia	—	1	—	—	8	1	—	1
Other parasitic	—	2	—	—	8	10	—	10
Total parasitic	—	**3**	—	—	—	**11**	—	**11**
Viral								
Hepatitis A	1	1	—	—	—	3	—	3
Other viral	3	4	2	—	5	14	—	14
Total viral	**4**	**5**	**2**	—	**5**	**17**	—	**17**
Confirmed etiology	49	55	6	1	45	164	4	168
Unknown etiology	64	161	11	3	70	317	19	336
Total 1997	**113**	**216**	**17**	**4**	**115**	**481**	**23**	**504**

[a]Includes Guam, Puerto Rico, and the U.S. Virgin Islands.

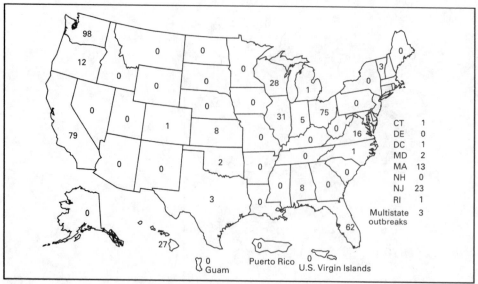

CT	1
DE	0
DC	1
MD	2
MA	13
NH	0
NJ	23
RI	1
Multistate outbreaks	3

* Includes Guam, Puerto Rico, and the U.S. Virgin Islands.

FIGURE 16.10 Number of reported foodborne-disease outbreaks by state—United States, 1997 (*Source:* Centers for Disease Control and Prevention).

monetary penalties for violations, and do a better job of monitoring test procedures (27).

ADDITIONAL CAUSES OF SPOILAGE

In addition to the biological, chemical, and physical hazards that may *contaminate* the food supply, other microbes, enzymatic activity and exposure to excessive moisture cause food *spoilage* by deteriorating the edible quality of food (see definitions). Diligence in care, preservation (Chapters 17), the use of additives (Chapter 18) and packaging (Chapter 19) are all methods of controlling undesirable spoilage or contamination.

DATING OF FOODS AS A MEANS OF ASSURING FOOD SAFETY

Food processors may place *open dates* on the food package, which provides the end-user, the foodservice establishment or consumer, with information regarding optimum time periods for food use. Dating is not a guarantee against spoilage or harmful contamination, so all related personnel in processing and foodservice operations, as well as consumers, must observe foods for their possible deterioration, and not use damaged products.

Open date labeling is *mandatory* for dairy products, but other foods may *voluntarily* have open date labeling. Foods may also display a *code date*, which can be read *only* by the manufacturer. Some examples of the types of dating that may appear on foods include the following:

- **"Best if used by" date**—informs consumers of the food's optimal period for retention of high quality
- **Expiration date**—such as on active dry yeast, indicates a deadline for recommended use
- **Pack date**—indicates when the food was packaged
- **Pull date**—for example, on milk, signifying the last day the food may be sold as fresh All food products should be made available for use only within established time frames.

RESPONSIBILITY FOR FOOD SAFETY

There are increasing numbers of "at-risk" populations that complicate the prevention of foodborne and waterborne illnesses, but the food supply should be safe. Who is responsible—governments, food companies, foodservice establishments, consumers? The answer is *all* of the above. A sample web page during which food safety experts edited and ranked food handling behaviors appropriate for preventing foodborne illnesses from pathogens, including Listeria monocytogenes, *Salmonella enteriditis*, Escherichia coli 0157:H7, Bacuillus cereus, Clostridium perfringens, Staphylococcus, Shigella ssp. Is shown in another reference. (28) Food handling behaviors of sticking to the basics is encouraged. (29)

Governments around the world regulate their own food supply (Chapter 20) to assure its safety and wholesomeness, by fostering science-based regulation, inspection and enforcement services, education and research. In the U.S., the FDA and the USDA's FSIS have a history of providing their numerous, well-researched documents (also available on their websites) on foodborne illness and risk assessment to both the food manufacturer and consumer. The President's Council on Food Safety website (www.foodsafety.gov/presidentscouncil) provides the latest in food safety news, recall information consumer advice, instructions on reporting possible foodborne illnesses and more.

Food manufacturing and processing industries, as well as *foodservice operations*, including hospitals, nursing homes and restaurants, must comply with those regulations. For example, as a means of food protection, foods companies have re-evaluated strategies to provide required plant sanitation and prevent product recalls. (A discussion of the potential for recalls for processors, including a 12-point risk reduction checklist is presented in *Food Engineering,* October 1998.) Increases in both time and financial resources allocated to food safety are apparent, as is the hiring of plant design engineers trained in sanitation (30).

In the food industry, a loss of human life, loss of brand loyalty, or loss of the company itself may propel personnel to maintain the right attitude, and do things right. Crisis management teams, and crisis management plans must emphasize prevention.

The Food and Drug Center for Food Safety and Applied Nutrition cites seven critical hindrances in maintaining a sanitary operation. These areas include the aforementioned microorganisms: bacteria and mold, chemical contamination, pests:

including birds, insects, and rodents, and as well, ignorance/carelessness. Thus, targeted employee training in these critical areas is crucial to food safety.

As the President of a food safety and sanitation consulting firm noted, "Sanitation is an attitude, not a process." "The bulk of sanitation cannot be done during production, that's the way the rule is and that's not going to change" (30). Also, food companies may literally move "sanitation" tasks from the third shift to the first or second shift, reflecting different priorities and the adoption of a greater emphasis on sanitation and the safety of their food products. Perhaps it is insufficient to just *say* that a food is safe. Data must support the claim.

Yet, it is the *consumer* who must ultimately be responsible for the consumption of safe foods that they themselves prepare, or that are processed/prepared by others in the food supply. The consumer must be vigilant and become educated on matters concerning food safety because food safety may be literally in the hands of the food preparer!

The large body of *food and nutrition professionals*, represented by The American Dietetic Association (ADA), has stated the following:

> "It is the position of The American Dietetic Association that the public has the right to a safe food and water supply. The Association supports collaboration among dietetics professionals, academics, and representatives of the food industry and appropriate government agencies to ensure the safety of the food and water supply by providing education to the public and industry, promoting technological innovation and applications, and supporting further research."

ALLERGEN-FREE

An issue that relates to food safety is the manufacture of allergen-free foods. As one author has said "Food safety is being redefined to include allergen-free as well as pathogen-free" (29). The FDA is responsible for ingredient labeling, and has given notice to food processors that narrow exemptions from ingredient labeling would not be tolerated. A food product *must contain what it states* on the label, and vice versa, it should *not* contain an ingredient it does *not* disclose. Life threatening allergens must be reported on the food label, and in uncertain cases, statements such as "may contain" are displayed as a safeguard.

The eight major foods to which people have allergies include: milk, eggs, peanuts, tree nuts (e.g., almonds, cashews), soy, wheat, fish, and shellfish. These are responsible for 90% of food allergic reactions, and therefore represent ingredients that should thus be isolated in the production process. Severe allergic reactions can cause anaphylaxis or death (Food Allergy Network, 31).

If an allergen is detected following product distribution, product recalls may be necessary. Data for the first few months of a recent year reveal 79 food product recalls, with 21 related to allergens (FDA, 32). Either an independent lab or allergen test kits may be used as part of industry's good manufacturing practices (GMPs).

The number of food product *recalls* due to allergens may not be as high as the actual number of food products containing alergens. According to the Director of the Office of Scientific Analysis & Support at FDA's Center for Food Safety & Applied Nutrition: "It may be because both FDA and food companies are looking harder for allergens, because allergic consumers are becoming more aware of the allergens in foods, and because of improved allergen-detection methods".

Some of the best paractices for allergen control relate to the following:

- R&D/Product Development
- Engineering and System Design with dedicated production lines
- Vendor certification of raw materials and ingredients
- Production scheduling to include longer production runs
- Rework segregated
- Labeling and Packaging with the right product going into the right package, and ingredients listing to match the actual food product!
- Sanitation. A HACCP-like approach
- Training (33)

CONCLUSION

The consumer expects safe food and protection from microbial, chemical, and physical hazards to the food supply. Foodborne illness may originate from bacteria, viruses, mold, parasites, and naturally occurring chemicals in food (such as fish toxins), accidental chemical contamination, toxic levels of additives or preservatives, and foreign objects. It may severely impact the health and welfare of a food company, hospital, restaurant, or the consumer at home.

The HACCP is a food safety system that focuses on foodborne disease prevention, and ensures a greater likelihood of food safety. Various segments of the food industry apply the HACCP system of food protection to their handling of hazardous ingredients. HACCP team members promote food safety by assessing potential hazards in the flow of foods through their operation and by establishing limits or controls for the identified hazards. HACCP is applied to all steps of handling, including processing, packaging, and distribution. This same process may be followed by foodservice operations.

The CDC monitors and reports FBDOs. Open and code dating are utilized. Food allergens are monitored by the FDA. It is the consumer (the one who consumes!) who must ultimately be responsible for the consumption of safe foods.

The USDA Food Safety Research Information Office (FSRIO) has created a new web site for the general public and food safety researchers. The site contains educational, professional, and foreign government links for food safety. www.nal. usda.gov/fsrio.

GLOSSARY

Biological hazard: Microbiological hazard from bacteria, viruses, fungi, and parasites.

Chemical hazard: Toxic levels of a specific chemical that may occur by accident, use of toxic levels additives, or toxic metals.

Contaminated: Presence of harmful substances.

Cross-contamination: Transfer of harmful microorganisms from one food to another by way of another food, hands, equipment, or utensils.

Emerging pathogens: Pathogens whose incidence has increased within the last few years or which threaten to increase in the near future.

Foodborne illness: Disease carried to people by food.

Fungi: Microorganisms that include mold and yeast.

HACCP: Hazard Analysis and Critical Control Point system of food safety.

Infection: Illness that results from ingesting living, pathogenic bacteria such as *Salmonella, Listeria,* or *Shigella.*

Intoxication: Illness that results from ingesting a preformed toxin such as that produced by Staphylococcus aureus, Clostridium botulinum, or Bacillus cereus.

Pathogenic: Disease-causing agent.

Physical hazard: Foreign object found in food; may be due to harvesting or manufacturing; may be intrinsic to the food (bone, shell, pit).

Potentially hazardous food: Natural or synthetic food in a form capable of supporting the rapid and progressive growth of infectious or toxigenic microorganisms; the growth and toxin production of *C. botulinum,* or in shell eggs, the growth of *S. enteritidis.*

Spoiled: Damage to the eating quality.

Spore: Thick-walled formation in a bacterium that is resistant to heat, cold, and chemicals; it remains in food after the vegetative cells are destroyed and is capable of becoming vegetative cell.

Temperature danger zone (TDZ): Temperature range within which most bacteria grow and reproduce 40–140°F (4–60°C).

Toxin: Poison produced by a microorganism while it is alive; may remain in food and cause illness after the bacteria is killed.

Toxin-mediated infection: Infection/intoxication illness that results from ingestion of living, infection-causing bacteria that also produce a toxin in the intestine, such as *C. perfringens* or *E. coli* 0157:H7.

REFERENCES

1. Food and Drug Administration. Department of Health and Human Services. Public Health Service.
2. Espy M. Ensuring a safer and sounder food supply. *Food Technology.* 1994; 48(9): 91–93.
3. Fung DYC. What's needed in rapid detection of foodborne pathogens. *Food Technology.* 1995; 49(6): 64–67.
4. Troller JA. *Sanitation in Food Processing,* 2nd ed. San Diego, CA: Academic Press, 1993.
5. Longree K. *Quantity Food Sanitation,* 3rd ed. New York: Wiley–Interscience, 1980.
6. Russell M. Improving the safety net. *Food Engineering.* 1994; 66(7): 51–56.
7. Mermelstein NH. High interest in testing for *E. coli* 0157:H7. *Food Technology.* 1994; 48(8): 100.
8. Nettleton J. Feasting on fear. *Food Technology.* 1994; 48(7): 25.
9. Nettleton J. Panic over pathogens. *Food Technology.* 1995; 49(3): 30.
10. Thonney PF, Bisogni CA. Government regulation of food safety: Interaction of scientific and societal forces. *Food Technology.* 1992; 46(1): 73–80.
11. USDA. Agricultural Research Service Washington, DC.

12. The Educational Foundation of the National Restaurant Association. Chicago, IL.

13. Watson DH. *Safety of Chemicals in Food: Chemical Contaminants*. New York: Ellis Horwood, 1993.

14. Katz F. Research priorities move toward healthy and safe. *Food Technology*. 2000; 54 (12): 42–46

15. Crawford LM, DVM. Food irradiation's advantages will not escape public attention. *Food Technology*. 52(1): 55.

16. Higgins KT. E-beam comes to the heartland. *Food Engineering*. 2000; 75 (10): 89–96.

17. Meyer RS, Cooper KL, Knorr D, Lelieveld HLM. High-pressure sterilization of foods. *Food Technology*. 2000; 54(11): 67–72.

18. Hussain SA, ConAgra Refrigerated Prepared Foods, Technical Services. Surak JG, Clemson University, Cawley JL, Northwest Anaytical. Butterball integrates SPC with HACCP. *Food Engineering*. 2000; 75(10): 82.

19. Pierson MD, Corlett DA, eds. *HACCP Principles and Applications*. New York: Chapman & Hall, 1992.

20. National Advisory Committee for Microbiological Criteria for Foods (NACMCF). *HACCP Principles for Food Production*. Washington, DC: USDA—FSIS Information Office.

21. *HACCP Reference Book*. Chicago, IL: The Educational Foundation of the National Restaurant Association, 1993.

22. Mancini L. Drafting the HACCP team. *Food Engineering*. 1994; 66(11): 83–88.

23. *HACCP Manual. A Program to Ensure Food Safety in the Supermarket—The Hazard Analysis Critical Control Point System*. Washington, DC: Food Marketing Institute, 1989.

24. Karr KJ, Maretzki AN, Knabel SJ. Meat and poultry companies assess USDA's Hazard Analysis and Critical Control Point system. *Food Technology*. 1994; 48(2): 117–122.

25. Puckett RP, Schneider G. Keeping it clean, playing it safe: What the HACCP program is all about. *Journal of the American Dietetic Association*. 1997; 97: 125.

26. Centers for Disease Control and Prevention. *CDC Surveillance Summaries*, 1993–1997. *Mortality and Morbidity Weekly Reports*. 2000; 49 (No. SS-1).

27. Eye on Washington. *Food Engineering*. 2000; July/August: 16.

28. Medeiros LC, Kendall P, Hillers V, Chen G, and DiMascola S. Identification and classification of consumer food-handling behaviors for food safey education. *J Am Diet Assoc*. 2001; 101: 1326–1332, 1337–1339.

29. Peregrin T. Teaching food-handling safety: stick to the basics. *J Am Diet Assoc*. 2001; 101: 1339.

30. Van Milligen D. Sanitation 101. *Food Engineering*. 2001; 73 (1): 55–60.

31. Dietitians face the challenge of food allergies. *Journal of the American Dietetic Association*. 2000; 100: 13.

32. Higgins KT. Food safety is being redefined to include allergen-free as well as pathogen-free. *Food Engineering*. 2000; 72(6): 75–82.

33. Morris CE. Best practices for allergen control. *Food Engineering*. 2002; 74 (3): 33–35.

BIBLIOGRAPHY

FDA Enforcement Report.

Flickinger B. The microbiology lab of the future. *Food Quality*. 1995; 1(4): 21–28.

Francis FJ. *Food Safety: The Interpretation of Risk.* Ames, IA: Council for Agricultural Science and Technology, 1992.

Institute of Food Technologists' Expert Panel on Food Safety and Nutrition. Scientific Status Summary, Foodborne illness: Role of home food handling practices. *Food Technology.* 1995; 49(4): 119–131.

LaVella B, Bostik JL. *HACCP for Food Service.* St. Louis, MO: LaVella Food Specialists, 1994.

National Restaurant Association. The Educational Foundation. *Applied Foodservice Sanitation,* 4th ed. New York: John Wiley and Sons, 1992.

Silliker Laboratories Group Inc., Educational Services Group, Homewood, IL.

Texas A&M University—Center for Food Safety, College Station, TX.

ASSOCIATIONS AND ORGANIZATIONS

The American Dietetic Association (ADA) National Center for Nutrition and Dietetics (NCND), Chicago, IL

American Public Health Association (APHA), Washington, DC

Association of Food and Drug Officials (AFDO), York, PA

Cooperative Extension Service (CES), throughout the United States

Council for Agriculture Science and Technology (CAST), Ames, IA

Food Marketing Institute (FMI), Washington, DC

Institute of Food Technologists (IFT), Chicago, IL

International Association of Milk, Food, and Environmental Sanitarians (IAMFES), Des Moines, IA

International Food Manufacturers Association (IFMA), Chicago, IL

International Council of Hotel, and Restaurant Industry Educators (CHRIE), Washington, DC

National Environmental Health Association (NEHA), Denver, CO

National Sanitation Foundation (NSF) International, Ann Arbor, MI

The Educational Foundation of the National Restaurant Association (NRA), Chicago, IL

United States Environmental Protection Agency, (EPA), Washington, DC

CHAPTER 17

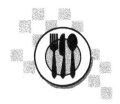

Food Preservation and Processing

INTRODUCTION

Preservation by heat, cold refrigeration, freezing temperature, or other means and application of the preservation techniques are introduced in this chapter. Storage conditions and preservation processes are subject to Food and Drug Administration (FDA) inspection and enforcement. Preservation from microbial, chemical, and physical contamination, as well as enzymatic activity, is necessary for preserving and extending the shelf life (time a product can be stored without significant change in quality) of food. Adequate packaging is important in preserving food (Chapter 19).

HEAT PRESERVATION

Heating or cooking foods as a means of preserving them or making them more palatable has been important for centuries. Heating is a vital form of food preservation and there are many different methods of heating processes available today.

Foods are heat processed for four main reasons:

- To eliminate pathogens (organisms that cause disease)
- To eliminate or reduce spoilage organisms
- To extend the shelf life of the food
- To improve palatability of the food

Methods of Heat Transfer

Heat may be transferred to a food by conduction, convection, or radiation. The following listing offers a brief discussion of each:

Conduction is the term used for the transfer of heat from molecule to molecule and is the major method of transfer through a solid. Examples of heat transfer by conduction include a saucepan resting on a hot ring. The heat is transferred by direct contact with the heat source. This is a relatively slow method of heat transfer.

Convection occurs when currents are set up in heated liquid or gas. For example, as water is heated in a saucepan, the warmer sections become less dense and therefore rise, whereas the cooler regions flow down toward the bottom of the pan. This sets up a flow or current, which helps to spread the heat throughout the liquid. Heating by convection is therefore faster than heating by conduction.

Radiation is the fastest method of heat transfer. This occurs when heat is transferred directly from a radiant heat source, such as a broiler or a campfire, to the food to be heated. The energy is transferred in the form of electromagnetic waves. Any surfaces between the heat source and the food being heated reduce the amount of energy transmitted by radiation. The rays fan out as they travel, and so the farther a food is from the heat source, the fewer rays it receives and the longer it takes to get hot.

Heat Treatment Methods

Heat treatment methods can be divided into two categories, depending on the amount of heat applied: The heat processing method may be *mild* or *severe*. The aims, advantages, and disadvantages of these two types of heat treatment are different. Depending on the objectives, a food processor may choose to use either a mild or a severe form of heat treatment to preserve a food product. Consumers rely on cooking to uphold conditions of food safety in the home. The two types of heat treatment will be discussed in detail; an overview of the main aims, advantages, and disadvantages of both is shown in Table 17.1.

TABLE 17.1 Overview of Mild and Severe Heat Treatments

Mild Heat Treatment	Severe Heat Treatment[a]
Aims	*Aims*
Kill pathogens	Kill *all* bacteria
Reduce bacterial count (food is *not* sterile)	Food will be commercially sterile
Inactivate enzymes	
Advantages	*Advantages*
Minimal damage to flavor, texture, and nutritional quality	Long shelf life
	No other preservation method is necessary
Disadvantages	*Disadvantages*
Short shelf life	Food is overcooked
Another preservation method must be used, such as refrigeration or freezing	Major changes in texture, flavor, and nutritional quality
Examples	*Examples*
Pasteurization, blanching	Canning

[a]See the section on canning.

Mild Heat Treatment.   Examples of *mild* heat treatment include pasteurization and blanching.

Pasteurization is a *mild* heat treatment used for milk, liquid egg, fruit juices, and beer. The main purpose of pasteurization is to achieve the following:

- Destroy pathogens
- Reduce bacterial count
- Inactivate enzymes
- Extend shelf life

Pathogens are microorganisms causing foodborne disease, either directly (foodborne infection), by releasing a substance that is toxic (foodborne intoxication), or via a toxin-mediated infection. All pathogens must be destroyed so that the food is safe to eat or drink; however, a pasteurized product is *not* sterile, the bacterial count in a pasteurized product is simply reduced. Any bacteria that are more heat resistant than those pathogens intended for destruction will not be destroyed, and they are able to grow and multiply in the food. They will cause spoilage of the food after a while, but that is usually obvious, as opposed to the unseen proliferation of pathogens causing contamination.

To increase the shelf life of a pasteurized product, it is necessary to refrigerate it to delay bacterial growth. For example, milk is pasteurized to ensure that it is safe to drink, but harmless bacteria are still present. If the milk is kept out on the kitchen counter on a warm day, the bacteria grow and produce lactic acid, and the milk turns sour within a day or two. However, milk can be stored in a refrigerator for at least a week, and sometimes longer, before it turns sour.

The mild heat treatment involved in pasteurization is usually sufficient to denature and inactivate enzymes. For example, milk contains the enzymes phosphatase and lipase, both of which are denatured during pasteurization (Chapter 11). To ensure that milk has been pasteurized properly, a colorimetric phosphatase test may be performed: if phosphatase is present, it turns a chemical reagent blue, indicating that the heat treatment has been insufficient. Absence of the blue color indicates that the phosphatase has been inactivated and the milk has been adequately pasteurized.

For detailed description of pasteurization of milk, see Chapter 11. Pasteurization of other products may differ in detail, but the principles are the same. For example, egg white or whole egg are heated to 140–144°F (60–62°C) and held for 3.5–4.0 minutes to prevent growth of *Salmonella*. Fruit juices are also pasteurized, the main aim being to reduce the bacterial count and to inactivate enzymes, as fruit juices do not *normally* carry pathogenic microorganisms.

Blanching is another *mild* heat treatment, used mainly for vegetables and some fruits prior to freezing. The main aim of blanching is to *inactivate enzymes* that would cause deterioration of food during frozen storage. This is essential, because freezing does not completely stop enzyme action, and so foods that are stored in the frozen state for many months slowly develop off-flavors and off-colors.

Blanching usually involves dipping the vegetable in boiling or near-boiling water for 1–3 minutes. Blanching treatments have to be established on an experimental basis, depending on size and shape and enzyme level of the different vegetables. For example, peas, which are very small, require only 1–1.5 minutes in water at 212°F (100°C), whereas, cauliflower or broccoli that are broken into small flowerets require 2–3 minutes. Corn on the cob is blanched for 7–11 minutes depending on size to destroy the enzymes within the cob itself.

Some destruction of bacteria is also achieved during blanching, and the extent depends on the length or the heat treatment. As with pasteurization, blanching does not produce a sterile product. Foods that have been blanched require a further preservation treatment to significantly increase their shelf life. Usually, foods are frozen after blanching.

Canning

Canning is a well-known method employed in food preservation. It involves hermetically sealing food in a container, and then inhibiting pathogenic and spoilage organisms with the application of heat. Nicholas Appert (1752–1841) is credited with the thermal process of canning, which was discovered (1809) as a result of a need to feed Napoleon's troops. One year later Peter Durand received a patent for the tin-plated can. Decades later, Louis Pasteur understood the principle of microbial destruction, and was able to provide the explanation for canning as a means of preservation. Samuel Prescott and William Underwood of the U.S. established further scientific applications for canning, including time and temperature inter- actions, in the late 19th century (for more information on canning, see Chapters 7 and 19).

Canning (Table 17.1) is an example of a food processing method that involves *severe* heat treatment. Food is placed inside a cylinder, or body of a can, the lid is sealed in place, and the can is then heated in a large commercial pressure cooker known as a retort. Heating times and temperatures vary, but the heat treatment must be sufficient to sterilize the food (1). Temperatures in the range 241–250°F (116–121°C) are commonly used for canning. Calcium may be added to canned foods as it increases tissue firmness.

The main purpose of canning is to achieve the following:

- Commercial sterility
- Extended shelf life (more than 6 months)

Commercial sterility is defined as "that degree of sterilization at which all pathogenic and toxin-forming organisms have been destroyed, as well as all other types of organisms which, if present, could grow in the product and produce spoilage under normal handling and storage conditions." Commercially sterilized foods may contain a small number of heat-resistant bacterial spores that are unable to grow under normal conditions. However, if they were isolated from the food and given special environmental conditions, they could be shown to be alive (2).

Most commercially sterile foods have a shelf life of 2 years or more. Any deterioration that occurs over time is due to texture or flavor changes, not due to microbial growth.

In the case of canning fruits and vegetables, the canneries may be located immediately near the field. The raw food is washed and prepared, blanched, placed into containers, perhaps under a vacuum (to mechanically exhaust the air), sealed, sterilized to destroy remaining bacteria, molds, yeasts [240°F (116°C)], then cooled, and labeled. Next, the can is sent to the warehouse for storage prior to distribution.

The Effect of Heat on Microorganisms

Heat denatures proteins, destroys enzyme activity, and, therefore, kills microorganisms. Bacteria are destroyed at a rate proportional to the number present in the food. This is known as the *logarithmic death rate*, which means that at a constant temperature, the same percentage of a bacterial population will be destroyed in a given time interval, irrespective of the size of the surviving population (Table 17.2). In other words, if 90% of the bacterial population is destroyed in the first minute of heating, then 90% of the remaining population will be destroyed in the second minute of heating, and so on. For example, if a food contains 1 million (10^6) organisms and 90% are destroyed in the first minute, then 100,000 (10^5) organisms will survive. At the end of the second minute, 90% of the surviving population will be destroyed, leaving a population of 10,000 (10^4) microorganisms. This is illustrated in more detail in Table 17.2.

If the logarithm number of survivors is plotted against the time at a constant temperature, a graph is obtained like the one shown in Figure 17.1. This is known as a **thermal death rate curve** (Figure 17.1). Such a graph provides data on the rate of destruction of a specific organism in a specific medium or food at a *specific* temperature.

An important parameter that can be obtained from the thermal death rate curve is the **D value** or **decimal reduction time.** The D value is defined as the time in minutes at a specified temperature required to destroy 90% of the organisms in a given population. It can also be described as the time required to reduce the population by a factor of 10, or by one log cycle.

TABLE 17.2 Logarithmic Death Rate

Time (min)	No. of survivors
1	1,000,000
2	100,000
3	10,000
4	1,000
5	100
6	10
7	1
8	0.1
9	0.01

Note: In this table, the decimal reduction time is 1 minute.

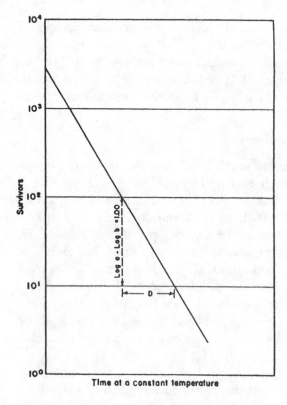

FIGURE 17.1 A typical thermal death–**rate** curve (*Source*: Stumbo, Thermobacteriology in Food Processing, 2nd ed. Academic Press, NY, 1973).

The D value varies for different microbial species. Some microorganisms are more heat resistant than others; therefore, more heat is required to destroy them. The D value for such organisms will be higher than the D value for heat-sensitive bacteria. A higher D value indicates greater heat resistance, because it takes longer to destroy 90% of the population.

Destruction of microorganisms is temperature dependent. Bacteria are destroyed more rapidly at higher temperatures; therefore, the D value for a particular organism decreases with increasing temperature. For a specific microorganism in a specific food, a set of D values can be obtained at different temperatures. These can be used to plot a ***thermal death time curve*** (Figure 17.2) with the logarithm of the time plotted on the Y axis and the temperature on the X axis.

A thermal death time curve provides data on the destruction of a specific organism at different temperatures. The heating time on the graph may be the D value or it may be the time to achieve $12D$ values, as will be explained later. The important thing to remember about the thermal death time curve is that every point on the graph represents destruction of the same number of bacteria. In other words, every time–temperature combination on the graph is equivalent in terms of killing bacteria. Such graphs are important to the food processor in determining the best

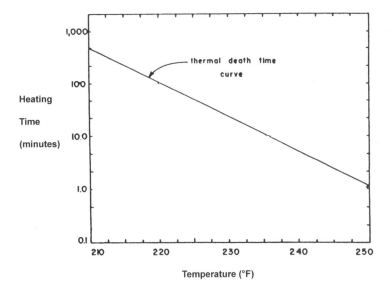

FIGURE 17.2 A typical thermal death–**time** curve
(*Source:* Adapted from Desrosier and Desrosier, Technology of Food
Preservation, 4th ed. AVI Publishing Co. Westport, CT, 1977).

time–temperature combination to be used in canning a particular product and
ensuring that commercial sterility is achieved.

The other parameters shown on the thermal death time curve are beyond the
scope of this book, and so will not be explained in detail here. (The z value indicates
the resistance of a bacterial population to changing temperature and the F value is a
measure of the capacity of a heat treatment to sterilize.)

Selecting Heat Treatments

All canned food must be commercially sterile and must therefore receive a heat
treatment that is sufficient to kill essentially all bacterial vegetative cells and spores.
However, such severe heat treatment adversely affects food qualities such as texture,
flavor, and nutritional quality. The food processor aims to ensure commercial
sterility, but to achieve this using the mildest heat treatment possible, so that the
food does not taste too "overcooked." In other words, the optimal heat treatment
will do the following:

- Achieve bacterial destruction (commercial sterility)
- Minimize adverse severe heat effects
- Be the mildest heat treatment necessary

To select a safe heat preservation treatment, it is important to know the time–
temperature combination required to inactivate the most heat-resistant pathogens
and spoilage organisms in a particular food. This depends on several factors:

1. *The heat penetration characteristics of the food.* The food in the center of the can must receive sufficient heat treatment to achieve commercial sterility. This may mean that the food toward the outside of the can is overcooked. How fast the heat penetrates to the center of the can depends on the size of the can, and also on the consistency of the food. Heat will reach the center of liquid foods, such as soup, much more quickly than solid foods such as meat.

2. *The pH of the food.* Bacteria are more heat resistant at neutral pH than they are in acid. Therefore, high-acid foods, such as tomatoes or fruits, need a less severe heat treatment to achieve sterility.

3. *The composition of the food.* Proteins, fats, and sugar in high concentrations all have a protective effect on bacteria, because they hinder the penetration of wet heat; thus, a more severe heat treatment is needed to sterilize foods that are high in protein, fat, or sugar.

4. The pathogenic and spoilage organisms likely to be present.

It is important to have thermal death time curve data available for the most heat-resistant microorganisms that may be present in the food. Such data must be obtained for the food to be processed, as the composition of the food affects the heat sensitivity of the bacteria. Thermal death time curves obtained in one food may not apply to the same bacteria in a different medium. Without obtaining thermal death time curves for the specific food, it is impossible to ensure commercial sterility.

As has already been mentioned, every point on the thermal death time curve is equivalent in terms of destruction of bacteria. An increase in temperature greatly reduces the time required to achieve commercial sterility. However, the color, flavor, texture, and nutritional value of foods are not as sensitive to temperature increase. Generally speaking, a 50°F (10°C) rise in temperature *doubles* the rate of chemical reactions but causes a *tenfold* increase in the thermal death rate. Therefore, a high-temperature short-time combination is preferred, in order to minimize adverse chemical changes in the food such as loss of flavor, texture, and nutritional quality.

The food processor wants to use the time–temperature combination that causes the least damage to food quality.

REFRIGERATION PRESERVATION

Our ancestors were familiar with placing food in cold cellars, holes in the ground, or natural caves, as these storage sites would assure uniform temperatures in storage, and preserve food. Ice became widespread as a means of cold preservation in the middle 1800s—food was stored in a closed, wooden "ice box" that contained a block of ice in a chamber above the food to keep it cold. *Mechanical* refrigeration was introduced in the later 1800s, and has undergone enormous developments since then.

Refrigerator and freezer temperatures both fail to sterilize food, but the latter temperatures are more effective in retarding bacterial growth. Refrigerated food is generally held at temperatures below 45°F (7.2°C) [41°F (5°C)] and is subject to *state* or *local* FDA or USDA requirements for handling, storage, and transport (3).

The microbiological and safety quality of extended shelf life refrigerated foods continues to be an issue for processors and the food preparer (4). A food may be better preserved in storage if it is stored under controlled atmospheric (CA) conditions. CA extends shelf life by reducing oxygen and increasing carbon dioxide in the atmosphere surrounding fruits (Chapter 7). Controlling gases in the atmosphere is also useful in providing longer storage of meats (Chapter 9) and eggs (Chapter 10). Meat preservation for example, involves controlling microbial growth, retarding enzymes, and preventing the development of rancidity through the oxidation of fatty acids.

Packaging materials may be used in conjunction with refrigeration to preserve foods (Chapter 19). Simply covering a food inhibits unwanted dehydration and contamination, yet choice of film material used also assists in prolonging shelf life.

Problems Associated with Refrigeration

Spoilage, or damage to the edible quality of food, is possible without maintenance of the proper temperatures and humidity, use of FIFO, and regular cleaning.

Cross-contamination, or the transfer of harmful substances from one product to another, is possible without adequate covering or placement of foods. Pathogens from an improperly placed raw product may contaminate other food.

Temperatures. If temperatures are *too cold*, "chill injury" to fresh vegetables or fruits, or sugar development in potatoes may result. Low-temperature storage increases the starch content of sweet corn (Chapter 7). *High* refrigerator temperatures or large containers of food that cannot cool quickly can lead to foodborne illness. Potentially hazardous foods must be kept at 41°F (5°C) or less, and if refrigerated after preparation, must be cooled to 41°F (5°C) or less in 4 hours or less. The Centers for Disease Control and Prevention (CDC) report that improper cooling (including improper cooling in the refrigerator) is, by far, the number one cause of bacterial growth leading to foodborne illness (see local jurisdiction).

Odor. Odors may be transferred from some foods, such as onions, to butter, chocolates, and milk. If possible, strong odor foods should be stored separately from other foods. Packaging may be utilized to minimize odor problems.

Freezing

Frozen food is held at colder temperatures than refrigeration. As opposed to refrigerator short-term storage, freezing is a long-term storage form that entails several months or a year. In freezing, water is unavailable for bacteria, thus they are dormant, and there is no multiplication of pathogens. Foods freeze as their water component turns to ice, or *crystallizes*.

With a *slow* freeze, *extra*cellular crystallization occurs prior to *intra*cellular crystallization; therefore, water is drawn from the inside of the cell as the external solute concentration increases. The result is that cell walls tear and shrink. At a cellular level, there is physical damage to the food as the water expands and the extracellular ice crystallization separates cells. Tissues survive a *rapid* freeze better than a slow freeze because water does not have time to migrate to seed-crystals and form large crystals.

Freezing Methods

Rapid freezing by commercial freezing methods includes the following procedures:

- Air blast tunnel freezing
- Plate freezing
- Cryogenic freezing

Air blast procedures utilize convection and cold air (Figure 17.3). With this method of freezing, foods are placed either on racks that are subsequently wheeled into an insulated tunnel, or on a conveyor belt, where very cold air is blown over the food at a quick speed. When *all* parts of the food reach a temperature of 0°F (−17.8°C), the packages are put into freezer storage. The products may be packaged prior to, or following freezing.

In *plate freezing,* the packaged food is placed between metal plates, which make full contact with the product and conduct cold, so that *all* parts of the food are brought to 0°F (−17.8°C). Automatic, continuous operating plate freezers can freeze the food and immediately deposit it to areas for casing and storage.

Cryogenic freezing may involve either *immersion* or *spraying* the food product with liquid nitrogen (LIN). LIN has a boiling point of −320°F (−196°C) and therefore freezes food more rapidly than other mechanical techniques. Food such as meats, poultry, seafood, fruits, and vegetables, prepared or processed foods, may be preserved by cryogenic freezing (Figures 17.4 and 17.5). Cryogenic techniques for freezing include use of tunnel freezers that use LIN sprayed onto food. The LIN vaporizes to nitrogen gas at −320°F (−196°C), at the end of the tunnel, and is then re-circulated to the tunnel entrance. LIN is approved by the FDA's Food Safety and Inspection Service (FSIS), for contact and freezing both meet and meat products, and poultry and poultry products.

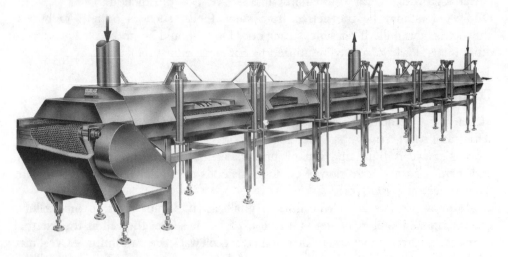

FIGURE 17.3 Example of air blast tunnel freezer
(*Source: 8 1996* Air Products and Chemicals, Inc.; photograph courtesy of Air Products and Chemicals, Inc).

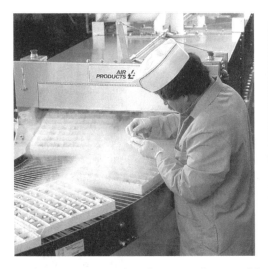
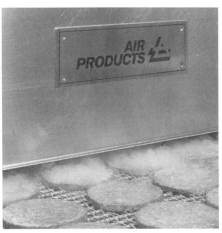

FIGURE 17.4 Examples of cryogenic freezing of foods
(*Source: 8 1996* Air Products and Chemicals, Inc.; photograph courtesy of Air Products and Chemicals, Inc).

At home, the consumer does not have these options and it is recommended that no more than 2–3 pounds of food per cubic foot of food be placed in the freezer at one time.

Problems Associated with Freezing

Most of the problems associated with freezing are due to the following:

- *Physical damage* due to formation of ice crystals
- Changes in texture and flavor caused by the *increased solute concentration* that occurs progressively as liquid water is removed in the form of ice.

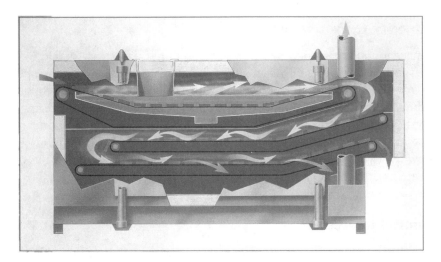

FIGURE 17.5 Example of the cryogenic immersion freezing process
(*Source: 8 1996* Air Products and Chemicals, Inc.; photograph courtesy of Air Products and Chemicals, Inc).

Both of these effects are minimized by fast freezing methods. Fast freezing minimizes formation of large crystals that would cause the most damage to cell structure and colloidal systems. Ice crystals can actually rupture cell walls, break emulsions, and cause syneresis in gels.

Increases in solute concentration can cause changes in pH, and denaturation of proteins, and increased enzyme activity, all of which may lead to deterioration of food quality. Fast freezing shortens the time period during which the concentration effects are important, thereby decreasing their effect on food quality.

Recrystallization may be a problem in maintaining a high-quality product. With refreezing, ice crystals enlarge because they are subject to fluctuating temperatures. Evidence of refreezing is frequently observed with large crystalline formation on the inside of the package.

Freezer burn is the dehydration that may accompany the freezing process. The surface of food may show white patches and becomes tough. This occurs due to sublimation of ice. Solid ice will become a moisture vapor, bypassing the liquid phase, and the vapor pressure differential between the food material and the atmosphere will lead to sublimation and desiccation. The use of moisture-proof freezer wraps is suggested for storage (Chapter 19).

Oxidation may lead to the development of off-flavor fats, as the double bonds of unsaturated fats are oxidized. Fruits and vegetables may brown due to enzymatic oxidative browning if enzymes are not denatured before freezing. Vitamin C (ascorbic acid) may be oxidized.

Colloidal substance change in freezing may occur due to the following:

- Starch syneresis—the freezing and thawing cycle may produce "weeping" because in thawing, less water is reabsorbed than what was originally present (Chapter 4).

- Cellulose—becomes tougher

- Emulsions—break down, are subject to dehydration and precipitation

Chemical Changes to Frozen Foods

Chemical changes to foods may occur as they are frozen. Off-odors may develop as acetaldehyde is changed to ethanol. As mentioned earlier, in oxidation, enzymatic oxidative browning is observable as phenols react with available oxygen, and ascorbic acid may become oxidized. It is recommended that blanching occur prior to freezing, as it may prevent oxidation. Pigments such as chlorophyll undergo degradation.

Eggs show an increased concentration of soluble salts in unfrozen portions if freezing is slow. Egg yolks show granule disruption due to an aggregation of low-density lipoproteins, forming a gummy product.

Moisture Control in Freezing

Drying occurs when a food gives up water to the atmosphere. Such dehydration also draws water from bacterial cells too, which is needed for subsequent growth outside of the freezer.

Added Sugar and Salt

The addition of salt or sugar lowers the freezing point, rendering water less available for microbial growth.

DEHYDRATION

Dehydration is a means of preservation that subjects food to some degree of water removal. The primary intent is to reduce moisture content and preclude the possibility of microbial growth such as bacteria, mold, and yeast. A decrease in relative humidity (RH) leads to a decrease in microorganism growth.

While traditional methods of drying are utilized around the world, new drying techniques are being developed. Methods used for drying foods include the following:

- Natural or sun drying—dries by direct sunlight or dry, hot air.

- Mechanical drying—dries with heated air blown in a tunnel, cabinet, or tray that contains the food (fluidized-bed drying, where hot air passes through the product and picks up moisture is a special type of hot air drying).

- Drum drying—dries the product on two heated stainless steel drums before it is scraped off. Milk, juices, and purees may be dried in this manner.

- Freeze drying—*freezes* and subsequently *vacuums* to evaporate moisture in the process of sublimation (ice is converted to a vapor without passing through the liquid phase); examples include instant coffee, meats, and vegetables.

- Puff drying—either by *heat* and subsequent *vacuum* (to increase the pressure difference between the internal and external environments), or a combination of vacuuming and steaming. The product may also puff as the temperature of the water in the food is raised above 212°F (100°C) and then external pressure is quickly released. Examples are some ready-to-eat puffed cereal products.

- Smoking—preserves by dehydrating, thus offering microbial control (Chapter 9) and also treats meat to impart flavor by exposure to aromatic smoke.

- Spray drying—dries the product as it is sprayed into a chamber concurrently with hot air. For example, eggs, instant coffee, and milk may be sprayed dried.

The result of dehydration is increased shelf life and a reduction in distribution costs due to less weight.

Deterioration may occur even in dried products. Detrimental color, flavor, or textural changes may result from enzymatic changes, and these may be controlled by deactivating enzymes, by blanching, or adding sulfur compounds prior to dehydrating. Nonenzymatic browning may occur in dried foods either due to caramelization or the Maillard browning. The Maillard reaction products may lead to significant unwelcome browning, development of bitter flavors, less solubility of proteins, as well as diminished nutritive value. Dry milks or eggs, and breakfast cereals participate in this reaction. Overall, oxidative spoilage, or chemical changes by oxidation of fats, is the primary cause of deterioration.

Factors needing control in dehydration include atmospheric conditions such as temperature, humidity, pressure, and portion size. The length of storage time is also a factor in the quality of the end product.

CONCENTRATION

Foods are **concentrated**, primarily to reduce weight and bulk. This makes transportation, shipping and handling easier and less expensive, and so it is economically advantageous. Many foods are concentrated, including fruit and vegetable juices and purees, milk products, soups, sugar syrups, jams and jellies, to name a few.

Concentration is not usually considered to be a method of preservation of a food, since the water activity is not reduced sufficiently to prevent bacterial growth (see Chapter 2). The exception to this is jams and jellies, which contain high levels of sugar. Additional preservation methods, such as pasteurization, refrigeration or canning, are therefore used to prevent spoilage of concentrated foods.

Methods of concentration

Some of the more common methods of concentration are:

- Open kettles—used to concentrate maple syrup, where the high heat produces the desired color and flavor. They are also used for jellies, jams, and some types of soups. The disadvantage of open kettles is the risk of product burn-on at the kettle wall due to high heat and long processing times.

- Flash evaporators—use heated steam (150°C), which is injected into the food, and later removed, along with water vapor from the food. This reduces heating time, but temperatures are still high, and so foods may lose volatile flavor constituents.

- Thin-film evaporators—enable the food to be continuously spread in a thin layer on the cylinder wall, which is heated by steam. As the food is concentrated (by removal of water vapor), it is wiped from the wall and collected. Heat damage is minimal due to the short time required to concentrate the food.

- Vacuum evaporators—used to concentrate heat-sensitive foods, which would be damaged by high heat. Operation under vacuum allows concentration to be achieved at much lower temperatures.

- Ultrafiltration and reverse osmosis—expensive processes that may be operated at low temperatures, and use selectively permeable membranes to concentrate liquids. Different membranes are required for different liquid foods. These processes are used to concentrate dilute protein dispersions such as whey protein, which cannot be concentrated by traditional methods without being extensively denatured (see Chapter 11). Ultrafiltration involves pumping the dispersion under pressure against a membrane that retains the protein, but allows smaller molecules such as salts and sugars to pass through. Reverse osmosis is similar, but higher pressures are used, and the membrane pores are smaller, and so they are able to hold back various salts and sugars, as well as larger protein molecules.

Changes During Concentration

The changes that occur during concentration arise primarily due to exposure of food to high heat. A "cooked" flavor may develop, and discoloration may occur. In addition, the product may thicken or gel over time, due to denaturation of proteins. This is a potential problem in evaporated milk (Chapter 11). Nutritional quality may also be lost. The extent of the changes depends on the severity of the heat treatment.

Concentration methods that employ low heat or short processing times cause the least damage to food. However, they are also the most costly, and may not always be the practical choice for the food processor, who must balance cost against quality.

ADDED PRESERVATIVES

Specific preservatives may be applied to a food to extend shelf-life:

- **Acid**—denatures bacterial proteins, preserving food, although not always sufficient to ensure sterility. Acid may be naturally present in foods such as citrus fruits and tomatoes. The combination of acid and heat provides more effective preservation.

- **Sugar and salt**—heavy syrups or brines compete with bacteria for water. By osmosis, the high percentage of water moves out of bacterial cells to equal the lower level of water in the surrounding medium. Other microorganisms, such as the fungi, yeast, and mold, are capable of growing in a high sugar or salt environment. Early U.S. settlers preserved meats using salt and sugar.

- **Smoke**—may contain a preservation chemical such as formaldehyde. Smoke retards bacterial growth due to surface dehydration. Smoking may also be used simply to impart flavor.

- **Chemicals**—subject to FDA approval. The burden of proof for usefulness and harmlessness is on industry. The chemical properties of the foods itself, such as pH and moisture content, affect the growth of microorganisms.

OTHER PRESERVATION TECHNIQUES

Fermentation—with the addition of nonpathogenic bacteria to a food, acid is produced, the pH is reduced, and the growth of pathogenic bacteria is controlled.

RADIATION

Foods may be heated by radiant energy including the use of microwave heat treatment, or the lesser heat of irradiation.

Microwave Heating

Microwave heating is a nonionizing, rapid method of cooking. It may be used for both processing and preservation. Some commercial uses of industrial microwave use that have been considered or put to use include baking, blanching, browning, coagulating, concentrating, cooking, curing, drying, fermenting, freeze drying, gelatinization, heating, pasteurizing, precooking, preservation, processing, proofing, puffing, roasting, separating, shucking, solvent removal, sterilizing, tempering, thawing, and vacuum drying (4–7).

It is reported that microwave heating inactivates vitamin B12, which is found in animal products and fortified vegetarian products. The nutrient plays an important role in maintaining the nerve tissue (9).

In combination with newer food packaging technologies, microwaveable foods are plentiful in the marketplace. General recommendations to be followed when heating by microwave include the following:

- Turn the container while cooking to avoid "hot spots" of concentrated energy in one spot
- Include a "rest period" or "standing time" beyond the designated cooking time, in order to continue cooking the food
- Beware of hot containers from conduction of heat from food to the container
- Select a low power setting for defrosting. Microwave energy is then sent intermittently into the frozen food.

Some definitions relating to the microwave method of heating include the following:

---

hot spots—the nonuniform heating of high-water foods

molecular friction—the heat generation method of microwave heating

skin—the surface dehydration and hardening as more microwave energy is absorbed at the surface of the food

shielding—protection of portions of food such as cylindrical ends of food, which readily overcook

thermal runaway—differential heating of food without thermal equilibrium

---

Irradiation

Irradiation is the administration of measured doses of energy that are product-specific. A positive biological effect it that it has a **bactericidal** effect, thus reduces the microbial load of a food, kills insects, controls ripening, and inhibits the sprouting of some vegetables (10,11).

Irradiation is a cold process of food preservation that does not add heat to the food. In the spectrum of energy waves, radio waves are at one end of the spectrum, microwaves are in the middle, and the gamma rays of irradiation are at the other end of the continuum. Gamma rays are passed through the food to be irradiated, and the food is thus sterilized and preserved as it passes through an irradiation chamber on a conveyor belt. Scientific evidence demonstrates that foods do not become radioactive and that no radiation residue remains in the food.

Irradiation is a process approved by the Food and Drug Administration, for use with specific foods, and only at **designated dosages** (Table 17.3) (12). Foods that may be irradiated include wheat, potatoes, spices, pork, red meat, fruit, poultry, dehydrated enzymes, or vegetable substances, including fresh produce (and bagged salads). So, in looking at dosages needed for pork, as an example, it is shown that a *low* dose is required to stop *reproduction* of *Trichinella spiralis* (the parasite responsible for causing trichinosis), but a much *higher* dose is needed in order to *eliminate* it from the pork.

Biologically speaking, there may be some negative effects of food preservation by irradiation. For example, the *carbohydrate* component of foods may become depolymerized, and as a result, contribute less gel strength to foods. *Fats* may become oxidized, and subsequently rancid in an irradiated food. Therefore, it is a standard operating procedure to irradiate fatty foods that are vacuum-packaged, and held at subfreezing temperatures. With regard to *protein*, it is found that use of *low* doses of radiation may not inactivate spoilage enzymes. *Vitamins* that are sensitive to irradiation in the presence of air, include vitamins A, E, and B_1 (thiamin).

Whole food items must be labeled if they are irradiated. A universal symbol of irradiation, namely the radura symbol, is used for recognition of irradiated food. In the United States, the words "Treated with Radiation" or "Treated by Irradiation" may also appear with the symbol. Spices do not require this labeling. Processed foods that contain irradiated ingredients, or restaurant foods prepared using irradiated ingredients, do not require an irradiation label.

Research has.been conducted on the sensory aspects of irradiated food. It is reported that, "The sensory appeal of foods which are processed with irradiation at levels that are approved for use is quite good. Researchers who have conducted experimental studies using sensory panelists to evaluate such foods found that food freshness, color, flavor, texture, and acceptability are not significantly different from unirradiated foods" (13). Due to its cold process of food preservation, the nutritive value of irradiated food is not significantly different from food subject to alternate methods of preservation, including canning.

Irradiation preserves food by killing insects and pests. It also kills microorganisms. With regard to food safety, food is made safer by the elimination of disease-causing bacteria such as *E. coli*, *Salmonella* and the parasite *Trichinella spiralis*. Irradiated food lasts longer and there are reduced losses due to spoilage (14).

Low doses of irradiation may be used to slow fruit ripening and control pests, without the use of pesticides. The process of irradiation leaves no residue.

Food irradiation facilities exist for the irradiation of foods, whereby the food product is sent off site for treatment. As well, in-line irradiation brings the technology to a company's own production line. A large defense contractor that radiates medical supplies is now using electron beams to pasteurize/irradiate meat, including prepared meats, and other foods (15). A patent was awarded to this corporation for development of a miniature version of their chamber that could incorporate the electronic pasteurization into food producer's processing line. Both cost and convenience issues need to be addressed by a company considering irradiation of its products.

While irradiation of meat and poultry has received the approval of every major government and health agency in the United States, consumer health activists have yet to give their stamp of approval. As a result, meat companies are proceeding at a less than full-steam-ahead rate with irradiation (16).

The General Accounting Office (GAO) reports to the U.S. House Committee on Commerce has stated that the benefits of irradiation outweigh any risks. " Food safety experts believe that irradiation can be an effective tool in helping to control foodborne pathogens and should be incorporated as part of a comprehensive program to enhance food safety."

Ohmic Heating

Ohmic heat processing of foods is relatively new for food manufacturers. In place of radiant heat, an electrical current is passed through food to heat it rapidly. A continuous heating system reaches the food as it passes between electrodes. An advantage of ohmic heating is that this system of heating prevents surface drying and overcooking while heating to control pathogenic microorganisms (17).

In ohmic heating, the *liquid* portion of the food, such as stew or soup, is heated rapidly and it conducts heat rapidly to the *inner* portion. In comparison, conventional heating tends to overprocesses the surrounding liquid as it conducts heat to the inner portion; thus, quality is diminished.

OTHER—DIRECT CONTACT PRODUCTS, ETC.

Other anti-microbial, direct contact products, including lactoferrin (naturally occurring protein in mammalian milk), cetylpyridinium chloride (a trade name "Cecure", for ready-to-eat [r-t-e], ready-to-cook and processed foods, not only meat) and acidified sodium chloride (ASC, for comminuted, formed r-t-e products, and produce) are promising (16).

NUTRITIVE VALUE OF PRESERVED FOODS

There is no question regarding the importance of preserving factors such as the appearance, texture, and flavor of food. Yet, in a discussion of food preservation, and the extension of a food's shelf life, preservation of nutritive value also becomes important. For example, prolonged or improper storage may have a deleterious effect on food due to the Maillard reaction. Perhaps water-soluble vitamins may be lost from a food, or high levels of sugar or salt may be added. These, and more, become issues to address with regard to nutritive value of preserved foods.

Irradiated fresh produce, such as bagged salad, may now be a healthful addition to the diet of the young, elderly, pregnant, and immunocompromised individuals. The microbial load can be drastically cut, assuring less likelihood of *Shigella* and *E. coli* (18).

SAFETY OF PRESERVED FOODS

The safety of preserved foods must be taken into account when seeking to store and extend the shelf life of foods. The processor/manufacturer's Good Manufacturing Practices (GMP's), the FDA's inspection, and the consumer's attentiveness, all contribute to ensuring that food is properly preserved, stored, and not held beyond acceptable time parameters.

CONCLUSION

Food is preserved by methods such as *heat*, either mild—such as blanching or pasteurization, or severe including canning; *cold*, either refrigeration or freezing; *dehydration*; use of *added preservatives,* or *radiation*, including microwave heat, irradiation, or *ohmic heating*. Storage conditions and preservation processes are subject to FDA inspection and enforcement. Consumer vigilance is also necessary in order to preserve food. Environmental control of oxygen and water availability, and enzymatic control extend shelf life of food, and assist in providing food safety.

GLOSSARY

Blanching: Mild heat treatment that inactivates enzymes that would cause deterioration of food during frozen storage.

Canning: An example of a food processing method that involves *severe* heat treatment. Food is placed inside a can, the lid is sealed in place, and the can is then heated in a large commercial pressure cooker known as a retort.

Commercial sterility: Severe heat treatment. A sterilization where all pathogenic and toxin-forming organisms have been destroyed as well as all other types of organisms which, if present, could grow in the product and produce spoilage under normal handling and storage conditions.

Concentration: Method of removing some of the water from a food, to decrease it bulk and weight. Concentration does not prevent bacterial growth.

Conduction: Transfer of heat from one molecule to another molecule; the major method of heat transfer through a solid.

Convection: Flow or currents in a heated liquid or gas.

D Value: Decimal reduction time; time in minutes at a specific temperature required to destroy 90% of the organisms in a given population.

Dehydration: A means of preservation with the primary intent to decrease moisture content and preclude the possibility of microbial growth such as bacteria, mold, and yeast.

Irradiation: The administration of measured doses of energy that are product-specific. It reduces the microbial load of a food, kills insects, controls ripening, and inhibits the sprouting of some vegetables.

Ohmic heat: In place of radiant heat, a continuous electrical current is passed through food to heat it rapidly, maintaining quality.

Pasteurization: Mild heat treatment that destroys pathogenic bacteria and most non-pathogens. It inactivates enzymes and extends shelf life.

Radiation: Fastest method of heat transfer; the direct transfer of heat from a radiant source to the food being heated.

Thermal death rate curve: Provides data on the rate of destruction of a specific organism in a specific medium or food at a specific temperature.

Thermal death time curve: Provides data on the destruction of a specific organism at different temperatures.

REFERENCES

1. Jackson J. *Fundamentals of Food Canning Technology*. Westport, CT: AVI, 1979.
2. Potter N, Hotchkiss J. *Food Science,* 5th ed. New York: Chapman & Hall, 1995.
3. Moberg L. Good manufacturing practices for refrigerated foods. *Journal of Food Production.* 1989; 52(5): 363–367.
4. IFT. Extending shelf of refrigerated foods: Microbiological quality and safety. 1998; 52(2).
5. Gerling JE. Microwaves in the food industry: Promise and reality. *Food Technology.* 1986; 40(6): 82–83.
6. Mudgett RE. Microwave properties and heating characteristics of foods. *Food Technology.* 1986; 40(6): 84–93.
7. Schiffman RF. Food product development for microwave processing. *Food Technology.* 1986; 40(6): 94–97.
8. Decareau RV. Microwave food processing throughout the world. *Food Technology.* 1986; 40(6): 98.
9. Watanabe F, Abe K, Fujita T, Goto M, Hiermori M and Nakano Y. Effects of microwave heating on the loss of vitamin B_{12} in foods. *J Agric Food Chem* 1988: 46: 206–210.
10. Thorne S. *Food Irradiation*. New York: Chapman & Hall, 1991.
11. Satin M. *Food Irradiation: A Guidebook*. Lancaster, PA: Technomic Publishers, 1993.
12. FT 52(1) Chart.
13. Texas A&M University—Center for Food Safety, College Station, TX.
14. Thayer DW. Wholesomeness of irradiated foods. *Food Technology.* 1994; 48(5): 132–135.
15. Higgins KT. E-beam comes to the heartland. *Food Engineering.* 2000; October: 89–96.
16. Gregerson J. Bacteria Busters. *J Am Diet Assoc.* 2001; 101: 62–66.
17. Parrott DL. Use of ohmic heating for aseptic processing of food particulates. *Food Technology.* 1992; 46(12): 68–72.
18. Stanley D. Safer salad is 'In the bag'. *Agricultural Research.* 1999.

BIBLIOGRAPHY

Air Products. Allentown, PA.

Buffler CR. *Microwave Cooking and Processing: Engineering Fundamentals for the Food Scientist*. New York: Chapman & Hall, 1993.

Charin SE. Dehydration of foods. In: Charm SE, ed. *Fundamentals of Food Engineering*. Westport, CT: AVI, 1978.

Charley H and Weaver C. *Foods: A Scientific Approach*, 3rd ed. New York: Merrill/Prentice Hall. 1998.

Dennis C, Stringer M. *Chilled Foods: A Comprehensive Guide*. Chichester: Ellis Horwood Ltd., 1992.

Des Rosier NW, Des Rosier JN. *Technology of Food Preservation*, 4th ed. Westport, CT: AVI, 1977.

Jul M. *The Quality of Frozen Foods*. New York: Academic Press, 1984.

Loaharann P. Cost/benefit aspects of food irradiation. *Food Technology*. 1994; 48(1): 104–108.

Lopez A. *A Complete Course in Canning, Vol. III*. Baltimore, MD: The Canning Trade Inc., 1987.

Mallet CP. *Frozen Food Technology*. New York: Chapman & Hall, 1993.

Pohlman AJ, Wood OB, Mason AC. Influence of audiovisual and food samples on consumer acceptance of food irradiation. *Food Technology*. 1994; 48(12): 46–49.

Vieira ER. *Elementary Food Science*, 4th ed. New York: Chapman & Hall, 1996.

Thayer DW. Food irradiation: Benefits and concerns. *Journal of Food Quality*. 1990; 13(3): 147–169. USDA.

CHAPTER 18

Food Additives

INTRODUCTION

According to the Food and Drug Administration (FDA), a food additive in its broadest sense is any substance added to food. *Legally,* the term refers to "any substance the intended use of which results or may reasonably be expected to result directly or indirectly in its becoming a component or otherwise affecting the characteristics of any food."

Additives are useful in controlling such factors as decomposition and deterioration, nutritional losses, loss of functional properties and aesthetic value, but may not be used to disguise poor quality. Their use is subject to regulation in the 1958 Food Additives Amendment to the Food, Drug and Cosmetic (FD&C) Act with exemptions for prior sanctioned items and Generally Recognized as Safe (GRAS) substances.

Food processors must petition the federal Food and Drug Administration for approval of a new food additive. FDA approval is then required for use at *specific* levels, only in *specific* products.

Vitamins and minerals are a special category of food ingredients. They are essential for nutrition but their use *apart from food* is often surrounded with controversy. Their use in foods has been increasing as they have been associated with the prevention and/or treatment of at least four of the leading causes of death in the United States. Existing additives, as well as new ones, are utilized in new product development.

DEFINITION OF FOOD ADDITIVES

The 1958 Food Additives Amendment to the Food Drug and Cosmetic Act of 1938 legally defined a food additive, and the Committee on Food Protection of the National Research Council (NRC) more simply and practically defined an additive as: "A substance or a mixture of substances, other than a basic foodstuff, that is present in a food as a result of an aspect of production, processing, storage, or packaging."

Exempt from food additive regulation are two groups: *prior sanctioned* substances, determined as safe for use prior to the 1958 amendment, such as sodium nitrite and potassium nitrite, and *GRAS* substances such as salt, sugar, spices, vitamins, and monosodium glutamate.

A food **additive** in its *broadest sense* is any substance added to food. *Legally,* additives are classified as *direct* if they are intentionally or purposely added to foods, in which case they must be named on food labels, or *indirect* if they are incidentally added to food in very small amounts during some phase of production, processing, storage, packaging, or transportation.

According to the FDA, food additives are substances added to foods for specific physical or technical effects. They may not be used to disguise poor quality but may aid in preservation and processing, or improve the quality factors of appearance, flavor, nutritional value, and texture (Chapter 1).

Although the consumer may be skeptical of, or perhaps in opposition to, an uncommon or unfamiliar chemical name of a food additive, in fact, all additives, including GRAS substances, such as salt, are chemicals. Food additives undergo rigorous toxicological analysis before their approval and use in foods.

The Joint FAO/WHO (Food and Agriculture Organization of the United Nations, and the World Health Organization) Expert Committee on Food Additives (JECFA) represents an international expert scientific committee that has met since 1956 to evaluate the safety of food additives.

FUNCTION OF FOOD ADDITIVES

General categories of food additives include preservatives, nutritional additives, sensory agents, and processing agents. As new food products are developed, new or existing food additives may be utilized.

Food manufacturers attempt to increase the life of their products by controlling and preventing deterioration; therefore, additives may be used to preserve, or combat *microbial* or *enzymatic deterioration*. All living tissue resists microorganism attack to some degree, and additives assist in microbial (pathogens and nonpathogens) protection. The use of additives at the point of manufacture or processing cannot stop *all* foodborne illness though, and cannot guarantee food safety for the population at large. For example, mishandling of food at restaurants and homes contributes a larger portion of foodborne illness than handling at food processing plants.

Ingredients may be included *to maintain* or *improve nutritional value*. Additives *enrich, fortify,* or restore what is lost in processing. They may add nutrients and correct deficiencies, such as when the first food additive, iodine was used to treat goiter, or when the minerals calcium and iron are added to food. Antioxidants such as lemon juice, BHT, BHA, and vitamins A and C are added to control the damaging effect of exposure to oxygen, or vitamin D is added to fortify milk. Many grain products are enriched or fortified with thiamin to prevent the disease beriberi, niacin to control the devastating pellagra, and more recently, with folate to prevent the reoccurrence of neural tube defect. Nutritional fortification is of tremendous benefit to many people.

In addition to food protection and nutrition fortification, additives, such as flavor and color sensory agents may be added to food so that it is made *more appealing*. Additives may be included in foods to *maintain product consistency*, to emulsify, stabilize, or thicken a food.

As mentioned, the first food additive in the United States was iodine, used to treat and prevent goiter, common in the Great Lakes and Pacific Northwest regions of the United States. Without seawater, the soil, water, and crops in these regions were deficient in iodine, and the problem of goiter in local populations was prevalent. It was added to salt (because it was commonly consumed and thus a good vehicle) in 1924 and iodized salt quickly became a common dietary source of iodine.

LEGISLATION AND TESTING FOR ADDITIVES

The *FDA* regulates the inclusion of additives to food products subject to interstate commerce or import, by authority of the Food Additives Amendment (1958) and the Color Additives Amendment (1960) to the Federal Food, Drug and Cosmetic Act of 1938. The *USDA* regulates additives of meat and poultry products.

Approval of Additives

In order to win approval for use of an additive, manufacturers must petition the FDA for approval of a new food additive and

- provide evidence of harmlessness of an additive at the intended level of use
- provide data from at least 2 years of feeding of at least two animals, male and female (usually dogs and rats)
- prove the safety, usually by utilizing an outside toxicology laboratory for testing

Manufacturers must show evidence that the additive is safe and that it will accomplish its intended effect. Although *absolute safety* of any substance can never be proven, there must be a *reasonable certainty* of no harm from the additive under its proposed use. In the approval evaluation, a "typical" intake is considered and additives are evaluated on a case-by-case basis.

Animal tests are conducted to show effects of large doses and lifetime or generational feedings, or *market basket patterns of consumption studies* are completed, which shows disappearance data of food that is produced and imported. The latter shows, on average, the 7-day intake of an adult male.

If the additive wins approval by the FDA, it is only for use at *specific levels* in *specific products*. For example, certain fat replacements may only be approved for addition to savory snacks. Then, subsequent to approval, periodic review of additives based on up-to-date scientific evidence occurs.

The FDA's Adverse Reaction Monitoring System (ARMS) monitors and investigates complaints that are associated with, and related to, food and color additives, specific foods, or vitamin and mineral supplements. The FDA also has an

Advisory Committee on Hypersensitivity to Food Constituents. Consumers should read product labels in order to determine specific ingredient information.

Delaney Clause

The **Delaney Clause** (named for the congressional sponsor Rep. James Delaney—NY) to the Food Additives Amendment states that no additive shown to cause cancer in man or laboratory animals, regardless of the dose, may be used in foods. Proposed additives are not acceptable for use in the food supply if they have been documented to be carcinogenic by *any* appropriate test. Such legislation continues to be reviewed, as both finer detection methods to detect minute amounts of a carcinogen, previously undetected, and improvements in additive testing over the years have become available.

This detection and improvement in testing has led to the question of what *is* an appropriate test. For example, is there *any* substance that is *totally* safe at *any* level of ingestion? Or will testing document the presence of carcinogens? The real issue may be in regard to *"risk versus benefit"* of an additive, for an additive may pose a ''risk,'' but a risk is *not* a threat to life. On the other hand, a ''benefit'' of using the additive is that there is an improvement in the condition of a food.

Currently, the FDA must abide by the mandate of the Delaney Clause in approving food additives, but this may change in the future. Overall, the goal of *any* ingredient testing is to provide a safe food supply for the public.

Nutrition Labeling Education Act (NLEA)

The Nutrition Labeling and Education Act of 1990 (Chapter 20) requires that all food labels *must list additives*, such as certifiable color additives by the common or usual name. Labels contain valuable information that allows people who may have food or food additive sensitivities to select appropriate food.

MAJOR ADDITIVES USED IN PROCESSING

Additives may be *naturally occurring* or *synthetic*. The additives most commonly used in the United States are **generally recognized as safe** (GRAS) flavor agents, along with baking soda, citric acid, mustard, pepper, and vegetable colors, that total greater than 98% by weight, of all additives in the United States.

Foods may contain ingredients that are added prior to retail sale. Vegetables and fruits, for example, may be treated with pesticides before harvesting, and dyes, fungicides, and waxes may be applied to retard ripening or promote sales. *Sodium nitrites* may be deliberately added to prevent *Clostridium botulinum* growth and preserve color, and *sodium phosphates* may be added for purposes of retaining texture and preventing rancidity.

An additive may serve multiple purposes and therefore be listed in several classes of additives. Some of the major additives used in processing are identified in the following text.

Anticaking Agents and Free-Flow Agents

Anticaking agents and free-flow agents inhibit or prevent lumping and caking in crystalline or fine powders, including salt and baking powder. Various silicates such as *aluminum calcium silicate, calcium silicate,* and *silicon dioxide,* as well as *tricalcium phosphate,* are examples of anticaking agents that may be added to powdered food.

Antimicrobials

Antimicrobials inhibit the growth of pathogenic or spoilage organisms. Most recognizable is *sodium chloride,* common table salt. Organic acids such as *acetic acid, benzoic acid, propionic,* and *sorbic acid* are utilized with low pH level food items. *Nitrites* and *nitrates* are used as antimicrobials in meat products to combat *C. botulinum,* while *sulfites* and *sulfur dioxide* are added to fruit juices and wine.

Antioxidants (Chapter 7)

The presence of oxygen may result in rancidity or deterioration of color, flavor, and nutritional values. Thus, antioxidants are added to combine with available oxygen to halt oxidation reactions. For example, antioxidants prevent or limit rancidity in fats and foods containing *fats,* stabilizing foods by preventing or inhibiting *oxidation of unsaturated fats and oils,* colors, and flavorings. Also, antioxidants prevent browning of cut *fruit,* by enzyme-catalyzed oxidation in *enzymatic oxidative browning* (Chapter 7).

Many antioxidants occur *naturally,* such as *ascorbic acid* (vitamin C), the *tocopherols* (vitamin E), *citric acid,* and some *phenolic compounds.* The most widely used *synthetic* antioxidants are *BHA* (butylated hydroxyanisole), *BHT* (butylated hydroxytoluene), *TBHQ* (tertiary butyl hydroxyquinone), and *propyl gallate.* These four synthetic antioxidants may be used alone or in combination with one another, or another additive to control oxidation. They may be used to prevent oxidation in fat-containing *food* (up to 0.02% of the fat level) or in *food packaging,* such as in whole grain cereal boxes.

Many meat processors add *sodium ascorbate* or *sodium erythorbate* (*ethorbic acid*) to cured meat to maintain processed meat color and to inhibit the production of nitrosamines from nitrites. (Nitrites are antioxidants that are also used as curing agents.) Ethylenediaminetetracetic acid (*EDTA*) may be used as an antioxidant or for other purposes in food (see Sequestering Agents).

Bleaching and Maturing Agents (Chapter 6)

As freshly milled flour ages, it whitens and improves in baking quality. Bleaching and/or maturing agents are added to flour either during or after the milling process to whiten and/or speed up the aging process. *Benzoyl peroxide* is added to bleach the yellowish carotenoid pigment to white, and *chlorine dioxide* is added to mature flour for better baking performance. *Bromates* may also be common as is *hydrogen peroxide* that is used to whiten milk for certain types of cheese manufacture.

Bulking Agents

Bulking agents such as *sorbitol, glycerol,* or *hydrogenatedstarch hydrolysates* are used in small amounts to provide body, smoothness, and creaminess that supplement the viscosity and thickening properties of hydrocolloids (colloidal material that binds water). They provide an oily or fatty mouthfeel and are frequently used in foods where sugar is reduced or absent. *Polydextrose* (Chapter 12) is an example of a bulking agent used when calories are limited in foods. It contains 1 cal g and is made from a mixture of glucose, sorbitol, and citric acid (89:10:1).

Coloring Agents

A color additive is any dye, pigment, or substance that imparts color when added or applied to a food, drug, cosmetic, or to the human body. The term "FD&C" is applied to *food color additives* approved by the FDA for food, drug, and cosmetic usage, "D&C" is used for approved *drug and cosmetic coloring agents,* and "External D&C" is granted to approved *color additives applied externally.* The *synthetic* coloring agents are assigned FD&C classifications by initials, the shade, and a number; for example, FD&C Red #40, and FD&C Yellow #5.

Coloring agents are added to foods because of the sensory appeal they provide, for the purpose of making processed foods look more appetizing. For example, colors are used in baked products, candies, dairy products such as butter, margarine, and ice cream, gelatin desserts, jams, and jellies in order to improve their appearance. It has been said that people "eat with their eyes" as well as their palates!

There are thousands of foods that use colors to make them look appetizing and attractive. The primary reasons for adding coloring agents include the following:

- Offsetting color loss due to exposure to air, light, moisture, and storage
- To correct natural variations in color or enhance color
- To provide visual appeal to wholesome and nutritious foods
- To provide color to foods that would otherwise be colorless, including "fun foods" and special foods for various holidays

Pigments may be derived from *natural* sources such as plant, mineral, or animal sources primarily the former (Table 18.1) and, if so, are *exempt* from FDA *certification* (see below), although they are still subject to *safety* testing prior to their approval for use in food. Some of the same ingredients added to foods for their health benefits, also offer "natural" (uncertified) coloring. These include anthocyanins, carotenoids, chlorophylls, foods such as beets (betalains), cabbage, tomatoes (lycopene), and a number of other flowers, fruits and vegetables.

Synthetic coloring agents are generally less expensive than natural colorants, are more intense, and have better coloring power, uniformity, and stability when exposed to environmental conditions such as heat and light. They may be water-soluble, or made water *in*soluble by the addition of aluminum hydroxide. Only small quantities of granules, a paste, powder, or solution are needed in foods to achieve the

TABLE 18.1 Colors Exempt from Certification (Uncertified)/Natural

Annato extract (yellow-reddish orange)	Grape color extract[a]
B-Apo-8′-carotenal[a] (orange)	Grape skin extract[a]
Beta-carotene	Paprika
Beet powder	Paprika oleoresin
Canthaxanthin	Riboflavin
Caramel color (brown)	Saffron
Carrot oil	Titanium dioxide[a]
Cochineal extract (red)	Turmeric (yellow)
Cottonseed flour, toasted, partially defatted, cooked	Turmeric oleoresin
Ferrous gluconate[a]	Vegetable juice
Fruit juice	

[a]Restricted to specific uses.

desired coloring effect. Each batch of synthetic food color must be tested by both the manufacturer and the FDA prior to gaining approval. Such testing assures safety, quality, consistency, and strength of the color additive.

The FDA permitted nine *"certifiable"* colors in the 1906 Food and Drug Law under a *voluntary* certification program; seven of those were approved for addition to *food* (Table 18.2). Certification became *mandatory* in 1938, with authority for testing passing to the USDA. Today, the term "certifiable" food color refers to color additives that are synthetic, or *man-made*, not natural.

In 1982, The National Institutes of Health concluded that there was no scientific evidence to support the claim that coloring agents or other food additives caused hyperactivity.

TABLE 18.2 Certifiable Colors–Synthetic

FD&C Blue No. 1 (bright blue)	FD&C Yellow No. 5 (lemon yellow)—tartrazine; second most widely used food dye
FD&C Blue No. 2 (royal blue)—Indigotine	
FD&C Green No. 3 (sea green)—minimally used	FD&C Yellow No. 6 (orange) Orange B[a]
FD&C Red No. 3 (orange-red)—erythrosine	Citrus Red No. 2[a]—used on some orange skins
FD&C Red No. 40 (cherry-red)—most widely used food dye	

[a]Restricted to specified uses other than foods.

Curing Agents (Chapter 9)

Curing agents impart color and flavor to foods. *Sodium nitrate* and *nitrite* contribute to the color, color stability, and flavor of cured meats such as bacon, frankfurters, ham, and salami. They also have antimicrobial properties to control *Clostridium botulinum* bacteria, and in fact, since nitrite use in cured meats became common, there have been no reported cases of botulism linked with cured meats. Nitrites also inhibit the growth of *C. perfringens, Staphylococcus aureus,* as well as other non-pathogens during storage of cured meats. (A nitrite concern is that nitrites reacts with certain amines to produce carcinogenic nitrosamines. Repeated testing of cured meat products showed that nitrosamines were absent or present at very low levels. In fact, endogenous human saliva usually contains more nitrite than has been detected in cured meat. Therefore, with these test results, the FDA permits use of nitrates, and nitrites at low levels, but has encouraged research on alternative ways of preserving meats.)

Dough Conditioners/Dough Improvers (Chapter 6)

Dough conditioners modify the starch and protein (thus, gluten) components of flour. They promote the aging process and improve both dough handling (such as in breadmaking machinery) and baking qualities (more uniform grain and increased volume). *Ammonium chloride, potassium bromate (bromination), diammonium phosphate,* and *calcium* or *sodium stearoyl lactylate* are processing aids that are examples of dough conditioners.

Some enzymes that provide food for yeast, and emulsifiers may be included in this class of additives. Conditioners may include iodates, a dietary source of iodine.

Edible Films (Chapter 19)

Edible films become part of food and are therefore subject to FDA approval. Examples include some *casings,* such as in sausage, and *edible waxes,* such as those applied to fruits and vegetables. The waxes function to improve or maintain appearance, prevent mold, and contain moisture while allowing respiration. Food may be coated with a thin layer of polysaccharides such as *cellulose, pectin, starch,* and *vegetable gums,* or proteins, such as *casein* and *gelatin* in order to extend shelf life.

Emulsifiers (Chapter 13)

Emulsifiers are a class of surface active agents that improve and maintain texture and consistency in a variety of foods. They contain both a hydrophobic molecular end, which is usually a long-chain fatty acid, and a hydrophilic end, and so, act as a bridge between two immiscible liquids, forming an emulsion. For example, they maintain a uniform dispersion by keeping water and oil fractions of a mixture together and they prevent large crystalline formations in products such as ice cream.

Lecithin, monoglycerides, diglycerides, and *polysorbates* (Polysorbate 60, 65, and 80) are examples of emulsifiers.

Enzymes

Enzymes are nontoxic protein substances that occur *naturally* in foods or may be produced by *microorganisms* or *biotechnology* to catalyze various reactions. They are easily inactivated by a specific pH and temperature. Although the presence of some enzymes may produce negative quality changes, other enzymes are often intentionally added to foods for their beneficial effect. Microorganisms are responsible for producing some of the enzymes desired in foods; thus, the microbes may be intentionally added to food.

Some examples of enzymes that are additions to other foods include *bromelain* (from pineapples), *ficin* (from figs), and *papain* (from papayas). These enzymes act as meat tenderizers of muscle tissue or connective tissue. *Amylases* hydrolyze starch in flour and are used along with acids in the production of corn syrup. *Invertase* is used to hydrolyze sucrose and prevent its crystallization. *Pectinases* clarify pectin-containing jellies or juices; *proteases* may be used as meat tenderizers, to create cheeses from milk (rennin), and to produce soy sauce. *Glucose oxidase* is added to foods such as egg whites in order to prevent the Maillard browning.

Fat Replacers (Chapter 12)

Fat replacers include carbohydrate, fat, or protein-based replacers. They include the following:

- Hydrocolloids, the long-chain polymers that thicken or gel
- Hemicelluloses, a plant polysaccharide
- β-Glucans, a subgroup of hemicelluloses (used in milk)
- Soluble bulking agents
- Microparticulated cellulose, egg, milk, or whey proteins (such as Simplesse®)
- Composite materials such as gums with milk or whey solids, or cellulose in combination with carboxymethyl cellulose
- Various functional blends of corn syrup solids, emulsifiers, modified food starch, nonfat milk solids, and vegetable protein
- Sucrose polyester (Olean®)

These ingredients are fat replacers that can be used alone, or in combination to provide a fatty or oily mouthfeel (1).

Firming Agents

Firming agents, such as *calcium chloride,* act on plant pectins to control the softening that may accompany the canning process of fruits or vegetables.

Flavoring Agents

Flavoring agents are the *largest single group* of food additives. Food and beverage applications of flavors include dairy, fruit, nut, seafood, spice blends, vegetables, and wine flavoring agents. They may complement, magnify, or modify the taste and aroma of foods. There are over 1200 different flavoring agents used in foods to create flavor or replenish flavors lost or diminished in processing, and hundreds of chemicals may be used to simulate natural flavors. *Alcohols, esters, aldehydes, ketones, protein hydrolysates,* and *MSG* are examples of flavoring agents.

Natural flavoring substances are extracted from plants, herbs and spice, animals, or microbial fermentations. They also include essential oils and oleoresins (created by solvent extract with solvent removed), herbs, spices, and sweeteners.

Synthetic flavoring agents are chemically similar to natural flavorings, and offer increased consistency in use and availability. They may be less expensive, and more readily available than the natural counterpart, although they may not adequately simulate the natural flavor. Some examples of synthetic flavoring agents include *amyl acetate,* used as banana flavoring, *benzaldehyde,* used to create cherry or almond flavor, *ethyl butyrate* for pineapple, *methyl anthranilate* for grape, *methyl salicylate* for wintergreen flavor, and *fumaric acid,* which is an ideal source of tartness and acidity in dry foods.

Flavor enhancers such as *monosodium glutamate* (MSG) intensify or "bring out," enhance or supplement, the flavor of other compounds in food; they have a taste outside of the basic sweet, sour, salty, or bitter. Monosodium glutamate was chemically derived from seaweed in the early 1900s, but is manufactured commercially by the fermentation of starch, molasses, or sugar.

MSG is a GRAS substance to which a small percentage of the public is severely allergic. Therefore, MSG must be identified on food labels when it is included in food. However, it may be a portion of another compound, such as "hydrolyzed vegetable protein" (which may contain up to 20% MSG); in that case, MSG is not stated on the label. In a summary of several decades of research, and one century of use, arguments *against* the GRAS status of MSG are overwhelmed by evidence *in support of* MSG.

Other examples of flavoring agents include the common salt (sodium chloride) and sugar (sucrose), corn syrup, aspartame (also a nutritive sweetener), autolyzed yeast (also a flavor enhancer), essential plant oils (such as citrus), ethyl vanillin and vanillin (a synthetic flavor compound), extracts (such as vanilla), glycine, mannitol (nutritive sweetener), saccharin (non-nutritive sweetener), and sorbitol (nutritive sweetener).

Fumigants

Fumigants are used to control pests and molds.

Humectants (Chapter 14)

Humectants are added to foods such as candy or shredded coconut in order to retain moisture content. The four polyhydric alcohols that are used to improve texture and retain moisture due to their affinity for water are *glycerol, mannitol* and *sorbitol* which also take moderately sweet, and *propylene glycol*. These may be functional in diet beverages, candy, stick chewing gum, and other foods to provide texture and sweetness. In order to prevent moisture absorption, *mannitol* may be "dusted" on chewing gum. *Glycerol monostearate* is another commonly used humectant.

Irradiation (Chapter 17)

Irradiation is subject to FDA approval as an *additive*. Only specific foods, dosages, and irradiation sources are approved to kill microorganisms such as *E. coli*, *Salmonella, Trichinella*, and insects.

Leavening Agents (Chapter 15)

Leavening agents leaven batters and doughs by producing or stimulating CO_2. Inorganic salts such as ammonium or phosphate salts such as *sodium acid pyrophosphate* may be combined with yeast, a biological leaven. *Sodium bicarbonate* (baking soda) or *ammonium bicarbonate* react with an acid to chemically produce CO_2.

Lubricants

Lubricants such as mineral hydrocarbons (nonstick cooking spray) may be added to food-contact surfaces to prevent foods from sticking and may become a part of the food.

Nutrient Supplements

Nutrient supplements are added to provide essential nutrients that are lost in processing or lacking in the diet. The addition of nutrients maintains or improves the nutritional quality of food. Common foods such as milk, cereal, flour, margarine, and salt contain added vitamins and minerals. For example, iodine may be added to salt, and B vitamins (including thiamin, riboflavin, niacin, folate) and iron are added to grain products. This improves the nutritional status of individuals who might not otherwise obtain essential nutrients. Oftentimes, the nutrients may be encapsulated for addition to food products, and thus more intact.

Some examples of nutrient supplementation include the following:

Alpha tocopherols (vitamin E) is an antioxidant and nutrient. It is commonly used in vegetable oil.

Ascorbic acid (vitamin C) is an antioxidant that reacts with unwanted oxygen, stabilizing colors, flavors, fats, and oils in foods. It maintains the red color of cured meats and prevents the formation of nitrosamines (from sodium nitrite). It is a nutrient that is added to beverages, breakfast cereals, and cured meats. *Sodium ascorbate* is a more soluble form of ascorbic acid that may be added to foods. *Sodium erythorbate* (*erythorbic acid*) achieves the same purpose without adding nutritional value.

Beta carotene is a nutrient and coloring agent that may be added to butter, margarine, or shortening.

B vitamins—thiamin, riboflavin, niacin, pyridoxine, biotin, and folate.

Calcium pantothenate, and other forms of calcium are added to supply calcium.

Ferrous gluconate is a nutrient and coloring agent. It may be added to foods such as black olives to create a jet black color. *Ferric orthophosphate, ferric sodium pyrophosphate,* and *ferrous fumarate* may be added to supply iron. *Ferrous lactate* is also a GRAS color fixative for ripe olives.

Phosphates in the form of *phosphoric acid* acidifies and flavors food; *sodium aluminum phosphate* is a leavening agent; *calcium* and *iron phosphate* act as mineral supplements to food.

Vitamins A and D are added to improve the nutritive value of foods such as margarine, reduced-fat and nonfat milks.

Minerals such as *iodine* and *zinc* may be added to foods.

pH Control Substances

Natural or synthetic *acid* or *alkali* ingredients change or maintain the initial pH of a product. For example, acidulents flavor, preserve, and regulate pH. The acid ingredients regulate by lowering the pH, and preserve foods by inhibiting microbial growth. Regardless of the acid level of food ingredients, food acids are incorporated into foods in order to maintain a constant acid level. *Natural acids* include the following: *acetic acid* or vinegar, *citric acid,* from citrus, that controls unwanted trace metals otherwise catalyzing oxidation reactions; *malic acid* (an organic acid from apples and figs) and *tartaric acid* (a weak acid). These acids may be added to foods to impart flavor and control tartness. *Lactic acid,* present in almost all living organisms, is an acidity regulator and is used in balancing the acidity in cheesemaking, as well as adding tartness to many other foods. The acid salt *calcium propionate* is added to control pH of breads. *Sodium lactate* (the salt of lactic acid) may be used in processed meat and poultry products.

Examples of *alkaline* ingredients include *sodium bicarbonate* (baking soda), an ingredient that balances the acid component of baking powder, *sodium hydroxide,* used in modified starches, and *potassium hydroxide.* Alkaline compounds are used to neutralize excess acid that could otherwise produce unwelcome flavors. In food they leaven and soften hard water.

Preservatives

Preservatives are classified as either *antimicrobial* agents that prevent microbial growth (bacteria, mold, yeast), or *antioxidants* that halt undesirable oxidative changes in food. They are used to delay natural deterioration, thus extending the shelf life of foods.

A preservative may be used alone or in combination with other additives or preservation techniques such as cold temperature storage, heat preservation, or dehydration (Chapter 17). Preservation is offered by the use of *salt* or *sugar,* which competes with bacteria for water and therefore lowers the water activity (A_w) of the food. *Calcium or sodium propionates* and *potassium sorbate* are additives used to control mold and bacterial growth, such as the bacilli that causes "rope" in breads. *Sodium benzoate* inhibits mold and yeast growth in condiments, fruit juices, and preserves.

Sulfur dioxide inhibits unwanted enzymatic oxidative browning in fruits and vegetables; it also prevents wild yeast growth in the wines used to produce vinegar and is legally used on grapes. However, a small number of individuals are severely allergic to sulfites, thus, they were banned in 1986 from addition to products not ubject to further cooking (e.g., many salad bar items).

Nitrites, such as *sodium nitrite,* are effective preservatives, preventing the growth of *C. botulinum,* adding flavor and retaining meat color in cured meats. *Antibiotics* are incorporated into animal feed and function as preservatives, but may *not* be added to human food. Some weak acids or *acid salts* and *chelating agents* (which tie up unwanted traces of metal) are utilized as preservatives.

Propellants

Propellants and aerating agents provide *pressure* needed for aerosol can products to be expelled and to *add air* to a product. Carbon dioxide, nitrogen, nitrous oxide, and other gasses may be used in aerosol containers, such as containers of "whipped topping".

Sequestrants

Sequestrants are known as chelating agents or metal scavengers. They are substances that *bind* or combine with trace amounts of unwanted metals such as copper and iron, making them unavailable for participating in negative reactions such as deterioration in food. They form *inactive complexes* with metallic ions during processing and storage, and therefore prevent metals from catalyzing reactions of fat oxidation, pigment discoloration, and flavor or odor loss, and from causing cloudy precipitates in beverages such as tea. They protect vitamins from oxidation.

Examples of sequestrants include citric and *malic acid, ethylenediaminetetraacetic acid (EDTA),* and *polyphosphates.*

Solvents

Solvents are used to separate substances by dissolving a substance in the solvent and removing the solvent.

Stabilizers and Thickeners

Stabilizers and thickeners function variously in food. For example, they provide consistency and texture to many foods. They are water-holding substances added to stabilize, gel, or thicken foods by absorbing some of the water present in foods. They increase viscosity of the final product, prevent ice crystal formation, or form gels. Stabilizers or thickeners are added for appearance and mouthfeel, to protect emulsions, and to contain volatile oils that would otherwise evaporate. Most are polysaccharides. They include the following:

- *Alginates* (from kelp).

- *Carrageenan* (a seaweed derivative).

- To provide visual appeal to wholesome and nutritious foods.

- *Cellulose* may be reacted with derivatives of acetic acid to form sodium carboxymethylcellulose (CMC), which is used to prevent sugar crystallization.

- *Dextrins*.

- The hydrocolloids (colloidal material that holds water); *gelatin* (the protein from animal bones, hoofs, etc.), *gums* such as arabic, guar, and locust beans, and *pectin*.

- Propylene glycol.

- *Protein derivatives* such as casein or sodium caseinate, and hydrolyzed vegetable protein.

- *Starches* (including amylose and modified starches) allow oils, water, acids, and solids to remain well mixed by the addition of natural or chemically modified starches.

Some stabilizers and thickeners are commercially available for use by the healthcare industry in preparation of food items such as pureed foods.

Surface Active Agents

Surface active agents are organic compounds that are used in food systems to reduce the surface tension or forces at the surface of a liquid. Dispersion into food mixtures is resisted if the forces attracting surface molecules of a liquid to one another is not reduced. Classifications of surface acting agents include wetting agents, lubricants, dispersing agents, and emulsifiers. For example, *wetting agents* reduce surface tension in chocolate milk mixes, so that particles to be mixed may absorb water more easily and mix into the milk. *Emulsifiers* enable two ordinarily immiscible substances to combine—for example, oil and water—and they also improve texture.

Sweeteners (Chapter 14)

Sweeteners are added to many foods and beverages. The disaccharide *sucrose* (table sugar) is a common food additive. *Fructose,* is one of the components of sucrose. It is two times as sweet as sucrose and will not crystallize out of solution as does sucrose. It is the most water-soluble sugar and is used to create a very sweet solution. It is hygroscopic and, therefore, may function as a humectant. *Lactose* (milk sugar) and *maltose* (malt sugar) are often food additives. *Corn syrup, high-fructose corn syrup, honey, maple syrup sugar,* and *molasses* are other examples of sweeteners used as food additives. *Invert sugar* is the 50:50 mixture of glucose and fructose produced by enzymatic or acid treatment of sucrose. Its use prevents sugar crystallization, for example, in the liquid center of chocolate-covered cherries.

Sweeteners, Alternative (Chapter 14)

Some low-calorie, artificial sweeteners, and sugar alcohols that are added to foods include the following:

Acesulfame K may be used alone or in combination with other sweeteners. It is a synthetic derivative of acetoacetic acid that is not metabolized by the body and is therefore excreted unchanged. Acesulfame is stable in heat and is many times sweeter than sucrose, with no bitter aftertaste.

Aspartame is a synthetic dipeptide (aspartic acid, phenylalanine). It is in products used by diabetics but cannot be used by phenylketonuric (PKU) individuals. It is not stable in heat unless encapsulated and cannot substitute for sucrose when the texture of the food depends on solids content.

Cyclamates of sodium, calcium, magnesium, and potassium that are approximately 30 times sweeter than sucrose (not used in the United States).

Saccharin is used as the calcium or sodium salt. It cannot be used as a substitute for sucrose when the texture of the food depends on solids content.

Sugar alcohols include *mannitol, sorbitol,* and *xylitol.*

NUTRIENT SUPPLEMENTS IN FOOD

As previously stated, the nutritive value of foods may be improved either by replacing nutrients lost in processing or lacking in the diet. The addition of *vitamins,* such as vitamin C, and *minerals,* such as calcium, is often made to common foods. Further detail appears in this section.

Food processors may choose to add any number of nutrient additives, at varying levels, to their food products. Products are enriched when nutrients that were *lost during processing* are replaced to levels comparable to the original levels. **Enrichment** is designed to prevent inadequacies in certain segments of the population, and it is the addition of nutrients to achieve established concentrations specified by the standards of identity (2). **Fortification** is the addition of nutrients (the same or different ones) at levels *higher* than those found in the original or comparable food. It can correct existing deficiencies in segments of the population, such as with the addition of calcium. Breakfast cereals, breakfast bars, and fruit drinks are prominent examples of fortification that provide needed nutrients to many individuals.

In addition to the enjoyment of eating, consumption of a varied diet offers many health benefits to the consumer, including nutrients such as vitamins and minerals as well as non-nutrient compounds (such as phytochemicals) that play an important role in reducing risks of certain diseases. For additional information, the reader is referred to the FDA's regulation of dietary supplements (3).

Endorsement of Nutrient Supplementation in Foods

The American Medical Association Council on Foods and Nutrition Board has set the following recommendations for endorsement of nutrient supplementation in foods:

1. The intake of the nutrient is below the desirable level in the diets of a significant number of people.
2. The food used to supply the nutient is likely to be consumed in quantities that will make a significant contribution to the diet of the population in need.
3. The addition of the nutrient is not likely to create an imbalance of essential nutrients.
4. The nutrient added is stable under proper conditions of storage.
5. The nutrient is physiologically available from the food.
6. There is a reasonable assurance against excessive intake to a level of toxicity.

Vitamins and Minerals Manufactured for Addition to Foods

There are many vitamins and minerals that are prepared for addition to foods. The *fat-soluble vitamins* that may be added to foods are the carotenoids, vitamin A precursors, the tocopherols (vitamin E), and vitamin D.

Among the *water-soluble vitamins,* ascorbic acid (vitamin C) may be added to foods in order to prevent oxidation, to prevent the formation of nitrosamines in cured meats, and to improve nutritive value, especially in beverages. The B-complex vitamins may be used as nutrient additives. *Thiamin hydrochloride* and *thiamin nitrate* (B_1), *riboflavin* and *riboflavin-5'-phosphate* (B_2), and several sources of *niacin*(B_3) are FDA approved and commercially available to processors for addition to foods.

Vitamin B_6 (pyridoxine, pyridoxal, and pyridoxamine), B_{12} (cyanocobalamin), pantothenic acid, folacin, and biotin are also manufactured for use in food. Recently, folic acid (folacin, folate) addition has been required by the FDA, for addition to flour and flour-based products. Folate has been shown to prevent neural tube defect (4).

Additionally, among *minerals,* there are three major minerals and six trace minerals used in foods. Of the major minerals, calcium, magnesium, and phosphorus may be added to a number of foods. Calcium is now more commonly added to orange juice. Copper, fluoride, iodine, iron, manganese, and zinc are trace minerals used as food additives. Chromium, potassium, molybdenum, selenium, and sodium may not have Reference Daily Intakes (RDIs), but rather safe and adequate intakes. Labels do not state these values, but may state "reduced sodium" and so forth if the statement is in compliance with NLEA regulations.

Functional Foods

Eating modified foods may supply health benefits beyond the traditional nutrients a food contains. Therefore, food products may be modified by the addition of nutrients not inherent to the original counterpart (5). A newly evolving area of food and food technology is **functional foods** (Chapter 20), which are defined as

> "Any modified food or food ingredient that may provide a health benefit beyond the traditional nutrients it contains" (6,7).

Phytochemicals

Phytochemicals (Chapters 7 and 20), non-nutrient substances from plants, (plant chemicals) may become useful as food additives because they may play an important role in reducing risk of cancers. They are naturally available in the diet and are currently in supplement form. Phytochemicals are defined as:

> "Substances found in edible fruits and vegetables that may be ingested by humans daily in gram quantities and that exhibit a potential for modulating human metabolism in a manner favorable for cancer prevention" (6).

Functional food components, along with phytochemicals, have been associated with the treatment and/or prevention of at least four of the leading causes of death in the United States—cancer, diabetes, cardiovascular disease, and hypertension. They have been associated with the treatment and/or prevention of other medical maladies including neural tube defect and osteoporosis, as well as abnormal bowel function and arthritis (8).

It is the position of the American Dietetic Association (ADA) that specific substances in foods (e.g., phytochemicals and naturally occurring components and functional food components) may have a beneficial role in health as part of a varied diet. The Association supports research regarding the health benefits and risks of these substances. Dietetics professionals will continue to work with the food industry and government to ensure that the public has accurate scientific information in this emerging field (ADA).

Nutraceuticals

The term nutraceutical (Chapter 20) is not recognized by the FDA and is outside FDA regulations because of the following:

Foods are defined as "products primarily consumed for their taste, aroma, or nutritive value."

Drugs are defined as "intended for use in the diagnosis, cure, mitigation, treatment or prevention of disease or to affect the structure or a function of the body" (10).

Nutraceuticals are defined by the Foundation For Innovation in Medicine as

> "Any substance that may be considered a food or part of a food and provides medical or health benefits, including the prevention or treatment of disease. Nutraceuticals may range from isolated nutrients, dietary supplements, and diets to genetically engineered "designer" foods, herbal products, and processed products, such as cereals, soups, and beverages" (9).

Formulating a New Product with Vitamin or Mineral Addition

Food processors may choose to use any additive, including nutrients or non-nutrient supplements, in the manufacture of food products. Regardless of what is used, they must comply with all Nutrition Labeling and Education Act (NLEA) regulations regarding the contents and stated **health claims** of their products. They must use vitamin and mineral additives judiciously (not just to enhance the values on their food label), and then only make label claims regarding nutritional benefits that are allowed (Chapter 20).

Food technologists formulate a new product with a number of considerations in mind regarding vitamin and mineral addition (2). Some considerations include the following:

- Overall product composition—such as pH, water activity, fat, fiber, protein, because the flavor and color of foods may change

- Ingredient interactions—of a vitamin or mineral combination

- Processing considerations—blanching, washing, stability to heat

- Shelf life and packaging—protection from oxidation or light

- Cost factors—price of the nutrient, overages due to loss, and costs of (the above) processing and packaging needs

A research dietitian with the USDA Agricultural Research Services has said:

"Open, academic research, including human testing of isolated food components (e.g., vitamins, minerals, amino acids, fatty acids, sugars, dietary fibers, and many other food components) has been fundamental to the development of nutrition science. Federal regulations (through FDA) and funding should be encouraged to promote human research and clinical testing of the health benefits of foods and food components, consistent with good science, safety, and the Nutrition Labeling and Education Act of 1990.

Although compounds in foods that must be concentrated to obtain physiologic effects should be regulated as drugs, foods and purified food constituents in amounts commonly consumed should not be classified as drugs simply because they are being tested for potential health effects or disease prevention. Research should not be discouraged by requiring investigative new drug procedures for substances in amounts available in the diet" (10).

CONCLUSION

Additives are "a substance or a mixture of substances, other than a basic foodstuff, that is present in a food as a result of an aspect of production, processing, storage or packaging." Additives function in foods to combat microbial and enzymatic deterioration, to maintain or improve nutritional value and product consistency, and to make food more aesthetically appealing. *Less* rancidity, spoilage, contamination, and overall waste, and *more* nutritional value and ease of preparation are possible with the use of additives. Many additives are natural food ingredients, used strictly for imparting flavor and color.

The Food Additives Amendment (1958) of the Federal Food, Drug and Cosmetic Act of 1938 contains legislation regarding the safety of additives. The Delaney Clause to the Food Additives Amendment requires testing of proposed additives in the United States for carcinogens. Salt, sugar, and corn syrup are the three most commonly used food additives in the U.S. food supply.

Major additives used in food processing include alternative sweeteners, anticaking agents, antioxidants, bleaching and maturing agents, bulking agents, coloring agents, curing agents, dough conditioners, emulsifiers, enzymes, fat replacers, firming agents, flavoring agents, fumigants, humectants, irradiation, leavening agents, lubricants, nutrient supplements, pH control substances, preservatives, propellants, sequestrants, solvents, stabilizers and thickeners, surface acting agents, and sweeteners.

The nutritional value of foods may be increased to exceed nutrient levels inherent in the traditional product. Food nutrients may be fortified or enriched. Specific vitamins and minerals are manufactured with the purpose of addition to foods. Functional foods are foods that are modified to provide a health benefit beyond the traditional product and may be used to treat/prevent disease. They along with phytochemicals and nutraceuticals are a newly evolving area of food and food technology.

GLOSSARY

Additive: Substance added to foods for specific physical or technical effects.

Delaney Clause: Clause added to Food Additives Amendment stating that no additive shown to cause cancer in man or laboratory animals could be used in foods.

Drugs: Intended for use in the diagnosis, cure, mitigation, treatment, or prevention of disease or to affect the structure or function of the body.

Enrichment: The addition of nutrients to achieve established concentrations specified by the standards of identity.

Foods: Products primarily consumed for their taste, aroma, or nutritive value.

Fortification: The addition of nutrients at levels higher than those found in the original or comparable food.

Functional foods: Any modified food or food ingredient that may provide a health benefit beyond that obtained by the original food; the term has no legal or general acceptance in the United States, but is accepted by some as food for specified health use.

Generally Recognized As Safe (GRAS): Substances in use, not shown to be unsafe.

Health claims: Describe an association between a nutrient or food substance and disease or health-related condition.

Nutraceuticals: The name given to a proposed new regulatory category of food components that may be considered a food or part of a food and may supply medical or health benefits including the treatment or prevention of disease; a term not recognized by the FDA.

Phytochemicals: Plant chemicals; natural compounds other than nutrients in fresh plant material that function in disease prevention; they protect against oxidative cell damage or facilitate carcinogen excretion from the body and exhibit a potential for reducing the risk of cancer.

REFERENCES

1. Glicksman M. Hydrocolloids and the search for the "Oily Grail." *Food Technology*. 1991; 45(10): 94–99.
2. Giese J. Vitamin and mineral fortification of foods. *Food Technology*. 1995; 49(5): 110–122.
3. Food and Drug Administration. Regulation of dietary supplements. *Federal Register*. 1993; 58: 3692.
4. Food and Drug Administration. Folate and neural tube defects. *Federal Register*. March 5, 1996; 61(44): 8750–8807.
5. Peter Pan Peanut Butter, Fullerton, CA.
6. Jenkins MLY. Research issues in evaluating "functional foods." *Food Technology*. 1993; 47(5): 76–79.
7. Goldberg I, ed. *Functional Foods: Designer Foods, Pharmafoods, Nutraceuticals*. New York: Chapman & Hall; 1994.
8. ADA Position of the American Dietetic Association: Phytochemicals and functional foods. *Journal of the American Dietetic Association*. 1995; 95(4): 493–496.
9. *The Nutraceutical Initiative: A Proosal for Economic and Regulatory Reform*. Cranford, NJ: The Foundation for Innovation in Medicine, 1991.
10. Hunt J. Nutritional products for specific health benefits—Foods, pharmaceuticals, or something in between? *Journal of the American Dietetic Association*. 1994; 94: 151–154.

BIBLIOGRAPHY

Accurate Ingredients. Syosset, NY.

Ashland Chemical. Columbus, OH.

Block G, Langseth L. Antioxidant vitamins and disease prevention. *Food Technology*. 1994; 48(7): 80–84.

Cooperative Extension. University of Illinois, Urbana, Champaigne, IL.

Dorko C. Antioxidants used in foods. *Food Technology*. 1994; 48(4): 33–34.

Dow Chemical. Midland, MI.

FIS Flavors Company. Solon, OH

Food and Drug Administration. *Food Risk: Perception vs. Reality*. Rockville, MD: Food and Drug Administration, 1990.

Food and Nutrition Board. *Food Additives: Summarized Data from NRC Food Additive Surveys*. Washington, DC: National Academy of Science, 1981.

Flavor Ingredients. Hampshire, IL.

Flavor Innovations. S. Plainfield, NJ.

Food Flavors. Derby, KS.

International Food Information Council Foundation, Washington, D.C.

Nolan AC. The sulfite controversy. *Food Engineering*. 1983; 55(10): 84.

Sloan AE. America's Appetite '96: The ten top trends to watch and work on. *Food Technology*. 1996; 50(7): 55–71.

Sloan AE. Prevents disease! Tastes great! *Food Technology*. 1994; 48(8): 96–98.

Sloan AE. Ingredients add more fun, flavor, freshness & nutrition. *Food Technology*. 1995; 49(8): 102.

Smith J. *Food Additive User's Handbook*. New York: Chapman & Hall, 1991.

CHAPTER 19

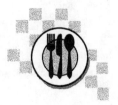

Packaging of Food Products

INTRODUCTION

Packaging is intended to preserve food against spoilage and contamination and extend its shelf life. The various packaging materials, including films and, package oxygen protect foods from such variables as light and moisture. Packaging may also maintain time-sensitive foods. Yet, packaging offers much more than these benefits to the manufacturer and consumer. It provides containment (holding the product), protection (quality, safety, freshness), information (graphics, labels), and utility of use or convenience (1).

Packaging materials for food include metal, glass, paper, plastics, foil, wood crates, cotton, or burlap (jute). Food may be vacuum packaged, subject to controlled or modified atmospheric packaging, or be aseptically packaged. Manufacturers must adhere to FDA regulations regarding both the method and materials of packaging.

Today, consumer-convenient packaging such as microwaveable packages, single-serve products, tubs, and zippered pouches, tamper evidence, and package atmosphere have become increasingly important as a packaging selection (2). Packaging functionality is a demand of both consumers and food companies alike, who want packaging/materials that meet their needs.

TYPES OF PACKAGING CONTAINERS

Packaging containers are classified as primary, secondary, and tertiary. A *primary* container is the bottle, can, drink box, and so forth that contains food. It is a direct-food-contact surface and is, therefore, subject to approval by the Food and Drug Administration (FDA), which tests for the possible migration of packaging materials into food.

Several primary containers are held together in *secondary* containers, such as corrugated fiberboard boxes (commonly, but not correctly, referred to as cardboard), and do not have direct food contact. In turn, several secondary containers are bundled into **tertiary** containers such as corrugated boxes or overwraps that prepare the food product for distribution or palletizing. They offer additional food protection during storage and distribution where errors, such as dropping and denting or crushing cartons, may occur. Tertiary containers prevent the brunt of the impact from falling on the individual food container.

PACKAGING FUNCTIONS

The functions of packaging are numerous and include such purposes as protecting *raw* or *processed* foods against *spoilage* and *contamination* by an array of external hazards. Packaging serves as a barrier in controlling oxygen and water levels, facilitates ease of use, offers adequate storage, conveys information, and provides evidence of possible product tampering. It achieves these goals by assisting in the following manners:

- Preserving against spoilage of color, flavor, odor, texture, and other food qualities
- Preventing contamination by biological, chemical, or physical hazards
- Controlling absorption and losses of O_2 and water vapor
- Facilitating ease of using product contents—such as packaging that incorporates the components of a meal together in meal "kits" (e.g., tacos)
- Offering adequate storage before use—such as stockable, resealable, pourable
- Preventing/indicating tampering with contents by tamper-evident labels
- Communicating information regarding ingredients, nutrition facts, manufacturer name and address, weight, bar code information, and so forth via package labeling
- Marketing—standards of packaging, including worldwide acceptability of certain colors and picture symbols vary and should be known by the processor. Packages themselves may promote sales. They may be rigid, flexible, metallized, and so forth, and may also carry such information as merchandising messages, health messages, recipes, and coupons.

PACKAGING MATERIALS

In choosing the appropriate packaging for their product, packers must consider many variables. For example, *canners* must make packaging choices based on cost, product compatibility, shelf life, flexibility of size, handling systems, production line filling and closing speeds, processing reaction, impermeability, dent and tamper resistance, and consumer convenience and preference (3). Processors who use *films* for their product must select film material based on its "barrier" properties that prevent oxygen, water vapor, or light from negatively affecting the food. As an example, the use of packaging material that prevents light-induced reactions, will control degradation of the chlorophyll pigment, bleaching or discoloration of vegetable and red meats, destruction of riboflavin in milk, and oxidation of vitamin C.

The most common food packaging materials include metals, glass, paper, and plastic. Some examples of these leading materials appear in the following text.

Metal

Metals such as steel and aluminum are used in cans and trays (Figures 19.1 and 19.2). A metal can forms a hermetic seal, which is a complete seal against gases and vapor entry or escape, and it offers protection to the contents. The trays may be reusable, or disposable recyclable trays, and either steamtable or No. 10 can size. Metal is also used for bottle closures and wraps.

Steel has a noncorrosive coating of tin inside, thus the name "tin can," whereas *tin-free steel* (TFS) relies on the inclusion of chromium or aluminum in place of tin. Steel is manufactured into the traditional *three-piece* construction can, which includes a base, cylinder, and lid, and also a *two-piece* can, consisting of a base and cylinder in one piece without a seam, and a lid. The latter are lightweight and stackable. Ninety-six percent of the close to 27 billion cans used annually in the United States are made of steel (4).

In addition to steel cans and trays, more than 25 billion beverage bottles crowns (closures with crimped edges) made of steel are used annually in the United States (4). The five primary types of steel vacuum closures include side seal caps, lug caps, press–twist caps, snap-on caps, and composite caps (Figure 19.3).

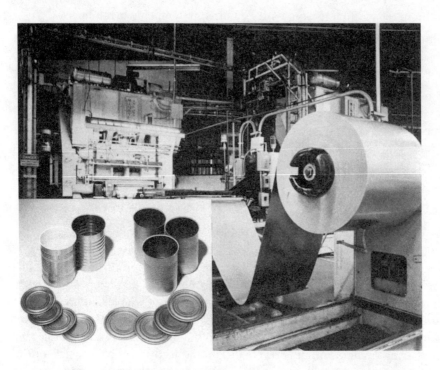

FIGURE 19.1   Steel (tin-free), and two-piece seamless cans with lids
(*Source:* American Iron and Steel Institute).

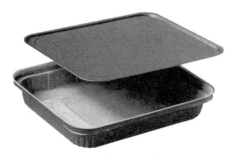

FIGURE 19.2   Steel steam table tray
(*Source:* American Iron and Steel Institute).

Aluminum is easily formed into cans with hermetic seals. It is also used in trays and for wraps such as aluminum foil, which provide an oxygen and light barrier. It is lighter in weight than steel and resists corrosion.

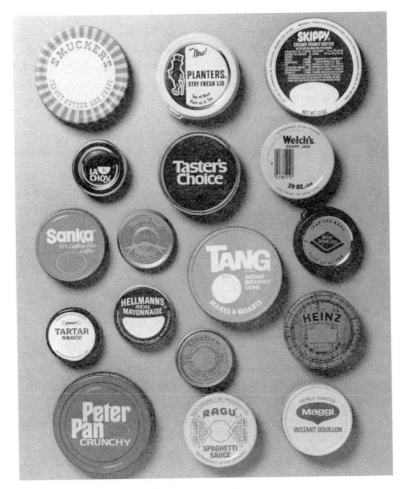

FIGURE 19.3   Examples of steel vacuum closures
(*Source:* American Iron and Steel Institute).

Glass

Glass is derived from metal oxides such as silicon dioxide (sand). It is used in forming bottles or jars (which subsequently receive hermetic seals) and thus protects against water vapor or oxygen loss. The thickness of glass must be sufficient to prevent breakage from internal pressure, external impact, or thermal stress. Glass that is *too* thick increases weight and thus freight costs and is subject to an increased likelihood of thermal stress or external impact breakage.

Technological advances in glass packaging have led to improvements in strength and weight, as well as color and shape. A resurgence of glass may be noted on supermarket shelves. The product is commercially sterile (see Chapter 16), yet the see-through glass tends to denote "fresh" to the consumer.

Glass coatings, similar to eyeglass coatings of silicons and waxes, may be applied to glass containers in order to minimize damage-causing nicks and scratches.

Paper

Paper is derived from the pulp of wood and may contain additives such as aluminum particle laminates, plastic coating, resins, or waxes. These additives provide burst strength (strength against bursting), wet strength (leak protection), and grease and tear resistance, as well as barrier properties that assure freshness, protect the packaged food against vapor loss and environmental contaminants, and increase shelf life.

Varying thicknesses of paper may be used to achieve thicker and more rigid packaging.

- *Paper* is thin (one layer) and flexible, typically used in bags and wrappers. Kraft (or "strong" in German) paper is the strongest paper. It may be bleached and used as butcher wrap or may remain unbleached and used in grocery bags.

- *Paperboard* is thicker (although still one layer) and more rigid. Ovenable paperboard is made for use in either conventional or microwave ovens by coating paperboard with PET polyester (see Plastic).

- Multilayers of paper form *fiberboard*, which is recognized as *"cardboard."*

When packaging serves as a *primary* container for food, it is a food-contact surface and must be coated or treated accordingly. For example, *paper* bags or wraps for bakery products may be laminated to improve burst or wet strength, grease and tear resistance, or prevent loss of moisture. *Paperboard* may be lined and formed to hold fluid milk. It may be formed into canisters with foil linings and resealable plastic overwraps, to provide convenience, protection and extended shelf life. *Corrugated paperboard* may be waxed in order to package raw poultry contents.

Dual-ovenable trays are designed to be *microwaveable* and able to be placed in a *conventional* oven. As with all new processing and packaging technology, the use of these trays is a new concept for many people, and may require written consumer education by food manufacturers.

Recycled papers may contain small metal fragments that could be unacceptable in packaging used for microwave cooking. The sparks, generated as the microwaves are reflected by metal, may start a fire in the microwave oven. Yet, paper may be manufactured to designated specifications and deliberately contain areas with small particles of aluminum, which form a "*susceptor*."

Susceptors are desirable for browning and crisping microwaveable foods such as baked goods, french fries (often placed in individual compartments of a susceptor), and pizzas. They are used in packages of microwaveable popcorn, for example, because the metal reflects microwaves, which subsequently heat the surface of the food.

When used in combination with metal, such as aluminum, paper may be used to produce fiber-wound tubing. An example of fiber-wound tube containers used for refrigerated biscuits is shown in Figure 19.4.

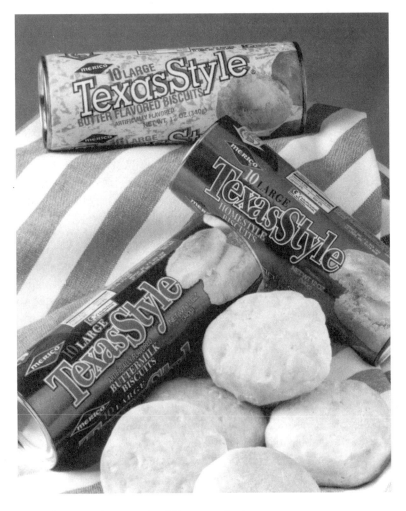

FIGURE 19.4   An example of fiber-wound tubes
(*Source:* The Earthgrains Company).

Metallized films and papers are increasingly chosen for food applications. The appearance, and its barrier properties to grease, and moisture are desirable for packaging specific foods. These materials contain plastic, which is discussed in the following chapter section.

Plastic

Plastic has shrink, nonshrink, flexible, semirigid, and rigid applications, and varies in its degree of thickness. Important *properties* of the many types of plastics that make them good choices for packaging material include the following:

- Flexible and stretchable
- Lightweight
- Low-temperature formability
- Resistant to breakage, with high burst strength
- Strong heat sealability
- Versatile in its barrier properties to O_2, moisture, and light

Basic hydrocarbon building blocks such as ethane and methane, which are derived from natural gas and petroleum, form organic chemical compounds called *monomers*. These are then chemically linked to form plastic molecular chains, or *polymers*. Their manufacture represents 1.5% of total U.S. energy consumed (5). Plastic has multiple *functions* as a packaging material, including use in bottles and jars, closures, coatings, films, pouches, tubs, and trays (1). It may also be used *in combination* with other packaging materials such as metal (for lining cans), paper (for moisture resistance), and glass (reduces bottle breakage).

Favorable views of plastic have developed as it was found that approximately 400% more material by weight would be needed to make packaging if there was *no* plastic (6), and that for every pound of plastic packaging that was used, 1.7 pounds of food waste were prevented (7). Additionally, *plastic grocery bags* require approximately 40% less energy to make than paper bags (8), and plastic bag packaging contributes up to 80% less solid waste by volume than paper sacks (9). It takes less than one-fourth pound of 2-liter plastic bottles to deliver 1 gallon of beverage, whereas it takes 4.3 pounds of 16-ounce glass bottles to deliver that same 1 gallon (8).

Choices of Plastics for Packaging. The food industry must provide packaging with barrier protection (against moisture, light, air, grease, etc.) and must "know what level of barrier performance is sufficient for the goods they are packaging" (10). *Insufficient* packaging, attributable in part to a high cost of materials, is not satisfactory, and *too much* performance (excesses in packaging contribution), with excessive barrier protection, is unnecessary.

Among the thousands types of plastics that are created, less than two dozen are polymers utilized in food packaging (see Table 19.1). Some of the more commonly used plastics for food products are discussed in the following:

TABLE 19.1   Example of the Repeating Units of Common Packaging Polymers

Repeating Units of Common Packaging Polymers	
Polymer	**Repeating Unit**
Polyester (PET)	$-\overset{\displaystyle H}{\underset{\displaystyle H}{C}}-\overset{\displaystyle H}{\underset{\displaystyle H}{C}}-O-\overset{\displaystyle O}{C}-\text{⊙}-\overset{\displaystyle O}{C}-O-$
Polyethylene (PE)	$-CH_2-CH_2-$
Polypropylene (PP)	$-CH_2-\overset{\displaystyle CH_3}{CH}-$
Polystyrene (PS)	$-CH_2-\overset{\displaystyle |}{CH}-$ ⬡
Polyvinyl Chloride (PVC)	$-CH_2-\overset{\displaystyle |}{\underset{\displaystyle Cl}{CH}}-$

Source: The Society of the Plastics Industry.

Polyethylene (PE): **Polyethylene** is the most common and the least expensive plastic, comprising 63% of total plastic packaging. It is a water-vapor (moisture) barrier and prevents dehydration and freezer burn. An example of the polyethylene pellets used in producing plastic, such as plastic bags, "zipper" seals, and plastic storage containers, is shown in Figure 19.5, and a view of the film coming off of the die is seen in Figure 19.6.

Polyethylene with ethyl vinyl acetate (EVA) creates "freezer wrap," which offers moisture-loss protection without getting brittle in low temperatures. Polyethylene terephthalate (PET) is used in "an increasing number of food and beverages" (11), including use as a tube which dispenses food. Some advantages of PET is that it with stands high temperature foods, and is lighter in weight than the glass that it replaces. Polyethylene naphthalate (PEN) received FDA approval in 1996 for use in food packaging. It provides a barrier against gas, moisture, and ultraviolet light. As bottled beverages, including waters, teas, and juices, continue to appear in the marketplace, the use of plastic bottle containers made of PET and PEN may be increasing.

Polypropylene (PP): Polypropylene has a higher melting point and greater tensile strength than polyethylene. It is often used as the inside layer of food packages that are subject to higher temperatures of sterilization (e.g., retort pouches or tubs).

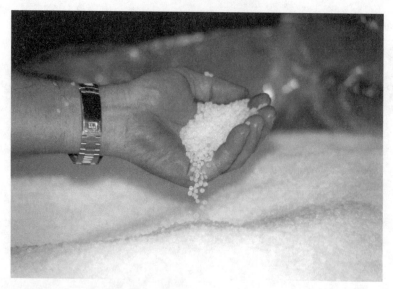

FIGURE 19.5 Polyethylene pellets
(*Courtesy of Rodeo Plastic Bag and Film, Inc., Mesquite, TX*).

Polystyrene (PS): **Polystyrene** is a versatile, inexpensive packaging material and represents 8% of total plastic packaging. When foamed, its generic name is expandable polystyrene (EPS). This styrofoam has applications in disposable packaging and drinking cups. It offers thermal insulation and protective packaging. EPS is used in "clam shell" fast-food packaging, egg cartons, bowls, cups, and meat trays and is the "peanuts" in packages. Approximately 30% less energy is required to form polystyrene cups than paperboard cups (12).

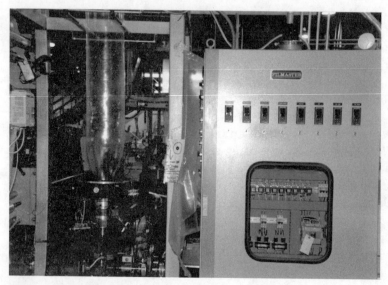

FIGURE 19.6 Blown film bubble coming off the die
(*Courtesy of Rodeo Plastic Bag and Film, Inc., Mesquite, TX*).

Polyvinyl chloride (PVC or vinyl): **Polyvinyl chloride** comprises 6% of total plastic packaging. It blocks out air and moisture, preventing freezer burn, and offers low permeability to gases, liquid, flavors, and odors. PVC prevents the transfer of odor and keeps food fresh by controlling dehydration and is capable of withstanding high temperatures without melting. PVC has good puncture resistance and "cling" properties. It is used to prevent splattering in microwave food preparation.

Polyvinylidene chloride (PVDC, Saran®): **Polyvinylidene chloride** is a thermoplastic resin used for household wraps and has excellent barrier properties. *Cryovac* is a Saran film used in vaccum-sealing (*Kryos* = cold *Vacus* = empty in Latin).

Many manufacturers specify proprietary molded and shaped bottles to hold the food contents. The appropriate plastic may be chosen to satisfy this highly specialized demand.

There are also *food-based* materials used to produce thermal plastic resins. They are made from natural sugars found in corn and other plants. For example, wheat starch and corn sugar are being developed for packaging purposes. As Australia's Cooperative Research Centers' Executive Director has noted, "The materials consist of wheat starch and are blended with other biodegradable materials so they will compost down fully in around 30–60 days" (13).

Other Packaging Materials

Cotton or **burlap** (jute) may be used for grains, flour, legumes, and some vegetables, primarily in transport.

Edible films are subject to FDA approval because they become part of the food. Natural edible films extend shelf life, although for shorter time than synthetic nonedible packaging materials. Edible films are a unique type of packaging material. As stated in a publication of the Institute of Food Technologist's Expert Panel on Food Safety and Nutrition:

> These films are ". . . defined as a thin layer of edible material formed on a food as a coating or placed (pre-formed) on or between food components. Its purpose is to inhibit migration of moisture, oxygen, carbon dioxide, aromas, and lipids, etc.; carry food ingredients (e.g. antioxidants, antimicrobials, flavor); and/or improve mechanical integrity or handling characteristics of the food" (14).

Antimicrobials may be included in films or containers. Antimicrobial activity may be due to the addition of specific substances, radiation, or gas-flushing. Irradiation sterilization of packaging materials may be forthcoming with FDA approval.

Examples of edible films include those used as the sugar shell on individual chocolate covered candies (M&Ms®), *casings,* such as in sausage, and *edible waxes,* such as those applied to fruits and vegetables. Serving in the role of edible films, the casings "contain," and the waxes function to improve or maintain appearance, prevent mold, and contain moisture while still allowing respiration. As well, food may be coated with a thin layer of polysaccharides such as cellulose, pectin, starch and vegetable gums, or proteins, such as casein and gelatin. Cut, dried, fruit pieces are often sprayed with an edible film prior to their inclusion into items such as breakfast cereal (See Active Packaging Technologies).

Bindings may be applied to a food's surface to be an adhesive for seasoning. Other coatings may significantly improve appearance (and reduce microbial contamination) by replacing egg washes, and acting as a glaze.

Foil is a packaging material that may be used in snack bags (chips, etc.) or as a laminate in aseptic packaging (see Aseptic Packaging). It is used as a wrapping for dry, refrigerator, or freezer storage. It provides a moisture-proof and vapor-proof barrier.

Laminates are multilayers of foil, paper, or plastics that may be utilized selectively according to the specific food packaging need. In combination, the various laminates may provide more strength and barrier protection than the individual laminate material. Laminates provide barriers useful in controlling O_2, water vapor, and light transmission, and they provide good burst strength. The laminates may resist pinholes and flex cracking. Retort pouches are examples of laminates used in packaging and contain polyester film, aluminum foil, and polypropylene.

Resins are used for sealing food packages. They must withstand the stress of processing and offer seal integrity that prevents product contamination.

Wood may be used in the manufacture of crates that contain fresh fruits and vegetables.

Bag-in-a-box is now offered in five-gallon bags with snap-on caps over a 1″ polyethylene spout. There is a high barrier film, with heat-resistance up to 190°F.

Regardless of the materials that are selected for use, *source reduction, reuse*, and *recycling* should be important considerations of packaging manufacturers. The food industry challenge is to provide the appropriate materials to accomplish packaging functions at reasonable cost.

CONTROLLING PACKAGING ATMOSPHERE

Reduced *temperature* remains as the primary means of food protection. However, controlling the known elements in the package environment, such as O_2, CO_2, water vapor, and ethylene concentration may also reduce spoilage and contamination (e.g., enzymatic, biological), thus extending shelf life (the time required for a food to become unacceptable from a sensory, nutritional, or safety perspective) (15).

The creation of a packaging environment with little or no oxygen has beneficial applications for the food industry. However, microbiological concerns arise simultaneously. As will be discussed, proper controls need to be in place for reduced oxygen packages.

The function of CO_2 addition in packaging is to inhibit growth of many bacteria and molds. The O_2 maintains respiration and color, and inhibits growth of anaerobic microorganisms. Nitrogen (N_2) is used to flush the package and rid it of air (O_2 specifically). Nitrogen also prevents a collapse of the loose-fitting packaging material.

Providing an example of the need to control packaging is, for example, fruits and vegetables. They continue to breathe and require oxygen after harvesting and processing, thus, the package must contain oxygen. Yet it needs to be controlled, as *too high* a level causes oxidation and spoilage and *too low* a level leads to anaerobic spoilage. In extending shelf life of fruit, oxygen levels should approximate 5%, and carbon dioxide at 1–3% (with refrigeration maintained at temperature-specific levels). Packaging environments must match the respiration rate as closely as possible.

The material that follows will address the internal package environment, and modification of gasses. The following are the significant manners of controlling packaging atmosphere:

- Vacuum packaging

- Sous Vide processing

- Flushing the packaging environment with specific, targeted gases

  MAP—one-time modification of gaseous environment
  CAP—continuous modification of gaseous environment

- Cook-Chill

- Other active packaging technologies

Vacuum Packaging

Vacuum packaging modifies the atmosphere surrounding the food by removing oxygen, and it extends shelf life. Further explained by the FDA, in its 1999 Guidelines for Reduced Oxygen Packaging (ROP), "Vacuum packaging reduces the amount of air from a package and hermetically seals the package so that a near-perfect vacuum remains inside. . . . A highly flexible plastic barrier is used by this technology that allows the package to mold itself to the contours of the food being packaged."

With the removal of oxygen, vacuum packaging controls rancidity that occurs with the oxidation of fatty acids. Vacuum-packaging machines are available for small-, medium-, or large-scale production capacity (Figures 19.7 and 19.8), and may be used to successfully package a variety of food sizes and forms such as small cheese blocks, large primal cuts of meat, or liquids.

The procedure used for vacuum packaging is to place the food in a flexible-film, barrier pouch, and put it inside a vacuum-packaging chamber, where oxygen is removed. This creates a skintight package wall and protects against the entry or escape of gases such as air and CO_2, or water vapor. It assures inhibition of microbial growth that would alter microbial and organoleptic properties such as appearance and odor. Water weight loss and freezer burn are also inhibited with this packaging method. The transparent, vacuum-packaging film allows product visibility from all angles. An example of vacuum-packaged food appears in Figure 19.9.

Controls Needed for Vacuum Packaging. The FDA recommends that local regulatory agencies prohibit vacuum packaging in retail stores unless the following six controls are all in effect:

- Foods must be limited to those that do not support growth of *Cl. botulinum* (as it is an anaerobe).

- Temperatures of 45°F (7°C) and below are maintained at all times. Anaerobic pathogens increase their growth rate exponentially with an increase in temperature.

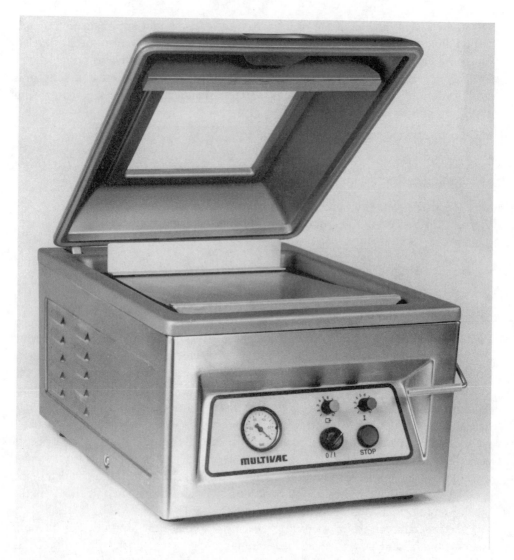

FIGURE 19.7 An example of small vacuum-packaging machinery (Courtesy of Multivac, Inc.).

- Consumer packages are prominently labeled with storage-temperature requirements and shelf life.
- Shelf life must neither exceed 10 days nor extend that labeled by the initial processor.
- Detailed, written in-store procedures must be developed, observed, and carefully monitored. These should be HACCP based (Chapter 16) and include records subject to review by regulatory authorities.
- Operators must certify that individuals responsible are qualified in the equipment, procedures, and concepts of safe vacuum packaging.

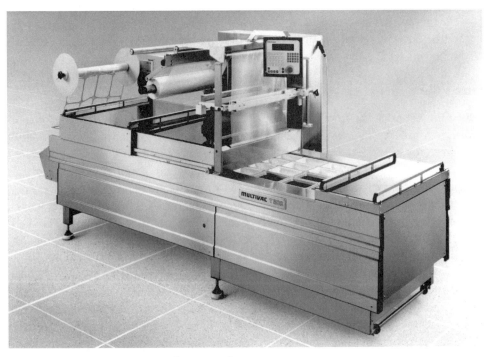

FIGURE 19.8   Large vacuum-packaging machinery
(Courtesy of Multivac, Inc.).

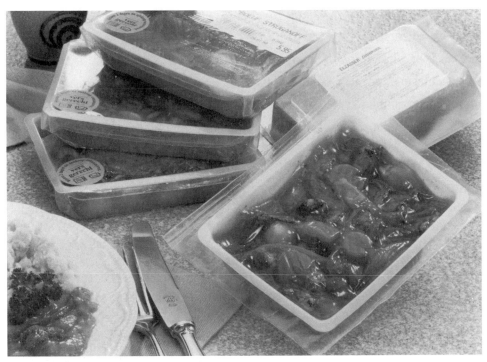

FIGURE 19.9   An example of vacuum-packaged foods
(Courtesy of Multivac, Inc.).

"Sanitation to maintain a low initial level is thus critical and must be combined with good manufacturing practice to prevent contamination with pathogens"(15).

Sous Vide

Sous Vide ("under vacuum") packaging involves mild, partial precooking of food prior to vacuum packaging. Once again, according to the FDA definition in the 1999 Guidelines for ROP, "Sous Vide is a specialized process of ROP for partially cooked ingredients alone or combined with raw foods that require refrigeration or frozen storage until the package is thoroughly heated immediately before service. The sous vide process is a pasteurization step that reduces bacterial load but is not sufficient to make the food shelf-stable." Since *some* of the ingredients may be partially cooked, and other ingredients may be raw, the product requires refrigeration or freezing, and then heating through prior to service.

The product package has its levels of *oxygen reduced* and CO_2 *raised* in the packaging environment in order to reduce the microbial (aerobic pathogens) load and extend the shelf life. Sous vide products are pasteurized, but *not* sterile, and may contain heat-resistant microorganisms and spores. Therefore, strict temperature regulation in production, as well as in the distribution process, is necessary to assure product safety. Food products must be kept cold to prevent the growth of bacteria.

According to FDA guidelines (FDA, 1999), guidelines related to the sous vide process include the following:

- Preparation of the raw materials (this step may include partial cooking of some or all ingredients);
- Packaging of the product, application of vacuum, and sealing of the package;
- Pasteurization of the product for a specified and monitored time/temperature;
- Rapid and monitored cooling of the product at or below 38°F (3°C) or frozen; and
- Reheating of the packages to a specified temperature before opening and service.

Modified Atmosphere Packaging

Modified atmosphere packaging (MAP) modifies the internal package atmosphere of food. It "is a process that employs a gas flushing and sealing process or reduction of oxygen through respiration of vegetables or microbial action. Modified Atmosphere Packaging is defined as packaging of a product in an atmosphere that has had a *one-time modification* of gaseous composition so that it is different from that of air, which normally contains 78.08% nitrogen, 20.96% oxygen, 0.03% carbon dioxide."

MAP is *primarily* applied to fresh or minimally processed foods that are still undergoing respiration, and it is used for the packaging of a variety of foods. Such foods include baked goods, coffees and teas, dairy products, dry and dehydrated foods, lunch kits, and processed meats (to keep the meat pigment looking desirable). It is also used for nuts, snack food applications, and pasta packaging. This type of packaging with high CO_2 levels inhibits many aerobic bacteria, molds, and yeasts.

MAP is one of the most widely used packaging technologies, as it functions to enhance appearance, minimize destructive waste, extend shelf life, and reduce the need for artificial preservatives. Its use thus expands a product's ability to reach new markets.

Following the packaging of foods, a machine vacuums out *all* of the package air, and then through the same package perforations, *evenly inserts* the new, desired gas combination. Since MAP contains the food under a gaseous environment that differs from air (some other percentage), it controls normal product respiration (consuming O_2, and generating CO_2, water vapor, and perhaps ethylene) and growth of aerobic microorganisms. For example, the change in CO_2 level shows an inhibitory effect on aerobic microorganisms. This effect is dependent upon conditions such as the level of CO_2 (a high level in proportion to air is more effective), moisture, pH, and temperature.

The initial mix of packaging atmosphere changes as a result of factors such as product respiration, the aerobic and anaerobic bacterial load, respiration of bacteria, permeation of gases through the packaging materials/seals, temperature, light, time and, so forth (15).

The addition of *nitrogen* gas, which is odorless, tasteless, colorless, nontoxic, and nonflammable, is introduced into the food package *after* all atmosphere has been removed from the pouch and vacuum chamber, and just *prior* to hermetic sealing of the package. It increases the package's internal pressure. This modification, by a pre-determined dose of liquid Nitrogen (LIN) offers protection from spoilage, oxidation, dehydration, weight loss and freezer burn, and extends shelf life, as nitrogen consumes oxygen.

Unlike vacuum packaging, the high barrier film (used to keep air out, and to prevent the modified atmosphere from escaping) used for MAP remains loose-fitting. This avoids the crushing effects of skintight vacuum packaging. When used in combination with aseptic packaging, which reduces the microbial load, MAP becomes a more effective technology. Most new and minimally processed foods use MAP in combination with aseptic technology and reduced temperature.

Controlled Atmosphere Storage and Packaging

Both controlled atmosphere (CA) in *storage* environments and **controlled atmosphere packaging** (CAP) are utilized in order to permit controlled oxygen and carbon dioxide exchange, thus preserving foods. As well, CAP is a prime alternative to pesticides and preservatives. When storage temperatures, and conditions of distribution vary in fresh and processed foods, CAP as well as MAP, assist in standardizing these variables and maintaining product quality.

The FDA defines CAP as "an active system which *continuously* maintains the desired atmosphere within a package throughout the shelf-life of a product by the use of agents to bind or scavenge oxygen or a sachet containing compounds to emit a gas." Controlled Atmosphere Packaging (CAP) is defined as a packaging of a product in a modified atmosphere followed by maintaining subsequent control of that atmosphere.

However, at any given time, and under variable environments, there is no continual "control" that the food technologist would describe as "ideal." The question then becomes, how much control *is* there in the package environment? Is it then more likely that the atmosphere is *modified*? This form of packaging also utilizes a high barrier film (or pouch), which may be EVOH high barrier polymers, or Polymid, a form of nylon.

Many packaged food products undergo respiration and microbial growth, requiring oxygen, while producing CO_2 and water. The carbohydrate molecule, in the presence of oxygen, $C_6H_{12}O_6 + O_2$ for example, yields $CO_2 + H_2O +$ heat. Therefore CA or CAP containers offer control by reducing the available O_2, elevating CO_2, and controlling water vapor, and ethylene concentration. The worldwide distribution and marketing of produce depends on CAP for high-quality food. A benefit is that less senescence and maintenance of nutritional value is observed.

C. botulinum is an anaerobic bacterium that grows in the absence of available oxygen. Therefore, it may grow in anaerobic packaging environments. To retard its growth in CAP food products, foods must have short-storage times and be held at cold temperatures. Control of water activity (A_w) and salt is also necessary to prevent growth as sodium competes with the bacteria for water absorption.

Food production has shown a rising use, thus the demand for various industrial gasses such as CO_2 and N_2. Perhaps this increase in demand may be attributed to more convenient foods, packagings that provide a longer shelf-life, CAP, and MAP.

Cook-Chill

Cook-chill is defined as a packaging procedure that also results in reduced oxygen levels. By FDA definition it "is a process that uses a plastic bag filled with hot cooked food from which air has been expelled and which is closed with a plastic or metal crimp." Such a system is one that may be frequently employed in hospital foodservice operations as an alternative to a more conventional food service operation.

Active Packaging Technologies

Active packaging began as "*smart*" *packaging* in 1980s, and was referred to as "*interactive*" *packaging* almost from the start. All three terms describe the same thing, which is packaging that could "sense" changes in the internal environment and respond by adapting as necessary. Sachets may be added to a package in order to control elements such as ethanol, oxygen, or microbes (16).

By its inherent design, packaging typically serves in a *passive* role by protecting food products from the external environment. It provides a physical barrier to external spoilage, contamination, and physical abuse in storage and distribution. Today, packaging more *actively* contributes to the product's development, controls maturation and ripening, helps in achieving the proper color development in meats, and extends shelf life (17). Thus it is considered to play an *active* (not passive) role in protecting foods (13,17). Yet, despite the many attributes and benefits of smart/interactive/active packaging, it generally does not actually "sense" the environment conditions, and change accordingly.

Examples of ***active packaging*** technologies are listed in the following text.

Active packaging for *fresh and minimally processed* foods provide the following:

- Edible moisture or oxygen barrier (to control loss of moisture and enzymatic oxidative browning in fresh cut fruits and vegetables and to provide controlled permeability rates matched to the respiration rate of the fruit) (Chapters 7 and 18).

- Edible antimicrobial (biocidal) polymer films and coatings (which may release controlled amounts of chlorine dioxide into the food, depending on temperature and humidity; or destroy E. *coli* 0157:H7 in meats, and prevent mold growth in fruits)

- Films that are scavengers of off-odors

- Oxygen scavengers for low oxygen packaging

Active packaging for *processed* foods provides the following:

- Edible moisture barrier

- O_2, CO_2, and odor scavenger

Other active packaging technologies include the following:

- Microwave doneness integrators (indicators)

- Microwave susceptor films to allow browning and crispness (french fries, baked products, popcorn)

- Steam release films

- Time–temperature indicators (TTI) which are unable to reverse their color when the product has been subject to time–temperature abuse

Specifically, the predictabilty of the behavior of a living, breathable fruit or vegetable, or even meat, is quite different from a non-food item that is packaged. There are numerous interactions between the food, any internal gas in the package atmosphere, and the material used for packaging. Sachets or films may release their intended effect at a controlled rate.

The FDA gave the "go-ahead" for a type of active packaging that releases chlorine dioxide gas to kill harmful bacteria and spoilage organisms (18).

Aseptic Packaging

In order to destroy any C. *botulinum* spores and extend the shelf life of low-acid foods, ***aseptic packaging*** may be utilized (Figure 19.10). Independent sterilization of both the *foods* and *packaging material,* with assembly under *sterile environmental* conditions, is the rule for aseptic packaging.

In an aseptic system of packaging, the packaging material consists of *layers* of polyethylene, paperboard, and foil (Figure 19.11). It is sterilized by heat (superheated steam or dry hot air) or a combination of heat and hydrogen peroxide, and then roll-fed through the packer to create the typical brick/block shape (Figure 19.12).

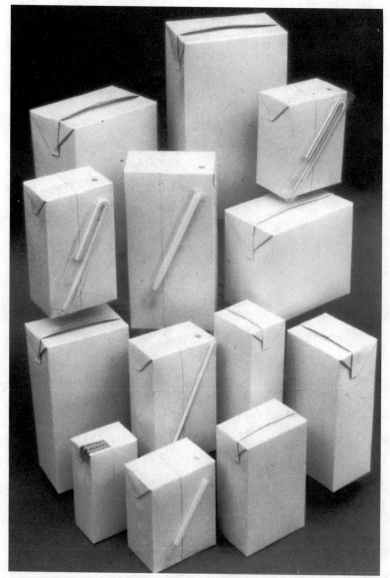

FIGURE 19.10 Different *Tetra Brik*® aseptic package sizes
(*Source:* Tetra Pak Inc.).

The container is filled with a sterile (no pathogens or spores) or commercially sterile (no pathogens, but *some* spores) liquid food product, and sealed in a closed, sterile chamber. Once packed, the product requires no refrigeration. Liquids such as creamers, milk, or juices may be packed in this manner. Triple or multiple packs of flavored milk and juice, with attached straws, are available on grocery shelves. The market leaders of aseptic packages have introduced easy-open, easy-pour features into their cartons. The plastic devices are injection molded and adhere to the package tops.

The sterility of packaging material has formerly relied on *chemical* technologies of sterilization (principally heat with hydrogen peroxide). *Nonchemical* techniques

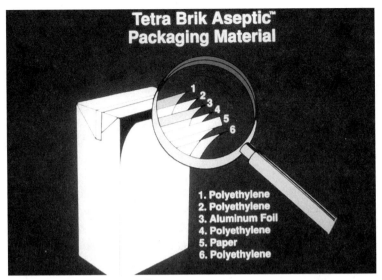

FIGURE 19.11 *Tetra Brik* ® *aseptic packaging material layers*
(*Source: Tetra Pak Inc.*).

have been explored in order to avoid chemical sterilant residues. Ionizing and nonionizing radiation have been tested for use in aseptic packaging.

Flexible Packaging

Flexible packaging is available for packaging use in the foodservice industry and is finding more applications at the *retail* level, including packaging for bagged cereals

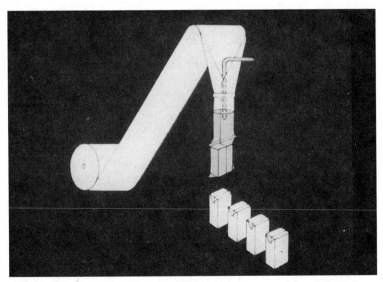

FIGURE 19.12   Illustration of roll-fed packaging material being formed into Tetra Briks
(*Source:* Tetra Pak Inc.).

and sliced deli meat. Nonrigid packaging containers such as stand-up pouches or tubes and zippered bags are examples of flexible packaging used for peanuts, peanut butter, or produce such as fresh-cut lettuce and peeled baby carrots. The same packaging might also need to be *resealable* to meet consumer demands and may require zipper handles or spouts with *easy open* screw-off tops.

"Flexible packaging uses less material, is more cost effective, and packaging speeds are getting higher. Large flexible packages have replaced cans and rigid packaging." Whether it is attributable to flexible packaging alone, or marketing, and so forth, one manufacturer of snack mix has said "Sales of the product more than doubled just by changing the package"(19).

Flexible packaging is adequate for the plethora of low-fat/no-fat food products such as salty snack foods that are available in the marketplace. It keeps these products fresh by providing flavor and aroma barriers, which keep outside odors out and flavors in. It is used for fresh fruits and vegetables and matches respiration rate as closely as possible.

Manufacturers are offering more food products in flexible packaging and find that "cost savings and environmental concerns are two of the driving forces behind the switch to flexible packaging"(20). "Faster, better, stronger, cheaper...the packaging industry continually tries to improve the process. Nowhere is this more apparent than in flexible packaging" (20).

FREEZER PACKAGING PROTECTION

Freezing foods is a means of preservation (Chapter 17), but foods may spoil due to desiccation or cavity ice if they are not adequately protected. Therefore, a moisture-barrier film, such as a freezer wrap, is needed in packaging material. Tear strength and wet strength are also needed in packaging material for freezer storage.

Freezer Burn

Pronounced desiccation occurs as water diffuses from the product to the atmosphere. This results in *freezer burn* with its resultant change in appearance, flavor, texture, and weight.

Cavity Ice

Cavity ice is the ice formation within the food package due to water condensation. Therefore, it is important to use moisture-proof and vapor-proof packaging.

TAMPER-EVIDENT BANDING AND SLEEVE LABELING

Tamper-evident banding and sleeve labeling may assist manufacturers and consumers by providing protection and offering the security that the package contents are unviolated. Today, tamper-evident neckbands and shrink-film sleeves are made in a number of colors and may be custom printed. Technology for full-body shrink-labels over glass and plastic bottles is more apparent, as it has become more

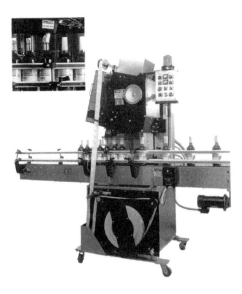

FIGURE 19.13 Example of machinery
applying a tamper-evident band
(*Source*: PDC International Corporation).

affordable and attractive. Pull-tabs and perforations provide ease of use. Figure 19.13 shows the application of tamper-evident banding, and Figure 19.14 provides an example of the tamper-evident banding that has been applied to a container. While the majority of rigid packaging includes tamper-evident attributes, not all food is packaged in this manner. Considering security issues, especially susceptible may be bakery and dairy products (21).

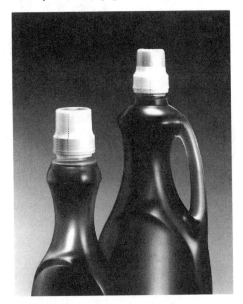

FIGURE 19.14 An example of a
tamper-evident band
(*Source*: PDC International Corporation).

MANUFACTURING CONCERNS IN PACKAGING

Selection of Packaging Materials

Environmental conditions in package transport and government regulations may dictate the materials a company uses in shipping food containers domestically or overseas. Many components of the food industry demand that packaging material is biodegradable, recyclable, strong, and waste-to-energy efficient. The food processor must choose materials that effectively preserve shelf life and are environmentally friendly and affordable. The packaging material needs to meet all criteria of shipment, labeling, marketing, and other purposes of packaging.

Migration from Packaging Materials

The packaging industry recognizes that the migration of substances from the packaging into the food *could* be harmful to the consumer or have an adverse effect on the acceptability of the food. Therefore, compliance with limits set on migration of packaging materials and control of additives at the point of manufacture must be ensured.

Plastics have a greater likelihood of imparting their "plastic taste," and odor to a food than paper. They may contain many additives, including antioxidants, antistatics, plasticizers (to improve the flexibility of some "cling" films), and stabilizers to improve the functional properties of the plastics. Although there has been no report of danger to human health from plasticizer additives, the plastics industry has reformulated some grades of films that contain plasticizers and continues to offer polyethylene plastic wraps with low levels of plasticizers. In addition to plastics, the printing *ink* on the package must be controlled, as it too imparts undesirable flavor to packaged food, and may stain the surface of material it contacts while hot (i.e., microwave oven).

Migration from packaging materials is more likely to occur at high temperatures with fatty foods; therefore, *industry* packaging of microwave foods is designed to be safe for microwave use at high temperatures. *Consumers* who use packaging films for cooking or reheating in the microwave should be aware that "microwave safe" criteria may not be established for packaging films that can have direct contact with food during reheating in a microwave. Therefore, using *glass* containers may be preferable choices for microwave reheating.

The use of recycled plastics and paper reduces control over contaminants that may be in the second-hand materials. Further research on the use of recycled materials must be conducted and brought forth, before it is recommended that recycled materials be used in food-contact applications (due to the possible migration of contaminants).

Packaging Lines at Processing Plants and Foodservice Operations

Packaging lines at processing plants may operate efficiently or be down and hold up production. When correctly managed, automated, computer-controlled production lines drastically increase the speed and productivity of many packaging machines, yet the repair of troubled computer controlled production lines requires significant expertise. Manufacturers' use of poor quality bottles, boxes, films, labels, and other materials may result in line stoppages which could result in reduced product quality if longer than expected holding of heat-sensitive ingredients is required (22).

Polyester films may be used to wrap dual-ovenable trays for meal delivery in some institutional foodservice settings such as schools. In the case of one institutional meal provider, serving almost 10 million meals per year, there was difficulty with the removal of heat-seal film from trays in clean-up operations. As a result, specially designed films were developed (23).

Survey of Important Issues in Food Packaging

A survey of food industry participants responsible for packaging (24) reveals that the three top issues in food packaging include *product safety, consumer convenience*, and *product shelf life*. They are the primary concern to 80, 73, and 70% of respondents, respectively. *Environmental concerns*, and *cost of materials* continue to be important issues (24). As mentioned, the use of food materials in packaging is possible, and it assists manufacturers in becoming more environmentally conscious. Another major concern of survey respondents is automation of their machinery—to give better handling and reduce labor costs.

A 1996 *Packaging Digest* survey reports that 95% of consumers rank the preservation of flavor and taste as the most important role for food packaging. Value for the money ranked second. More than 8 out of 10 wanted tamper-evident packaging (3).

PACKAGING OF THE FUTURE

Packaging offering single servings for toddlers through teens, working adults, to seniors in healthcare, has multiplied in recent years. For example, older Americans, who may exhibit a decreased manual dexterity, benefit from the use of more simple screw tops on gabletop liquid food containers.

It may all be relative to the day and age in which consumers live, but convenience is a desirable attribute of food and its packaging. In a recent year, there were over 14,000 new food and beverage introductions, many to provide convenience. The introduction of microwaveable, push tube, push-ups, for example, now represent a new packaging category of convenience. It can only be assumed that the future will contain many more packaging advances in order to supply convenience to the consumer.

A look at some predictions for packaging of the future is provided in the following subsections.

Paperboard

Paperboard packaging of the future may offer more benefits to the consumer and retailer. When surveyed by the Paperboard Packaging Council (PPC) and the Institute of Packaging Professionals (IoPP), packaging experts responded with some innovations that might be just a few years away. The five top predictions for the paperboard packaging of the future are that paperboard packaging might contain the following:

- Temperature sensors—to indicate doneness on consumer foods such as meals

- Freshness sensors—using colors that change, or displaying warnings to indicate when a product is no longer safe to consume

- Pilferage protection—by mini antitheft computer chips built into bar codes on paperboard cartons

- Holographics—used on paperboard packaging material for merchandising. Holographic effects are achieved by the utilization of an embossable metallized film combined with paperboard in a specially designed process.

- Taking cartoons—by the use of computer voice chips a box can talk to consumers (25).

The Association of Industrial Metallizers, Coaters and Laminators (AIMCAL) has given many technical and marketing awards to food packaging with holograms.

Future packaging ideas include packaging that eliminates the need for inner bags in ready-to-eat cereal boxes. Considerations for the acceptance of this packaging type include barrier protection, recycle ability, printability, and ease of use. In Europe, such packaging ideas include *Performa Barr* (26), a bleached sulphate board with a core of CTMP (chemi thermo mechanical pulp) that provides package bulk and stiffness. It consists of a clay outside coating which affords printability, and an inside coating of three layer plastic. The inside coating composite includes 1) oxygen and aroma barrier protection, 2) sealability and moisture resistance, and 3) a middle layer that is designed to hold the composite together. Once developed, uses may expand to other foods.

Aseptic and Modified Atmosphere Packaging Combinations

Together, aseptic and modified atmosphere packaging, two popular forms of packaging, may reduce microbial load (by heating the product) and make MAP a more effective treatment.

> " ...the two categories, not labeled as such for consumers to identify, continue to grow because their results fit contemporary consumer demand. The fact that the two seemingly unrelated technologies are being integrated to complement each other should suggest that we have entered into a new era of food science and technology in which disparate disciplines are—and must be—combined to synergistically achieve the optimum outcome of quality, convenience, and safety in our food supply" (27).

PACKAGING AS A COMMUNICATION AND MARKETING TOOL

Packages contain and protect food during storage, shipment, and sale, and serve other functions, as discussed, such as provide convenience, and utility of use. They also *communicate* important consumer information on their labels (Chapter 20). For example, information regarding ingredients, nutrition facts, manufacturers' name and address, contents weight, bar coding, and so forth, appear on package labels. The food processor must be aware of worldwide differences in acceptability of packaging format, including use of colors and picture symbols, before a product is marketed in another culture.

Packaging serves as a *marketing tool*. The package and label design are significant in attracting potential customers and many labels may carry recipes, coupons, mail-in offers, or announcements of special upcoming events. It may be that a change in packaging greatly increases sales. Yet changes must not confuse consumers who have built product loyalty by familiarity over the years. For example, milk cartons may not be readily accepted if changed, yet a difference in packaging material, such as cereal without a cardboard box, might be well accepted, and profitable.

It is reported by a university marketing professor (26) that consumers use more of a product at a time when it comes in a *larger* package. This may be attributed to 1) the buy-more, use-more phenomenon, as consumers perceive food products as less expensive when purchased in larger quantity (although this is not always true), 2) less concern with running out, and 3) desire to finish the food product as the large size occupies excessive shelf space (28). At the other end of the spectrum, *single* servings of products are also popular in the marketplace.

Although labels are discussed in another chapter of this text (Chapter 19), they will be mentioned here, in packaging. Paper and perhaps full sleeve, heat shrink PVC labels may be applied to food containers. They offer graphics, assistance as a marketing tool, provide tamper-evidence, information and more.

CONCLUSION

Primary, secondary, and tertiary packaging protects raw and processed food against spoilage and contamination while offering convenience and product information to the consumer. A variety of packaging materials, such as metal, glass, paper, and plastics or combinations of these, are used for packaging if they meet with FDA approval.

Packaging films and atmospheres may be selected according to a food product's storage and distribution needs. They may eliminate damaging levels of oxygen, light, temperature, as well as preventing water-vapor loss, while at the same time, protecting the food from spoilage and contamination. Compliance with limits set on migration of packaging materials and control of additives in the materials must be ensured.

Recycling and a variety of packaging technologies, including vacuum packaging, flushing the package with gas, or active packaging, may be used to contribute to effective packaging of food, and more developments loom on the horizon.

Packaging of freezer foods requires protection from spoilage. Tamper-evident banding is a protection against external hazards and may be viewed as essential by the manufacturer and consumer. The package label may communicate important information to the consumer serving as a marketing tool. Packaging today provides protection for food products that was unavailable a year ago, or even yesterday. More advances are on the horizon.

Glossary

Active packaging: Packaging that makes an active, not passive contribution to product development or shelf life by such techniques as providing an oxygen barrier, or odor and oxygen scavenger.

Aseptic packaging: Independent sterilization of foods and packaging with assembly under sterile conditions.

Cavity ice: Ice formation with the frozen food package due to water condensation and freezing.

Controlled atmosphere packaging (CAP): Controls O_2, CO_2, water vapor, and ethylene concentration.

Flexible packaging: Nonrigid packaging such as stand-up pouches, tubes, or zippered bags.

Freezer burn: Desiccation of frozen food product as the water diffuses from the frozen food to the atmosphere.

Modified atmosphere packaging (MAP): Or Gas Flush Packaging—Modification of O_2, CO_2, water vapor, and ethylene concentration by flushing with nitrogen gas.

Polyethylene: Most common, least expensive plastic film used in packaging material.

Polystyrene: Plastic type that is typically foamed to create expandable polystyrene or styrofoam.

Polyvinyl chloride (PVC or vinyl): Plastic packaging film.

Polyvinylidene chloride (PVDC or Saran®): Plastic packaging film.

Primary container: A direct food contact surface as in bottle, can, or drink box that contains a food or beverage.

Secondary container: Does not have food contact, but holds several primary containers in materials such as corrugated fiberboard, boxes, or wraps.

Sous vide: Mild, partial precooking to reduce the microbial load, followed by vacuum packaging to extend the shelf life.

Tamper-evident banding: Sleeves or neckbands providing protection and offering security by indicating evidence of tampering with the product.

Tertiary container: Holds several secondary containers in corrugated fiberboard boxes, overwraps, and so forth.

Vacuum packaging: Removes all atmosphere from the pouch and creates a skintight package wall.

References

1. The Society of the Plastics Industry (SPI) Washington, DC.
2. Ferrante MA. The brave new world of packaging technology at Pack Expo 96. *Food Engineering.* 1996; 68(10): 99–102.
3. Sloan AE. The silent salesman. *Food Technology.* 1996; 50(12): 25.
4. Steel Cans. A Steel-in-Packaging Report from the Committee of Tin Mill Products Producers. American Iron and Steel Institute.
5. Franklin Associates, Ltd. A comparison of energy consumption by the plastics industry to total energy consumption in the United States, 1990.
6. Society for Research into the Packaging Market (Germany), Packaging without plastic; ecological and economic consequences of a packaging market free from plastic, 1990.

7. Testin RF, Vergano PJ. Plastic packaging opportunities and challenges, January 1992.

8. Factoring source reduction into recycling costs, Proceedings of Recycle '93, Sixth Annual Forum (Davos, Switzerland), 1993.

9. Franklin Associates, Ltd. Resource and environmental profile analysis of polyethylene and unbleached paper grocery sacks, 1990.

10. Russell M: High-performance films. *Food Engineering.* 1995; 67(9): 139–146.

11. Le Maire WH. The PET revolution comes to food. *Food Engineering.* 1994; 66(8): 62.

12. Franklin Associates Ltd., Resource and environmental profile analysis of foam polystyrene and bleached paperboard containers, 1990.

13. Higgins KT. Not just a pretty face. *Food Engineering.* 2000; 72(5): 74–77.

14. Krochta JM, DuMulder-Johnston C. Edible and biodegradable polymer films: Challenges and opportunities. A Publication of the Institute of Food Technologists' Expert Panel on Food Safety and Nutrition. *Food Technology.* 1997; 51(2): 61–74.

15. Labuza TP. An introduction to active packaging for foods. *Food Technology.* 1996; 50(4): 68–71.

16. Brody AL. Smart packaging becomes Intellipac®. *Food Technology.* 2000; 54(6): 104–106.

17. Pszczola DE. Packaging takes an active approach. *Food Technology.* 1995; 49(8): 104.

18. Higgins KT. Active packaging gets a boost. *Food Engineering.* 2001; 73(10): 20.

19. Ferrante MA. Flexible packaging. Striking it right. *Food Engineering.* 1999; 71(2): 57–61.

20. Ferrante MA: Keeping it flexible. *Food Engineering.* 1996; 68(9): 143–150.

21. Higgins KT. Security takes center stage. *Food Engineering.* 2001; 73(12): 20.

22. Russell M. Peak packaging performance. *Food Engineering.* 1994; 66(10): 100–107.

23. Dallas County Sheriff's Department. Dallas, Texas.

24. Martin K. Safety & convenience take center stage. *Food Engineering.* 1999; 71(11): 79–86.

25. Paperboard Packaging Council, Washington, DC.

26. Regal Molle Group. Norway

27. Brody AL. Integrating aseptic and modified atmosphere packaging to fulfill a vision of tomorrow. *Food Technology.* 1996; 50(4): 56–66.

28. *Tufts University Diet & Nutrition Letter.* The bigger the package, the more you eat. 1997; 14(11): 1–2.

BIBLIOGRAPHY

American Packaging Corporation, Philadelphia, PA.

Blumenthal MM. How packaging affects food flavor. *Food Technology.* 1997; 51(1): 71–74.

Dow Chemical Co., Midland MI (PVDC).

DuPont Co. Wilmington, DE (PET, eng. grade).

Eastman Chemical Co., Kingsport TN (PCT, PET std. grade).

Innovation Packaging, Macedonia, NY.

Potter N, Hotchkiss J. *Food Science,* 5th ed. New York: Chapman & Hall, 1995.

Regal Moell Group. Norway.

Reynolds Metals Co. Flexible Packaging Division, Richmond, VA.

Tetra Pak. Chicago, IL.

PART VIII

Government Regulation of the Food Supply

CHAPTER 20

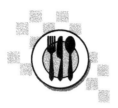

Government Regulation of the Food Supply and Labeling

INTRODUCTION

Consumers want the assurance that they are receiving a safe and sanitary food supply. They want deceptive claims and fraudulence to be nonissues for them to face in their everyday life. Therefore, for many centuries, governments throughout the world have regulated the food supply. Federal, state, and local government, their regulation, and the educational materials they offer, assist in providing a safe food supply.

One of the major regulatory agencies protecting the food supply is the Food and Drug Administration (FDA). Their basic purpose is to protect the public from foodborne illness (Chapter 16). FDA regulations known as "Good Manufacturing Practices" or GMPs are in operation at food plants. Maintaining the plant sanitation and food safety are ongoing duties of the food processing plant personnel.

Food supplies subject to interstate transport, food packaging, and labeling are also regulated as are grading standards and ordinances that specify sanitation for foodservice establishments. Intrastate transport is regulated by each state's Department of Agriculture. State and local health departments may adopt their own food-service regulations.

The United States Department of Agriculture (USDA) has responsibility for inspecting animal products, including meat, poultry, eggs, meat, and poultry processing plants, as well as voluntary grading.

The FDA Code of Federal Regulations (CFR) is cited several times in this chapter, with the hope of better portraying and understanding the government ruling on an issue.

THE FOOD AND DRUG ADMINISTRATION

The FDA is a public health agency. The agency regulates 25 cents of every dollar spent annually by American consumers—over $1 trillion worth of products (FDA) and does so at a taxpayer cost of several dollars per individual. The FDA inspects food—that it is safe and wholesome, also cosmetics, medicines and medical devices, radiation-emitting devices (such as microwave ovens), animal feed, and drugs.

FDA Federal Food, Drug and Cosmetic Act—1938

The FDA's *Federal Food, Drug, and Cosmetic Act of 1938* (FD&C Act) is the main law regulating the food supply in the United States. It replaced the 1906 Federal Food and Drug Act, or "Pure Food Law." With regard to food, this law regulates the processing of many food products, and the labels of processed or packaged food (see Labels) subject to interstate commerce or import. Since the origin of this law, there have been several amendments. Additionally, a federal Code of Regulations is written to cover specific regulations for the food industry.

The agency has several thousand researchers, inspectors, and legal staff in approximately 150 cities throughout federal, regional, and local offices in the United States, including scientists (over 2000), chemists (900), and microbiologists (300). Agents of the FDA may work with public affairs or small business as well as laboratory personnel. They monitor the manufacture, import, transport, and storage of products both prior to and following sale on the market. Products are examined for construction and labels must be truthful. In industry, the agency interprets laws, inspects products, and regulates food manufacturing plants.

Some of the varied activities of federal FDA agents include advising state and local agencies in general duties through the handling and preventing of disasters. The FDA has both a regulatory arm of enforcement, and cooperative programs of partnership with industry, the latter, for example, helps train employees in preventing foodborne illness. Due to budgetary constraints and a current transition of the FDA to a Hazard Analysis Critical Control Point focus (Chapter 16), the role of this government agency is in flux, yet the goal of the agency remains to protect the public.

Voluntary correction of public health problems is necessary, but when warranted, *legal sanctions* may be brought to bear against manufacturers or distributors. Recalls of faulty products are generally the fastest and most effective way to protect the public from unsafe products on the market.

Amendments to the Food, Drug and Cosmetic Act

Several major amendments to the Food, Drug and Cosmetic Act that were introduced and became law include the following:

- *1954 Pesticide Chemical Amendment*: The use of pesticides is subject to FDA approval. Raw agriculture products are prohibited from containing pesticide residues above a certain level.

- *1958 Food Additives Amendment*: With this amendment, the burden of proof for usefulness and harmlessness of an additive was shifted to industry. Exempt from this proof were Generally Recognized as Safe (GRAS) substances already in common use with no proof of cancer (see GRAS substances, below).

- The *Delaney Clause* (1966) of the Food Additives Amendment states that an additive (Chapter 18) cannot be used if it leads to cancer in man or animals, or if the carcinogen is detectable by any appropriate test. In recent years, a much-debated question on the necessity of the Delaney Clause has arisen. For example, what *is* an appropriate test to determine the level of a food additive that induces cancer? Finer detection of minute amounts of agents responsible for cancer has become available. There is *no* food item that is, or can be, totally safe at *any* level of ingestion. Thus, the question is: At what level is the presence of a carcinogen indicative of the need to remove that item from the food supply? The future will offer more debate and regulation of this matter.

- *1960 Color Additives Amendment* (Chapter 18): The use of food colors is subject to FDA approval.

- *1966 Fair Packaging and Labeling Act*: Requires all consumer products in interstate commerce to contain accurate information on the package, facilitating better control of misinformation. Consumers benefit in that they can use the label information on packages, in making purchasing and value comparisons.

GRAS Substances.   According to the General Provisions of the Code of Federal Regulations, Title 21 (21CFR582), Sec. 582.1, generally recognized as safe substances are discussed as follows:

> "It is impractical to list all substances that are generally recognized as safe for their intended use. However, by way of illustration, the Commissioner regards such common food ingredients as salt, pepper, sugar, vinegar, baking powder, and monosodium glutamate as safe for their intended use."

In 1990, the *Nutrition Labeling and Education Act (NLEA)* was passed by Congress, and the FDA then wrote regulations for compliance covering extensive labeling changes, including mandatory nutrition labels, uniform use of product health claims, and uniform serving sizes. This was an attempt to protect the consumer against misinformation and fraud.

The FDA has mandatory standards for interstate transport of food. Those standards are identified in the following:

Standard of Identity.   The FDA describes food and lists both required and optional ingredients that are included in manufacture. When *initially* introduced as law, if a food product followed a Standard of Identity in its manufacture, those same *required* and *optional ingredients* were *not* listed on labels, as it was understood that the consumer was familiar with ingredients that composed basic foods. Examples of products that follow a Standard of Identity included foods such as mayonnaise, white bread, and jelly.

In time, it became apparent that this familiarity with foods was not widespread. As a result, *after* 1967, *optional ingredients* of foods had to be included on labels, even if the product followed the Standard of Identity.

Since 1991, manufacturers have been required to state *all* ingredients on the product label, including required and optional ingredients. This change to the complete identification of food ingredients benefits consumers who are unfamiliar with food ingredients that make up a food, as well as those with food allergies or intolerances. Additionally, a standard is revised as new additives are approved for food use.

Standards of Minimum Quality. The FDA states the minimum quality standards for specific characteristics in a food, such as color, defects, and tenderness. A food must state "below standard in quality" if the minimum level of a particular quality descriptor is not obtained. Substandard does not signify safety hazards.

Processors of canned vegetables and fruits follow this standard. Color, tenderness, blemishes, clarity of liquid, and product size are some of the criteria used at the wholesale and retail level for evaluation.

Standard of Fill of Container. This FDA standard ensures that the headspace/void volume of packaged food offered for sale does not interfere with the weight of the product as stated on the label. It assures that the product offers the correct weight even if the package is only partially full. For example, packages of cereal, crackers, and potato chips may not appear full due to extra air space in the package that is needed to prevent food breakage, yet, this fact is taken into account, as the food is sold by *weight,* not by *volume.* Food products packed in a liquid medium, such as canned fruits or vegetables, must contain the stated weight of the product.

Adulterated and Misbranded Food

The FDA seeks to control *adulterated* and *misbranded* food sales in the United States. Adulterated and misbranded foods are defined as follows:

Adulterated food may not be offered for sale. A food is adulterated if it:

- Is poisonous or harmful to health at detrimental concentrations.
- Contains filth or is decomposed
- Contains a food or coloring agent that is not approved or certified
- Was prepared or packed under unsanitary conditions, making it contaminated
- Is derived from a diseased animal
- Contains any excessive levels of residue
- Was subject to radiation, other than where permitted
- Has any valuable constituent omitted
- Substitutes a specified ingredient with an unspecified ingredient
- Is damaged or conceals defects
- Is increased in bulk weight or reduced in its strength, making it appear better than it is

According to the FDA, food is *misbranded* if it:

- Is labeled falsely, or misleadingly
- Is offered for sale under the name of another food
- Is an imitation of another food, without stating "imitation" on the label
- Is packaged (formed or filled) so as to be misleading
- Fails to list the name and address of the manufacturer, packer, and distributor, and a statement of net contents on the label
- Fails to declare the common name of the product, and the names of each ingredient or has label information that is not legible and easily understood
- Is represented as a food for which there is a Standard of Identity but the food does not conform with an accurate statement of quantity or ingredients
- Is represented to conform to a quality standard or to a fill of container and does not conform
- Is represented with a nutritional claim or for special dietary use but the label fails to provide information concerning dietary properties of the food, as required by law
- Lacks proper nutrition labeling

The FDA Modernization Act of 1997

The FDA Modernization Act of 1997 (FDAMA) was passed by the Senate and the House, and signed into law in 1998. It amends the FD&C Act, and the biological products provisions of the Public Health Service Act (PHS Act), with the intent "... to improve the regulation of food, drugs, devices, and biological products, and for other purposes." The Act *eliminates* the FDA's *mandatory pre-market approval* for use of the majority of substances that come into contact with food, or may migrate into it. Instead, manufacturers must provide 120 days of notification to the FDA. Among other sections that address drugs, devices, and biological products, the FDAMA contains nine *food* petitions as separate sections of the ruling.

- Flexibility for Regulations Regarding Claims—Section 301
- Petitions for Claims—Section 302
- Health Claims for Food Products (authoritative statements, yet not FDA)—Section 303
- Nutrient Content Claims (significant information, 120 days)—Section 304
- Referral Statements (such as "see side panel for nutrition information")—Section 305
- Disclosure of Irradiation (size of statement, and use of symbol)—Section 306
- Irradiation Petition (to control food contamination with pathogens)—Section 307

- Glass and Ceramic Ware (regarding FDA's ban on ceramics)—Section 308
- Food Contact Substances (including additives' safety)—Section 309

Additionally, the FDA enforces The *Public Health Service Act* to maintain sanitary standards at retail foodservice establishments, and in milk processing and shellfish operations. The FDA monitors food for safety and wholesomeness on interstate carriers such as planes and trains. The FDA also has a Seafood HACCP (Chapter 16) program, which is aimed at controlling pathogens and foodborne illness from seafood.

THE UNITED STATES DEPARTMENT OF AGRICULTURE

The USDA is another major government agency regulating the food supply in the United States. It is responsible for inspection of meat, poultry, agricultural products, including milk, eggs, fruit and vegetables, and meat and poultry processing plants. While the **inspection service**, including bacterial counts, is mandatory, the **grading service** is voluntary and is paid for by the manufacturer, marketer, or packer. Accommodations such as a desk, telephone, and parking space should be made available for the USDA inspector who is routinely present at a plant to assure safe food handling and plant sanitation.

Using a meat example for government regulation, the USDA, or the individual State Departments of Agriculture (which must meet federal standards), inspects meat and stamps it with an abbreviation of "Inspected and Passed," containing a number that identifies the plant. Every *carcass*, but not every *cut* of meat, requires this stamp (made using nontoxic vegetable dye) as proof of sanitary quality and wholesomeness, and it is required for shipment in interstate commerce. The label stating "*wholesome*" indicates that no signs of illness were found, *not* that the meat is free from pathogenic microorganisms.

The *Federal Meat Inspection Act of 1906, Federal Poultry Products Inspection Act of 1957* and the *Wholesome Poultry Products Act of 1968* are enforced by the Food Safety and Inspection Service (FSIS) of the USDA. The inspection, labeling, and handling of poultry and poultry products are similar to the meat inspection process. *Processed* poultry products do *not* undergo a mandatory inspection.

The FSIS conducts activities such as the following to ensure the safety of *meat and poultry* products consumed in the United States:

- USDA inspectors and veterinarians conduct slaughter inspection of all carcasses at meat and poultry slaughtering plants for disease and other abnormalities and sample for the presence of chemical residues.
- USDA conducts processing inspection for sanitation and cleanliness, labeling, and packing at facilities where meat and poultry is cut up, boned, cured, and canned.
- Scientific testing in support of inspection operations is performed by USDA/FSIS laboratory services to identify the presence of pathogens, residues, additives, disease, and foreign matter in meat and poultry.

- Inspection systems in countries exporting meat and poultry products to the United States are reviewed by USDA as part of the import–export inspection system.

- USDA is placing increased emphasis on pathogen reduction and hazard analysis and critical control point (HACCP) in the entire meat and poultry production chain. This involves developing new methods for rapid detection of pathogenic microorganisms, new production, and inspection practices to reduce bacterial contamination, and educating consumers on safe food-handling practices.

- USDA's Meat and Poultry Hotline is a toll-free service where consumers, educators, researchers, and the media can speak with experts in the field of food safety.

The USDA also has a Food and Consumer Service (FCS) that administers food assistance programs such as the following:

- Food Stamp Program
- Food Distribution Program on Indian Reservations and the Trust Territories
- Special Supplemental Food Program for Women, Infants and Children (WIC)
- Farmers Market Nutrition Program
- Commodity Supplemental Food Program
- National School Lunch Program
- School Breakfast Program
- Special Milk Program
- Child and Adult Care Food Program
- Summer Food Service Program
- Nutrition Program for the Elderly
- Food Distribution to Charitable Institutions, Soup Kitchens, and Food Banks
- Nutrition Assistance Programs
- The Emergency Food Assistance Program (TEFAP)

To face the complex nutrition issue in the 21st century, there may need for researchers, policy makers, private and public sector organizations, to define and implement a strategy for action agenda. This was the case in the White House Conference on Food, Nutrition and Health in 1969.

Currently there are many nutrition programs, as mentioned, such as The Food Stamp Program, Special Supplemental Food Program for Women, Infants and Children, and so forth. There is also Dietary Guidelines, NLEA, etc., and these are "building blocks" over the past few decades, yet they do not represent a *national nutrition policy* (1).

FOOD SECURITY

In the aftermath of the September 11 terrorist attacks on the U.S., the FDA has urged industry to take necessary steps to ensure better food security. For example, farms, processors, grocery stores and restaurants can better protect the nation's food supply by requiring criminal background checks of all workers, and closely checking all food and water sources. New guidelines were issued by the FDA, and addressed by the ADA (FDA, ADA).

The USDA's FSIS now has a Food Biosecurity Action Team (F-BAT). It's intent is to protect agriculture and the food supply, ensure employee safety, have adequate capacity and security at agency laboratories, ensure that essential USDA functions can continue, and to be able to pass on necessary information (to employees, consumers, industry, the media, Congress and other agencies) in a single, consistent message (USDA).

The FSIS has decided that during food recalls, distribution lists which are usually confidential, may be made available to state and federal agencies. Such lists would not be subject to public disclosure.

In a land of plenty, with an increasing concern with managing personal weight, the USDA has released the 2000.

DIETARY GUIDELINES FOR AMERICANS

Aim for fitness:
>   Aim for a healthy weight.
>   Be physically active each day.

Build a healthy base:
>   Let the Pyramid guide your food choices.
>   Choose a variety of grains daily, especially whole grains.
>   Keep food safe to eat.

Choose sensibly:
>   Choose a diet that is low in saturated fat and cholesterol and moderate in total fat.
>   Choose beverages and foods to moderate your intake of sugars.
>   Choose and prepare foods with less salt.
>   If you drink alcoholic beverages, do so in moderation.

The USDA and Health and Human Services (HHS) publication emphasizes both *lifestyle* and dietary measures for health. *Food Technology* reports: "So, the news for the food sector is to continue to improve processes and formulations where appropriate, and help consumers avoid foodborne illness and excess, while keeping excitement at the table" (2). Other nations have adopted similar dietary guidelines for their population.

STATE AND LOCAL HEALTH DEPARTMENTS

As mentioned, the federal agencies (FDA, USDA) regulate *interstate* food supplies, and state agencies such as state Food and Drug Administrations, and state Agriculture Departments, regulate *intrastate* food supplies. In some states, the State Health Department has complete authority over all food operations, whereas in other states, county or city health departments adopt their own food-service regulations.

ADDITIONAL AGENCIES REGULATING THE FOOD SUPPLY

The **Federal Trade Commission** (FTC) protects against unfair and deceptive advertising practices of products, including food.

The **National Marine Fisheries Service** (NMFS) of the Commerce Department is responsible for voluntary grading of seafood.

The **Occupational Health and Safety Administration** (OSHA) regulates health hazards in the workplace (such as food manufacture, processing, or retail food service) and determines compliance with regulations.

The **Environmental Protection Agency** (EPA) sets environmental standards. This agency regulates air and water pollution by a plant, toxic substances, pesticides, and use of radiation.

GENERAL LABELING

Complete information about food must be supplied on food packages. It must include the following:

- Name of product; name and place of business
- Net weight—ounces (oz.), or pounds and ounces
- Ingredients—listed *by weight in descending order* on *ingredients list* (not Nutrition Facts portion) of label
- Company name and address
- Product date if applicable to product
  - Open date labeling—voluntary types able to be read by the consumer
  - Expiration date—deadline for recommended eating (i.e., yeast)
  - "Best if used by" date—date for optimum quality, QA, or freshness
  - Pack date—date food was packaged
  - Pull date—last day sold as fresh (i.e., milk, ice cream, deli)
  - Code date—read only by manufacturer
- Nutrition information—"Nutrition Facts" on nearly all labels
  - Nutrient content claims substantiated
  - Health claims used only as allowed
- Other information
  - Religious symbols—such as Kosher (if applicable)
  - Safe handling instructions—such as on meats
  - Special warning labels—alcohol, aspartame that may affect select consumers
  - Product code (UPC)—bar code

NUTRITION LABELING

Food products intended for human consumption are subject to mandatory **nutrition labeling,** regulated by the FDA. As a result of the *Nutrition Labeling and Education Act of 1990* (NLEA), there are regulations that specify information food processors must include on their labels, including "Nutrition Facts" (Figure 20.1). The purpose of the NLEA is the following:

- Assist consumers in selecting foods that can lead to a healthier diet
- Eliminate consumer confusion
- Encourage production innovation by the food industry

NLEA regulations became effective in August of 1994, and approximately 595,000 food products had to meet these regulations, according to the FDA and USDA.

Consumers benefit from the educational component of the labeling law, as the information on labels is easy to read and may be useful in planning healthful diets. The label provides consumers with consistency in the presentation of nutrition facts under *mandatory* "Nutrition Facts," which appears on *most* products offered for sale in the United States. *Voluntary* information for cuts of meat, raw fish, and the 20 most commonly eaten fruits and vegetables may appear on package bags, brochures, or posters at the point of sale. Labeling values for produce and fish have been revised since initially required, and further revisions will be proposed every 4 years.

The FDA has set 139 *reference serving sizes* for use on "Nutrition Facts" labels that more closely approximates amounts consumers actually eat than previous labeling. The serving size indicates values, such as the number of ounces in a beverage or the ounces and number of cookies or crackers per serving, the nutrient content of a food is based on this reference-serving size, and stated on the label (Figure 20.2). Depending on personal intake, the individual nutrient consumption may be *more* or *less* than that one serving. A food is labeled as a *single* serving if the amount of food is greater than 50% and less than 200% of the designated single-serving size.

With passage of the NLEA, the FDA set regulations stating that a food label must express nutrient information in terms of recommended daily intake, in grams (or milligrams) or as a percentage, thus the "**% Daily Values**" or "DV." It shows how a serving of the food fits into a total day's diet.

Two sets of values were included in the establishment of Daily Values. One is the *Reference Daily Intakes (RDI),* which is based on former "U.S. RDA" (derived from 1968 RDA) labeling values. The second is *Daily Reference Values (DRV)* for nutrients, such as fat, sodium, cholesterol, and total carbohydrates including dietary fiber and sugars, which do not have an RDA but have a significant health impact. The DV reference values are based on a 2000- or 2500-calorie diet, and consumers ingesting more or less calories should adjust numbers accordingly.

Many values are provided on nutrition labels. For example, the total calories and calories from fat, the total fat, and saturated fat (perhaps monounsaturated and polyunsaturated fat if the processor wants to include these) are stated. Cholesterol and sodium are stated in milligrams.

The New Food Label at a Glance

The new food label will carry an up-to-date, easier-to-use nutrition information guide, to be required on almost all packaged foods (compared to about 60 percent of products up till now). The guide will serve as a key to help in planning a healthy diet.*

Serving sizes are now more consistent across product lines, are stated in both household and metric measures, and reflect the amounts people actually eat.

The **list of nutrients** covers those most important to the health of today's consumers, most of whom need to worry about getting too much of certain nutrients (fat, for example), rather than too few vitamins or minerals, as in the past.

The label of larger packages may now tell the number of calories per gram of fat, carbohydrate, and protein.

New title signals that the label contains the newly required information.

Calories from fat are now shown on the label to help consumers meet dietary guidelines that recommend people get no more than 30 percent of the calories in their overall diet from fat.

% Daily Value shows how a food fits into the overall daily diet.

Daily Values are also something new. Some are maximums, as with fat (65 grams or less); others are minimums, as with carbohydrate (300 grams or more). The daily values for a 2,000- and 2,500-calorie diet must be listed on the label of larger packages.

Nutrition Facts

Serving Size 1 cup (228g)
Servings Per Container 2

Amount Per Serving

Calories 260 Calories from Fat 120

	% Daily Value*
Total Fat 13g	**20**%
Saturated Fat 5g	**25**%
Cholesterol 30mg	**10**%
Sodium 660mg	**28**%
Total Carbohydrate 31g	**10**%
Dietary Fiber 0g	**0**%
Sugars 5g	
Protein 5g	

Vitamin A 4% • Vitamin C 2%
Calcium 15% • Iron 4%

* Percent Daily Values are based on a 2,000 calorie diet. Your daily values may be higher or lower depending on your calorie needs:

	Calories:	2,000	2,500
Total Fat	Less than	65g	80g
Sat Fat	Less than	20g	25g
Cholesterol	Less than	300mg	300mg
Sodium	Less than	2,400mg	2,400mg
Total Carbohydrate		300g	375g
Dietary Fiber		25g	30g

Calories per gram:
Fat 9 • Carbohydrate 4 • Protein 4

* This label is only a sample. Exact specifications are in the final rules.

FIGURE 20.1 Nutrition Facts label
(*Source:* Food and Drug Administration, 1994).

Real-Life Serving Sizes

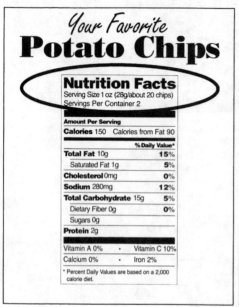

- Serving sizes are now more consistent across product lines.
- Serving sizes are now stated in both household and metric measures.
- Serving sizes now more closely reflect the amounts people actually eat.

FIGURE 20.2   Labels and serving sizes
(*Source:* Food and Drug Administration, 1994).

The total carbohydrate, sugar, and dietary fiber is also reported, as is protein, which is expressed as a quantity that takes into account the *completeness* of amino acids (Complete = having all essential amino acids in the needed amount). Food processors have the option of reporting protein as a % DV on a label, and, if they do, they must determine the *quality* of the protein to ascertain which daily value of protein to use as a comparison.

Consumers may be attempting to limit or attain specific quantities of certain nutrients in their diet. For example, a consumer may desire to limit fat or cholesterol; or they may want to increase their intake of vitamins and minerals commonly needed in the United States, such as vitamins A and C, calcium, and iron. A nutrition label can help the consumer know what nutrients are in food.

Examples of *terms* allowed on food *labels* appears in Table 20.1 They are consistent among products and manufacturers, food processors must abide by these definitions on their *product labels*.Yet, when merchandising a product through the *various forms of advertisement*, there exists *no* FDA regulation of terms.

In order to make the approved health claims (Table 20.2, Figure 20.3) a food (except for sugar alcohols and dental caries, etc. that are not appropriate) must

TABLE 20.1   Some Examples of Terms Allowed on Food Labels

General Desriptive Terms
- *free—negligible amount of the nutrient*
  - good source of—between 10 and 19% of the Daily Value of the nutrient
  - healthy—low-fat, saturated fat, cholesterol, and sodium food with at least 10% of the Daily Value for vitamins A and C, protein, iron, calcium, or fiber
  - low—not meeting Daily Values with frequent consumption
  - high—20% or more of the Daily Values for a nutrient per serving
  - light or lite—one-third fewer calories, or one-half the fat of the comparison food
  - more—at least 10% more of the Daily Value than a comparison food
  - less—at least 25% or less of a nutrient than the comparison food

Energy/Calories
- *free—fewer than 5 cal per serving*
  - low calorie—40 cal or less per serving
  - reduced calorie—at least 25% fewer calories per serving than a comparison food
  - light—one-third less calories than the comparison food

Fat And Cholesterol
- *Fat*
- *fat-free—less than 0.5 g fat per serving*
  - low fat—3 g or less fat per serving
  - percent (%) fat-free—only if low fat or fat-free, calories based on 100-g portions
  - less fat—25% or less fat than a comparison food
  - light—50% less fat than a comparison food

Saturated Fat
- *saturated fat-free—less than 0.5 g of saturated fat and trans fatty acid per serving.*
  - low saturated fat—1 g or less saturated fat per serving
  - less saturated fat—25% or less saturated fat than a comparison food

Cholesterol
- *cholesterol-free—less than 2 mg cholesterol and 2 g or less saturated fat per serving*
  - low cholesterol—20 mg or less cholesterol and 2 g or less saturated fat per serving
  - less cholesterol—25% or less cholesterol than a comparison food, and 2 g or less saturated fat per serving
  - extra lean—less than 5 g of fat, 2 g saturated fat, and 95 mg cholesterol per serving and per 100 g of meat, poultry, and seafood
  - lean—less than 10 g fat, 4.5 g saturated fat, and 95 mg of cholesterol per serving and per 100 g of meat, poultry, and seafood

Carbohydrates: Fiber and Sugar
- *high fiber—5 g or more fiber per serving, with 3 g or less of fat per serving (low fat) unless a higher level of fat is specified*
  - sugar-free—less than 0.5 g sugar per serving

Sodium

- *sodium-free—less than 5 mg sodium per serving*
  - low sodium—140 mg or less per serving
  - light—50% less sodium, in a low-calorie or low-fat food
  - very low sodium—35 mg or less per serving

---

contain no more than 20% of the Daily Value for total fat, saturated fat, cholesterol, or sodium, and the food must naturally contain at least 10% of the Daily Value for either vitamins A and C, protein, fiber, calcium, or iron.

In early surveys, conducted several months after implementation of the NLEA for the American Oil Chemists' Society, it was found that 40% of U.S. consumers seldom, if ever, used nutrition food labels in deciding which foods to buy (3). Twenty-one percent responded that they used nutritional information "frequently" in deciding which products to buy, and 20% "occasionally" used such information. Four percent of those surveyed said that the May 1994 label format was less useful than the format used prior to May 1994. It was reported that 73% of those that used Nutrition Facts label information regularly view the listing of *fat* content, and 53% of label readers regularly read *calorie* content. Today, training has attempted to provide more familiarity with the "Nutrition Facts" label, and thus greater use.

In making the labeling transition, information intended to assist consumers in making informed food choices did not come cheaply to food processors. The product analyses, as well as label redesign and printing costs, were incurred. In a survey conducted by the National Food Processors Association in 1992, it was estimated that $1.28 billion would be spent by the food industry as it implemented NLEA in an 18-month period.

TABLE 20.2 Examples of Approved Model Heath Claims Used on Food Labels

- Calcium and lower risk of osteoporosis
- Sodium and a greater risk of hypertension (high blood pressure)
- Saturated fat and cholesterol and a greater risk of coronary heart disease (CHD)
- Dietary fat and a greater risk of cancer
- Fiber-containing grain products, fruits, and vegetables and a reduced risk of cancer
- Fruits, vegetables, and grain products that contain fiber (particularly soluble fiber) and a reduced risk of CHD
- Fruits and vegetables and a reduced risk of cancer
- Folate and reduced risk of neural tube defect
- Sugar alcohols and reduced risk of tooth decay
- Soluble fiber from whole oats and psyllium seed husk and reduced risk of CHD
- Soy protein and reduced risk of CHD
- Whole grains and reduced risk of CHD and certain cancers
- Plant sterol and plant stanol esters and reduced risk of CHD
- Potassium and reduced risk of high blood pressure and stroke

The New Food Label at a Glance

Claims: While descriptive terms like "low," "good source," and "free" have long been used on food labels, their meaning — and their usefulness in helping consumers plan a healthy diet — have been murky. Now FDA has set specific definitions for these terms, assuring shoppers that they can believe what they read on the package.

Health Claims: For the first time, food labels will be allowed to carry information about the link between certain nutrients and specific diseases. For such a "health claim" to be made on a package, FDA must first determine that the diet-disease link is supported by scientific evidence.

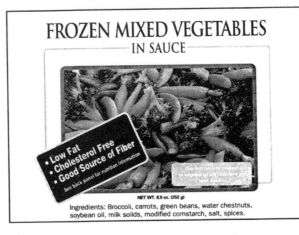

FROZEN MIXED VEGETABLES
IN SAUCE

- Low Fat
- Cholesterol Free
- Good Source of Fiber

See back panel for nutrition information

NET WT. 8.9 oz. (252 g)

Ingredients: Broccoli, carrots, green beans, water chestnuts, soybean oil, milk solids, modified cornstarch, salt, spices.

Ingredients still will be listed in descending order by weight, and now the list will be required on almost all foods, even standardized ones like mayonnaise and bread.

"While many factors affect heart disease, diets low in saturated fat and cholesterol may reduce the risk of this disease."

Health claim message referred to on the front panel is shown here.

FIGURE 20.3   The food label at a glance.
(*Source:* FDA)

Methods of analyses for nutrition labeling are available to food processors from the AOAC International and the Food Chemicals Codex (FCC). "Whole food" and "ingredient" databases assisted in providing the necessary nutrient information for labels (4). Yet, "even with all the methodology available, food scientists can still be at a loss if they are analyzing a complicated matrix such as canned spaghetti" (5).

Legislation for more simple wording, and common sense labeling, is supported by The Food Allergy Initiative (FAI), The Food Allergy & Anaphylaxis Network, and The Center for Science in the Public Interest (CSPI). It has been suggested that perhaps labels should just say "wheat" or say "milk products." This is in part due to food allergies. Some additional information on food allergens may be found in the chapter on food safety (Chapter 16).

Examples of approved **health claims** appear in Table 20.2. Currently, the FDA is considering greater flexibility in the use of health claims on foods, but other claims outside of these may not be used on food products. Health claims for dietary supplements is being constructed (www.cfsan.fda.gov).

PHYTOCHEMICALS, NUTRACEUTICALS, FUNCTIONAL FOODS, MEDICAL FOODS, AND LABELING

The focus of this section of the text is on food *labeling*, yet considering the frequency with which terms such as phytochemicals, nutraceuticals, and functional foods are used on labels, a brief explanation of terms is provided (see Food Additives, Chapter 18). In foods company, the food scientist who develops new products, the technical staff, and the marketer of these foods, must stay abreast of the health concerns of consumers who are making dietary changes in managing their personal healthcare. An expertise in consumer food acceptability, food engineering, food laws, ingredient technology, nutrition, and more, positions the food company for product success.

Phytochemicals (plant chemicals) are important non-nutrients in food that may be responsible for disease prevention. Many frequently consumed foods including grains, legumes, seeds, fruits and vegetables, as well as green tea are *naturally* a source of phytochemicals. When a product contains *added* phytochemicals (Chapters 7 and 18), it may be stated on the food package that the product contains phytochemicals, but no *nutritional* claim may be made other than stating the already-approved (Table 20.2) nutritional or medical benefits that are based on sound scientific data.

A food term used in product literature is **nutraceuticals** (Chapters 7 and 18). It is the name given to a proposed new regulatory category of food components that may be considered a food or part of a food and may supply medical or health benefits including the treatment or prevention of disease, yet the FDA does not recognize the term. Such foods may also be known as designer foods or functional foods; for example, margarines that contain plant sterols to lower serum cholesterol, are a food with medical benefits.

The term **functional foods**, has no legal or general acceptance in the United States. It is defined by the Institute of Medicine's Food and Nutrition Board (IOM/FNB), and accepted by some, as a modified food or food ingredient for specified health use (6–8).

The idea of functional foods originated in Japan, in the mid 1980's and was aimed at solving medical problems such as high blood pressure. Products must meet eligibility requirements of the Japanese Ministry of Health and Welfare to bear the approval stamp FOSHU—Foods for Specified Health Use. Today, in the U.S., foods are created to target diseases such as cancer, diabetes, heart disease, and more. It must be pointed out that while research shows beneficial properties of specific substances, such as iron, and vitamins, their survival in the food manufacturing process, and their contribution to appearance, texture, and flavor are important considerations. It is also important that usage of functional food components considers the risk:benefit ratio, and follows acceptable scientific guidelines with regard to toxicity (9).

With availability of these types of foods, greater health benefits may be provided by the formulation of food products with added nutrients/nutrient combinations (10).

As foods that provide health benefits beyond basic nutrition, the promotion of health and disease prevention through consumption of functional foods has been promoted. Specifically, intakes of tea, broccoli, fatty fish, garlic, purple grapes, oats, soy foods tomatoes/tomato products and yogurt were reported in a study by the Functional Foods of Health Program at the University of Illinois. The result of training was that a high percentage of participants were interested in measures to ensure good health, and that an intent to consume a greater amount of functional foods was indicated (11).

Medical foods are those regulated by the FDA Office of Special Nutritionals on a case-by-case basis and are used as enteral foods (not administered into a vein parenterally, but not traditional foods) to improve nutritional support of the *hospitalized* patient.

Medical foods may either supplement the diet or be the sole source of nutrition and are used based on medical evaluation. In 1988, Congress provided the first legal definition of "medical food" as food formulated to be consumed or administered enterally under the supervision of a physician and which is intended for the specific dietary management of a disease or condition for which distinctive nutritional requirements based on recognized scientific principles are established by medical evaluation (U.S. Congress 1988).

Currently, such medical foods may not be subject to NLEA labeling regulations, as they are not considered the same as foods for *special dietary use*. The fact that both categories of foods often overlap, poses new FDA policy/regulatory discussion.

The USDA recognizes medical foods as non-prescription nutrition used for dietary management of a disease or condition (It deserves mention here that Hippocrates once suggested: "Let food be your medicine, and medicine your food!").

LABELING FOR FOODSERVICE

The inclusion of material in this section is intended to clarify labeling requirements of food served for immediate consumption. While this section addresses the *menu,* and not *labels* on packaged foods, it may be of less concern to the food scientist. Yet, foods eaten at a foodservice operation represent a significant portion of the buying public's consumption, and therefore deserve attention.

The FDA encourages foodservice operations to provide nutrition and health claims to consumers, and further regulations may be forthcoming. Yet, nutrition analysis testing and Nutrition Facts labeling are not required of foodservice (12).

Nutrient content or health claims appearing on menus must be substantiated by the foodservice operation, either verbally or in written form, to consumers who request such information, as claims must meet established FDA criteria As specified in the CFR, a reliable cookbook or computer software program may be used as a reference, and preparation methods must support the claim, or the menu item must be removed from the menu.

The Code of Federal Regulations (21CFR101) specifies the following with regard to labeling for foodservice:

> "A nutrient claim used on food that is served in restaurants or other establishments in which food is served for immediate human consumptionor which is sold for sale or use in such establishments shall comply with the (same) requirements of this section ... except that ...

> "In lieu of analytical testing, compliance may be determined using a reasonable basis for concluding that the food bears the claim meets the definition for the claim.

This reasonable basis may derive from recognized data bases for raw and processed food, recipes, and other means to compute nutrient levels in the foods or meals and may be used provided reasonable steps are taken to ensure that the method of preparation adheres to the factors on which the reasonable basis was determined (e.g., types and amounts of ingredients, cooking temperatures, etc.). Firms making claims on foods based on this reasonable basis criterion are required to provide to appropriate regulatory officials on request the specific information on which their determination is based and reasonable assurance of operational adherence to the preparation methods or other basis for the claim."

"A term or symbol that may be in some contexts constitute a claim … may be used, provided that the use of the term or symbol does not characterize the level of a nutrient, and a statement that clearly explains the basis for the use of the term or symbol is prominently displayed and does not characterize the level of the nutrient. For example, the term such as "lite fare" followed by an asterisk referring to a note that makes it clear that in this restaurant, "lite fare" means smaller portion sizes than normal; or an item bearing a symbol referring to a note that makes clear that this item meets the criteria for the dietary guidance established by a recognized dietary authority would not be considered a nutrient content."

"Such claim is exempt from the requirements for disclosure statements … " (FDA).

According to a 1994 survey of the Research and Development Directors of 150 of the 400 largest foodservice corporations (13,14), "most companies were neutral about their willingness to use nutrition labeling." There were *menu-related* obstacles to nutrition labeling, such as menu variations, including use of daily specials, limited page space, and loss of flexibility. There were also *personnel-related* obstacles, such as difficulty in training employees and a shortage of time.

Nutrition expertise (15) and labeling assistance could be provided by registered dietitians, as 20% of the largest restaurant chains "employed a registered dietitian who could assist with the development of health-related menu offerings" (16). Nutrition and labeling in food service is further discussed in other sources (17–20).

The National Center for Nutrition and Dietetics of the American Dietetic Association has a hot-line number (800-366-1655) that offers messages and personally answers consumer questions about food labeling (21).

Supermarket Savvy Information and Resource Service® is an example of a service that provides new product information. A newsletter is included as one part of its service. It is written for the health professional and designed to provide information about new products (especially the healthier ones) so that the health professional can answer his/her clients' questions about new foods and guide his/her clients to better food choices in the supermarket and health/natural foods store (22).

CONCLUSION

Government regulation, industrial compliance, and consumer education are means of ensuring a safe food supply to consumers. The FDA is a public health agency that regulates food, cosmetics, medicines, medical devices, and radiation-emitting products, such as microwave ovens. The Food, Drug and Cosmetic Act of 1938 and its amendments were introduced to regulate the processing of many products subject to interstate commerce or import.

Food inspections are the responsibility of the FDA, with meat product inspection regulated by the USDA. Food packaging and labeling is regulated by the FDA and USDA for their respective products. The USDA administers the Food Safety and Inspection Service and numerous food programs.

The NLEA is an attempt to protect the consumer against fraud and misinformation. Labeling terms, "Nutrition Facts," and health claims are regulated by the FDA. The purpose of the NLEA is to assist consumers in selecting foods that can lead to a healthier diet, eliminate confusion, and encourage production innovation by the food industry. With greater knowledge of nutrients nutrient interactions, and promotion of health, greater health benefits may be provided with the formulation of new food products.

GLOSSARY

Daily value (90 DV): Two sets of values used on nutrition labels, including Reference Daily Intakes (RDI), based on former U.S. RDAs and Daily Reference Values (DRV) of nutrients that do not have an RDA but have a significant health impact.

Functional foods: Any modified food or food ingredient that may provide a health benefit beyond that obtained by the original food; the term has no legal or general acceptance in the United States but is accepted by some as food for specified health use.

Generally Recognized As Safe (GRAS): Substances (food ingredients) generally recognized as safe for their intended use.

Grading service: Conducted as a voluntary service of the USDA, paid for by packers.

Health claims: Describe an association between a nutrient or food substance and disease or health-related condition.

Inspection service: Of the USDA or state Department of Agriculture inspects and stamps inspected meat with a circle containing the abbreviations for "inspected and passed."

Medical foods: Food formulated to be consumed or administered enterally under the supervision of a physician and which is intended for the specific dietary management of a disease or condition for which distinctive nutritional requirements based on recognized scientific principles are established by medical evaluation (U.S. Congress 1988).

Nutraceuticals: The name given to a proposed new regulatory category of food components that may be considered a food or part of a food and may supply medical or health benefits including the treatment or prevention of disease; a term not recognized by the FDA.

Nutrition labeling: For the purpose of assisting consumers in selecting foods that can lead to a healthier diet, to eliminate consumer confusion, and to encourage production innovation by the food industry. Labeling expresses nutrients in terms of Reference Daily Intakes (RDI) and Daily Reference Values (DRV), both comprising the Daily Values.

Phytochemicals: Plant chemicals; natural compounds other that nutrients in fresh plant material that function in disease prevention; they protect against oxidative cell damage or facilitate carcinogen excretion from the body to reduce the risk of cancer.

Standard of Fill of Container: FDA standard that the volume of packaged food offered for sale does not interfere with the weight of the product as stated on the label.

Standard of Identity: FDA list of required and optional ingredients that are included in manufacture.

Standards of Minimum Quality: FDA minimum quality standards for specific food characteristics–color, etc.

Wholesome: The carcass and viscera of the animal were examined and no signs of illness were indicated, and conditions met sanitary standards.

REFERENCES

1. Crockett SJ, Kennedy E, Elam K. Food Industry's role in national nutrition policy: Working for the common good. *J Am Diet Assoc.* 2002; 102:478–479.
2. Katz F. 2000 IFT Annual Meeting and Food Expo. How food technologists react to the new Dietary Guidelines for Americans. *Food Technology.* 2000; 54 (8): 64–68.
3. Good news and bad on labels. *Food Engineering.* 1995; 67(6): 22.
4. Johnson GH, Mehrotal. Nutrition labeling databases: The food industry view. *Food Technology.* 1995; 49(5): 156–161.
5. Flajnik CM. Validating analyses for nutrition labeling. *Food Technology.* 1995; 49(6): 59–62.
6. Goldberg I. *Functional Foods.* New York: Chapman & Hall, 1994.
7. Hasler CM. Functional foods: Their role in disease prevention and health promotion. A Publication of the Institute of Food Technologists' Expert Panel on Food Safety and Nutrition. *Food Technology.* 1998; 52 (11): 63–70.
8. Sloan AE. The top ten functional food trends. *Food Technology.* 2000; 54(4): 33—62.
9. Pszczola DE. Addressing functional problems in fortified foods. *Food Technology.* 1998; 52(7): 38–46.
10. Staff Report. Combining nutrients for health benefits. *Food Technology.* 2001; 55 (2): 42–47
11. Pelletier S, Kundrat S, Hasler C. Effects of an educational program on intent to consume functional foods. *J Am Diet Assoc.* 2002; 102: 1297–1300.
12. Final labeling regulations implementing the NLEA of 1990. *Federal Register.* 1993; 58: 2066–2536.
13. Almanza BA, Nelson D, Chai S. Obstacles to nutrition labeling in restaurants. *Journal of the American Dietetic Association.* 1997; 97: 1157–1161.
14. R & I 400: ranking. *Restaurants and Institutions* 1993; 103: 25, 30, 34, 38, 44, 46, 48, 50.
15. Position of the American Dietetic Association: Nutrition in foodservice establishments. *Journal of the American Dietetic Association.* 1991; 91: 480–482.
16. Clay JM, Emenheiser DA, Bruce AR. Healthful menu offerings in restaurants: A survey of major US chains. *Journal of Food service Systems* 1995; 8: 91–101.
17. Mermelstein NH. Nutrition labeling in foodservice. *Food Technology.* 1993; 47: 65–68.
18. Court ruling backs menu health/nutrition claim requirements. *Food Institute Reports.* July 8, 1996; 27: 1.
19. Boger CA. Food labeling for restaurants. *Cornell Hotel Restaurant Administration Quarterly.* 1995; 36: 62–70.
20. Sneed J, Burkhalter JP. Marketing nutrition in restaurants: a survey of current practices and attitudes. *Journal of the American Dietetic Association.* 1991; 91: 459–462.

21. The National Center for Nutrition and Dietetics of the American Dietetic Association, Chicago, IL.
22. McDonald L, ed. Publisher of the SUPERMARKET SAVVY® *Information and Resource Service,* Houston, TX.

BIBLIOGRAPHY

Center for Food Safety and Applied Nutrition. www.cfsan.fda.gov (search for Health Claims)
Dudek J, Keenan C. NLEA—Two years later. *Food Quality.* 1996; 2(5): 20—21.
Food and Drug Administration. Focus on food labeling. *FDA Consumer. Food Labeling, Questions and Answers. Vol II.* Washington, DC: U.S. Dept. of Health and Human Services, 1995.
Medical Foods Inc. Cambridge, MA.
The Food Marketing Institute. Consumer Affairs Department. Washington, DC.
The United States Department of Agriculture.
Thonney PF, Bisogni CA. Government regulation of food safety: Interaction of scientific and societal forces. *Food Technology.* 1992; 46(1): 73–80.
The New Food Label at a Glance.
www.oregonstate.edu. – search for portion sizes.

INDEX

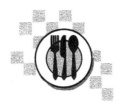

Fungi 350, 376
Furanose: 37, 45

Gel: 25, 28, 53, 60, 64, 67, 72
Gelatin 148, 185
Gelatinization 50, 51, 60
Gelation or setting of gelatinized starch
    pastes during cooling: 54
Gelation: 55, 60
General labeling 458
General structure of amino acids: 132
Generally Recognized As Safe (GRAS) 403,
    418, 452, 468
Geneva or systematic nomenclature 250
Germ: 74, 94
Gluten 77, 94, 317, 338
Gluten-forming potential 317, 338
Glycosidic bond: 38, 45
Government regulation of the food supply
    and labeling 450
Grading of meat 161
Grading of vegetables and fruits: 114
Grading service 455, 468
Grain of dough 320, 338
Grain of meat 148, 185
Granule: 47, 60
GRAS substances 452
Gums: 68, 71, 72

HACCP 355, 376
HACCP examples 358, 360–362
Halal Certification 160, 185
Hard water: 27, 28
Hard-to-Place Foods 316
Harvesting and postharvest changes: 109
Health claims 417, 418, 463, 468
Heat of crystallization 306, 310
Heat preservation 379
Heat treatment methods 380
Hemicellulose: 99, 124
High-altitude baking 336
High-methoxyl pectin: 63, 72
Homogenization 221, 240
Hormones and antibiotics 164
Hydrocolloid: 69, 72, 269, 275
Hydrogen bonds: 21, 28
Hydrogenation 258, 275
Hydrolysis

Hydrolysis of peptides and proteins: 140
Hydrolytic rancidity 260, 275
Hydrophilic 132, 145, 280, 293
Hydrophilic/lipophilic balance or HLB 286,
    293
Hydrophobic 132, 145, 280, 294
Hydroxyl group: 35, 45
Hygroscopicity 302, 310

Ice cream 231
Imbibition: 50, 60
imitation milk 234, 240
Infection 345, 376
Ingredients in specific bread
    products 329
Inspection service 455, 468
Inspections and grading for egg quality 192
Interactions involved in protein
    structure and conformation: 138
Interesterification or
    rearrangement 259
Interfacial tension 266, 275, 280, 294
Interfering agent 308, 310
Intoxication 346, 376
Inversion 302, 301
Invert sugar. 39, 45, 302
Irradiation 117, 394, 398
Isoelectric point: pI; 138, 145
Isomer 249, 275

Junction zone: 65, 72

Ketose: 37, 45
Kneading 335, 338
Kosher Inspection 158, 185

Label terms: 123
Labeling for Foodservice 466
Labeling of vegetables and fruits: 122
Lactose 215, 238
Lactose intolerance 238, 240
Latent heat of fusion: 23, 27, 29
Latent heat of vaporization: 23, 29
Leavening 320, 332, 338
Leavening process of baked products 323
Lecithin 247, 275
Legislation and testing for additives 402
Legume 177